Injury Prevention *and* Rehabilitation *for* Active Older Adults

Kevin P. Speer, MD

Southeastern Orthopedics Sports Medicine and Shoulder Center
Raleigh, North Carolina

EDITOR

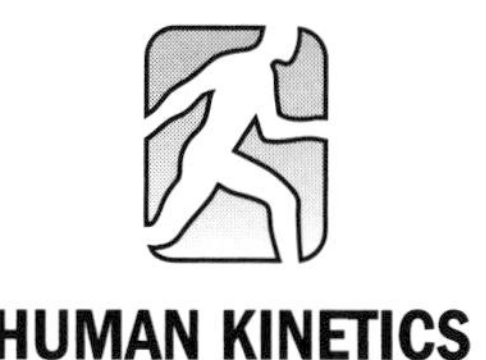

HUMAN KINETICS

Library of Congress Cataloging-in-Publication Data

Injury prevention and rehabilitation for active older adults / Kevin P. Speer, editor.
p. ; cm.
Includes bibliiographical references and index.
ISBN 0-7360-4031-5 (hardcover)
1. Older athletes--Wounds and injuries. 2. Older athletes--Rehabilitation. 3. Musculoskeletal system--Aging.
[DNLM: 1. Athletic injuries--prevention & control--Aged. 2. Athletic Injuries--rehabilitation--Aged. 3. Aging--physiology. 4. Exercise--Aged. 5. Sports Medicine. QT 261 I565 2005] I. Speer, Kevin P.
RC1218.A33I55 2005
617.1'027--dc22

2004020851

ISBN: 0-7360-4031-5

The Web addresses cited in this text were current as of November 22, 2004, unless otherwise noted.

Acquisitions Editor: Loarn D. Robertson, PhD; **Developmental Editor:** Elaine H. Mustain; **Assistant Editor:** Sandra Merz Bott; **Copyeditor:** Joyce Sexton; **Proofreader:** Anne Rogers; **Indexer:** Robert Howerton; **Permission Manager:** Dalene Reeder; **Graphic Designer:** Robert Reuther; **Graphic Artist:** Dawn Sills; **Photo Manager:** Kelly J. Huff; **Cover Designer:** Keith Blomberg; **Photographer (cover):** PhotoDisc/Getty Images; **Photographer (interior):** Figures 1.1, 1.4-1.7 courtesy of Hardayal Singh; figures 3.5-3.11 courtesy of W. Ben Kibler; photos on pp. 60-62, 63 (right column), 64 (left column bottom, right column), and 65, figures 4.2-4.5 courtesy of Carol Figuers; figures 6.2-6.4, 6.9 courtesy of Edward McFarland; figures 7.4-7.6 courtesy of Todd Ellenbecker; chapters 8, 9, 10 photos courtesy of Jonathan Isaacs, Joshua Rittenberg, Srino Bharam, respectively; figures 11.2-11.3, 11.5-11.98, 11.12-11.13 courtesy of Douglas Martini; figures 6.9, 12.2-12.3 courtesy of Sandra Shultz; figure 12.4 Daniel Grogan; figures 12.5-12.6, 12.9-12.10, 12.11b, 12.12-12.16 courtesy of Ryan Simovitch; figures 12.7-12.8 courtesy of Meir Nyska and Gideon Mann; photos on pages 63 (left column) and 64 (left column's top, middle photos), figures 6.7, 6.10, 12.11a Kelly J. Huff; **Art Manager:** Kelly Hendren; **Illustrator:** Craig Newsom; **Printer:** Sheridan Books

Printed in the United States of America 10 9 8 7 6 5 4 3 2 1

Human Kinetics
Web site: www.HumanKinetics.com

United States: Human Kinetics
P.O. Box 5076
Champaign, IL 61825-5076
800-747-4457
e-mail: humank@hkusa.com

Canada: Human Kinetics
475 Devonshire Road Unit 100
Windsor, ON N8Y 2L5
800-465-7301 (in Canada only)
e-mail: orders@hkcanada.com

Europe: Human Kinetics
107 Bradford Road
Stanningley
Leeds LS28 6AT, United Kingdom
+44 (0) 113 255 5665
e-mail: hk@hkeurope.com

Australia: Human Kinetics
57A Price Avenue
Lower Mitcham, South Australia
5062
08 8277 1555
e-mail: liaw@hkaustralia.com

New Zealand: Human Kinetics
Division of Sports Distributors NZ Ltd.
P.O. Box 300 226 Albany
North Shore City
Auckland
0064 9 448 1207
e-mail: blairc@hknewz.com

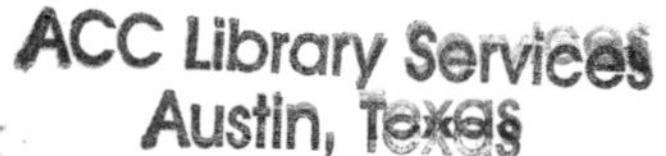

This book is dedicated to my senior patients who have taught me that the pursuit of sport and recreational activity is a lifelong pursuit and worthy of all the efforts that clinicians can muster to keep them as active as they would like to be.

Contents

About the Contributors

Kevin P. Speer, Editor
Southeastern Orthopedics Sports Medicine and Shoulder Center
Raleigh, NC

Venu Akuthota, MD
Assistant Professor
Department of Rehabilitation Medicine
Director, Spine Center
University of Colorado Health Sciences Center
Denver, CO

Franca B. Alphin, MPH, RD, LDN
Assistant Clinical Professor
Department of Community and Family Medicine
Student Health Services
Duke University Medical Center
Durham, NC

Srino Bharam, MD
Attending Staff
Department of Orthopaedic Surgery
St. Vincent's Medical Center
New York, NY

Lauren A. Carlson, MPH
Center for the Evaluative Clinical Sciences
Dartmouth Medical School
Hanover, NH

Efsthathios Chronopoulos, MD
Instructor
University Department of Orthopaedics
Hospital "Agia Olga"
Athens, Greece

Mark E. Easley, MD
Assistant Professor of Orthopaedic Surgery
Duke University Medical Center
Division of Orthopaedic Surgery
Durham, NC

Todd S. Ellenbecker, MS, PT, SCS, OCS, CSCS
Clinic Director
Physiotherapy Associates Scottsdale Sports Clinic
National Director of Clinical Research
Physiotherapy Associates
Scottsdale, AZ

Rafael F. Escamilla, PhD, PT, CSCS
Associate Professor
California State University, Sacramento
College of Health and Human Services
Department of Physical Therapy
Sacramento, CA

Carol C. Figuers, PT, EdD
Associate Clinical Professor
Division of Physical Therapy
Department of Community and Family Medicine
Duke University School of Medicine
Durham, NC

Jonathan Isaacs, MD
Assistant Professor
Department of Orthopaedic Surgery
Assistant Professor
Division of Plastic Surgery
Virginia Commonwealth University Medical Center
Richmond, VA

Utku Kandemir, MD
Former Sports Medicine Fellow
Department of Orthopaedic Surgery
University of Pittsburgh
Pittsburgh, PA

W. Ben Kibler, MD
Lexington Clinic Sports Medicine Center
Lexington, KY

Tae Kyun Kim, MD
Assistant Professor
Department of Orthopaedic Surgery
College of Medicine
Seoul National University
Seoul, Korea

L. Scott Levin, MD, FACS
Chief
Division of Plastic, Reconstructive, Maxillofacial and Oral Surgery
Professor of Plastic and Orthopaedic Surgery
Durham, NC

Douglas J. Martini, MD
Cary Orthopaedic & Sports Medicine Specialists, PA
Cary, NC

Edward G. McFarland, MD
Vice Chairman
Associate Professor
Department of Orthopaedic Surgery
Division of Sports Medicine and Shoulder Surgery
The Johns Hopkins University
Baltimore, MD

Daryl C. Osbahr, BS
Medical Student
University of North Carolina at Chapel Hill School of Medicine
Chapel Hill, NC

Hyung Bin Park, MD
Assistant Professor
Department of Orthopaedic Surgery
College of Medicine
Gyeongsang National University
Chinju, Korea

Marc J. Philippon, MD
Assistant Professor, Director of Sports Medicine/Hip Disorders
Department of Orthopaedic Surgery
University of Pittsburgh
Sports Medicine Center
Pittsburgh, PA

Joel M. Press, MD
Rehabilitation Institute of Chicago
Medical Director
Center for Spine, Sports, and Occupational Rehabilitation
Associate Professor
Department of Physical Medicine and Rehabilitation
Northwestern University Feinberg School of Medicine
Chicago, IL

Joshua D. Rittenberg, MD
Rehabilitation Institute of Chicago
Center for Spine, Sports, and Occupational Rehabilitation
Assistant Professor
Department of Physical Medicine and Rehabilitation
Northwestern University Feinberg School of Medicine
Chicago, IL

Amy E. Ross, MPT
Staff Physical Therapist
Rehabilitation Institute of Chicago
Center for Spine, Sports, and Occupational Rehabilitation
Chicago, IL

Ryan W. Simovitch, MD
Resident, Orthopaedic Surgery
Duke University Medical Center
Division of Orthopaedic Surgery
Durham, NC

Hardayal (Hardy) Singh, MD
Southeastern Orthopedics Sports Medicine and Shoulder Center
Raleigh, NC

Atsushi Yokota, MD
Department of Orthopaedic Surgery
Osaka Medical College
Osaka, Japan

Preface

Sports medicine is not exclusively defined as a medical specialty or as a surgical specialty. It is not merely the treatment and care of competitive athletes. Rather, sports medicine is a philosophy defined by the attitude of the patients and the clinician. Sports medicine involves the care of patients who have sustained injuries or conditions that limit the activities that they wish to pursue. A sports medicine clinician engages the patient in attempting to return to the desired activity. The most obvious model of sports medicine is the care of young competitive athletes. These patients are motivated to return to their sports, not to retire from their sports. This is true in spite of significant challenges, both clinical and therapeutic. This definition of sports medicine can just as easily be applied to the active older patient who encounters difficulty with recreational activities and pursuits.

We have entered an era in which a large part of the global population is aging. By current estimates, the number of people age 65 and older in the United States will be 53,348,000 by the year 2020. This is some 50% more than citizens in that demographic today in the United States. In the United States more and more people are retiring with enough savings that they can engage in elective recreational lifestyles, including golf, tennis, swimming, hiking, weightlifting, and various other forms of aerobic and anaerobic exercise. There is a consensus of opinion on the value of moderate exercise in the senior population: Most age-related declines in musculoskeletal function can be markedly reduced by participation in moderate exercise.

The "graying" of sports medicine involves senior patients who do not want to moderate or alter activity or recreational pursuits. They want to return to the activities that they cannot perform as a result of injury or chronic conditions. For example, arthritis is seen in 47% of older patients. These senior patients don't want or need clinicians who recommend moderation in activity as a solution to their problems. These patients want clinicians who will treat them and consider their goals as they would if they were treating a 20-year-old competitive athlete. Herein lies the great challenge in treating active older patients. Returning them to their previous level of activity involves a myriad of considerations that exceed those of the young athlete. Foremost among these considerations are the biologic changes that occur in all musculoskeletal tissues as we age. Recovery from injury or surgery is greatly complicated by reduced healing in these tissues. In addition, the general rehabilitation efforts that are routinely employed can cause tissue breakdown or microtraumatic injury to the actual site that is being treated.

The book is written is for all health care providers who take on the challenge of injury and dysfunction in active older patients who seek to attain their previous levels of activity. These challenges include biologic, senescent, and physiologic factors. In exploring these challenges in the active older patient, this book seeks to fulfill a need that previously has not been addressed. Providers, from the person of casual interest to the physician and professor, can all benefit from the information and collective explanations presented in this text. It is my hope that this book contributes to the body of literature to help all health care providers in advancing the field of sports medicine as it takes on the challenges of the active older patient and athlete.

PART

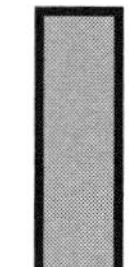

GENERAL ISSUES IN SPORTS MEDICINE FOR ACTIVE OLDER ADULTS

CHAPTER

1

Senescent Changes in the Human Musculoskeletal System

Hardayal Singh, MD

Locomotion and other abilities of the human body involving movement are made possible by the unique characteristics of certain tissues and structures: bone, joint configuration, ligaments, cartilage, tendons, and muscle tissue. These tissues collectively make up the musculoskeletal system. The components of this system have a common origin in undifferentiated mesenchymal cells. To understand pathology or disease involved in injury or old age, one must know what is normal for a younger individual. This helps one understand how changes (both macroscopic and microscopic) ultimately affect not only strength but also joint movement, locomotion, balance, and coordination. The aim of this chapter is to characterize these differences in order to explain differences in treatment options or approaches to an older individual with a degenerative disease as compared to a normal younger counterpart, with or without injury.

Aging is a complex, natural phenomenon that results in decline in most physiological systems and functions of the body. That there is an age-related decline in proprioception, lean muscle mass, balance, and overall quality of life is well known. These senescent changes also affect the musculoskeletal system and are an inevitable part of a confluence of change in the human body with aging. The following are some of the general physiological changes related to aging that affect neuromuscular function, directly or indirectly:

- Change in proprioception
- Altered sense of balance
- Increased propensity to falls
- Decreased coordination
- Effects on sight, hearing, and taste
- Cortical atrophy, decline in neurotransmitter levels
- Biochemical and functional changes in neuromuscular function
- Cataracts, macular degeneration, glaucoma
- Decrease in lean muscle mass
- Decreased ability of the reparative process after injury
- Overall decrease in cell function
- Decrease in work capacity
- Decreased bone mass
- Decrease in organ function (cardiac output, renal/liver function, etc.)

This chapter focuses on changes in the musculoskeletal system with age, comparing these senescent changes with what is typically seen in a young, healthy patient.

BONE AND ASSOCIATED CARTILAGE

Bone is a well-organized composite tissue composed of organic and inorganic structures. Organic structures include mainly type I collagen (>90%), osteocalcin, osteopontin, and growth factors. The collagen has a well-organized triple helix structure, providing tensile strength primarily to the bone. Compressive strength is provided mainly by hydroxyapatite, which is embedded in the structure of the collagen fibrils. Hydroxyapatite is the major constituent of the nonorganic structure of bone.

Cartilage is the "covering" of bone in and around the joints. One of its many functions is to provide a smooth gliding surface for joint motion. This is possible because cartilage provides the lowest possible amount of friction between biological structures. The loss of cartilage is what defines osteoarthritis. The natural deterioration of cartilage with age contributes to increasing friction between the joint surfaces, which further accentuates arthritis.

Bone

Bone contains outer and inner structures. The outer, stronger structure is the cortical bone, which through its densely organized lamellation functions mainly to provide mechanical strength. The inner cancellous bone functions primarily as a metabolic activity unit of the bone. Its relatively great number of lacunae or interior spaces aids in bone turnover functions, among many others.

Normal Structure and Function

Control of bone metabolism is performed for the most part by three types of cells: osteoblasts (bone-"forming" cells), osteoclasts (bone-"eating" cells), and osteocytes (the cells of matrix). It is postulated that signaling pathways between these cells help to regulate the balance between bone formation and resorption, and this modulates the development and activity of osteoclasts. Vitamin D, calcitonin, parathyroid hormone, kidney and liver function, and regulation of calcium ultimately control bone metabolism.

Bones are generally classified into four types according to shape: long, short, flat, or irregular. The functions of these bones depend on their location, shape, and size. For example, the biggest bone (femur) serves mainly as a mechanical support for ambulation against gravity and lower extremity strength, whereas one of the small bones of the hand (pisiform) may serve to add stability to the bones surrounding it.

Bone not only functions as a structural support for the body but also produces red blood cells within its marrow. In addition, bone serves as a reservoir for calcium in the body and has a major function in calcium homeostasis. Among other functions is storage of inorganic salts, including hydroxyapatite, phosphorus, and lead. Bone also functions to buffer blood against excessive pH changes by absorbing or releasing alkaline mineral salts. In summary, bone functions to support and protect the soft tissue structures; is a mainstay in movement; and plays a vital role in producing cells for blood and immune system formation, calcium and electrolyte balance, and acid–base balance.

Senescent Changes

It is well understood that structures composing the joint undergo a gradual decrease in blood supply with aging. This can lead to arthritic changes (decrease in space, osteophyte formation, etc.) with an effect on

Bone

	Young	Aging
Blood supply	Increased	Decreased
Osteoblast	Increased	Decrease in quantity and quality
Osteoclast	In equilibrium	Increased leading to increased bone destruction
Growth factor	Increased amount	Decreased
Joint space	Adequate	Decreased
Density	High/low (depending on demand)	Decreased
Immobilization	Adequate	Decreased
Force required to produce bone fractures	High energy	Low energy
Remodeling	High	Low potential
Calcium metabolism	Adequate	Compromised or decreased

joint function and motion. The overall homeostatic characteristic of skeletal tissue also declines with age.

Bone healing and osteogenic potential are also compromised after a fracture in an adult as compared to a younger person. This is primarily due to a decrease in the number of bone-forming osteoblasts during aging. Fractures heal much more slowly in adults than in children in terms of the quality of various stages of fracture healing and activity of osteoblasts (Lane, Russell, and Khan 2000). Immobilization after a fracture in a cast or after surgical fixation, along with a decrease in the expression of and response to growth factors and cytokines, further slows down this process.

Next we review three major pathological processes that occur in bone as a result of senescence.

Osteoporosis

As a person ages, the bone mass tends to decrease and the microarchitecture of bone tissue deteriorates, leading to increased bone fragility and fracture risk (Lane, Russell, and Khan 2000). This can be a subclinical event. Osteoporosis can be regarded as a silent and progressive disorder. According to one estimate, the number of femoral neck fractures due to osteoporosis in the elderly population (Baby Boomers) will double (250,000 to 500,000) by the year 2040. Postmenopausal women are especially vulnerable. Osteopenia may not be visible on plain X-rays until 30% to 50% of bone mineral loss has occurred—a loss that may be attributable to a combination of enhanced activity of osteoclasts and decreased activity of osteoblasts. Other medical conditions related to age such as cancer, diabetes, disuse, immobilization, and overall deterioration in various organ systems, as well as drug use and smoking, may further increase the development of osteoporosis. Additionally, various metabolic disorders and metabolic bone diseases can result in bone mineral loss and greater risk of bone fractures.

Osteonecrosis

Osteonecrosis (ON), also known as avascular necrosis, is a disease characterized by a poorly understood derangement of the osseous circulation (Mont et al. 2000). The derangement may be temporary or permanent depending on etiology and the person's age. Permanent loss of blood supply causes the bone in the joint to lose its structural strength, leading to collapse of joint surfaces. Besides a decrease in the blood supply to the bone with age, however, there are other causes of ON. These include injury or trauma, steroid usage, alcohol usage, systemic diseases like systemic lupus erythematosus or Gaucher's disease, and blood disorders like sickle cell disease. People with a minor level of ON (from any cause) during their younger years can present with arthritis of the joint as they age. This condition can be extremely debilitating.

Although ON is regarded as a multifactorial disease, age can play a large role in its etiology. Osteonecrosis has been staged from almost normal (stage 0) to complete destruction of articular cartilage and collapse of the bone with formation of severe osteoarthritis of the joint (stage 5).

Osteoarthritis

Osteoarthritis (OA) is the most common form of arthritis, affecting about 40 million people in the United States. Osteoarthritis is the leading cause of physical disability, increased need for health care, and impaired quality of life (Centers for Disease Control and Prevention 1997). Despite its prevalence, however, little is known regarding the etiology, pathogenesis, and progression of the disease. It is a non-inflammatory degenerative joint disease characterized by articular cartilage degradation, subchondral sclerosis, osteophyte formation, and changes in the soft tissues. (See the next section for discussion of cartilage metabolism.) Systemic factors, age, gender, mechanical stress, obesity, genetics (Herndon, Robbins, and Evans 1999), and local factors may control the site and severity of disease.

The prevalence of OA increases with age, perhaps due to a decrease in the cellular response to growth factors. The fundamental event resulting in the destruction of articular cartilage may be an imbalance between the catabolic and anabolic processes. As the protective capability of cartilage decreases, the underlying subchondral and periarticular bone experiences increased stress. This leads to senescent changes including lack of joint space, crepitus, lack of adequate function or motion, pain, and osteophyte formation. Newer techniques to treat OA involve autogenous cartilage implantation, autogenous osteochondral grafting, hyaluronic acid injection, and even gene therapies (Herndon, Robbins, and Evans 1999; LaPrade and Swiontkowske 1999).

Cartilage

Cartilage, which contains no blood vessels or nerves, is usually found in close association with bone. The main collagen type in cartilage, type II, is a tough, semi-transparent, elastic, flexible connective tissue. The cartilage cells (chondrocytes) lie scattered in the matrix. Cartilage is covered by a dense fibrous membrane, the perichondrium.

In mammals, the skeleton first forms as cartilage tissue. Cartilage acts as a model and is gradually replaced by bone in a process known as ossification. Not all cartilage is replaced by bone—the joint surfaces, the tip of the nose, the external ear, trachea, and larynx, for example, remain as cartilage.

Structure and Function

Cartilage has a very important function within the musculoskeletal system. It provides a smooth gliding surface for the joints by reducing friction (figure 1.1). The loss of this cartilage is what leads to OA of a joint. Cartilage also forms a base from which bone grows longitudinally, and acts as a major site of shock absorption and dissipation of joint forces.

Cartilage consists of water, extracellular matrix (ECM), and its main cell type, the chondrocyte. As well as lacking blood vessels and nerves, cartilage lacks lymphatic vessels (Brown and Branch 2000) and derives its nutrition from synovial fluid within the joint. The ECM primarily consists of water (70-80%), proteoglycans, and collagen (several types of collagen have been identified in cartilage but, as already noted, the major type is type II). Proteoglycan molecules, which are negatively charged, help to hold water within cartilage. The proteoglycans comprise glycosaminoglycan chains (keratan sulfate and chondroitin sulfate). This organization of proteoglycans within the collagen produces a strong, highly organized matrix.

The articular cartilage can be divided into distinct zones: the superficial zone (10-20%), middle zone (30-60%), deep zone (30-40%), calcified zone, and subchondral bone. The superficial zone, also known as the tangential zone, is the thinnest of the articular cartilage layers, with the highest content of collagen and the lowest amount of proteoglycans. The collagen is mainly arranged in a fashion tangential and parallel to the articular surface. Thus this layer is best geared to resist shearing forces on the joint. It also enhances the gliding surface of the joint and with its flattened chondrocytes helps in gliding and distribution of shear forces. Since this is the layer in contact with the joint and its forces and is the thinnest layer, it is the first to show pathological changes leading to OA.

The middle zone, also known as a transitional zone, acts to distribute shearing forces acting on the superficial layer to the compression forces acting in the deeper layer. It is composed mainly of proteoglycans and has a mixture of collagen arranged in both parallel and perpendicular directions to the joint. This layer contains more chondrocytes than the superficial zone.

The deep zone, also known as the deep radial layer, is the largest of the articular cartilage layers. With its collagen and chondrocytes arranged in a more perpendicular fashion in relation to the joint surface, it mainly functions to resist compression forces. The chondrocytes are more rounded in this layer as compared to the superficial layer, which also helps to dissipate joint forces evenly to the subchondral bone.

Deeper in relation to these layers is the calcified zone or the tidemark layer. This layer, the boundary between the calcified and noncalcified layers, separates the cartilage from the deeper subchondral bone.

The organization of layers helps the articular cartilage function as each layer contributes to overall cartilage function. This structural makeup also enhances the viscoelasticity of the cartilage as it experiences various loads. Figure 1.2 illustrates the viscoelastic properties of articular cartilage, which can be attributed to interactions between the proteoglycan subunit and type II collagen.

Disruption of the superficial architecture of articular cartilage is the foundation for the pathological process of OA (figure 1.3). Surface irregularities and fissures penetrate deeper into the cartilage, eventually prompting a critical point at which cartilage cells respond to

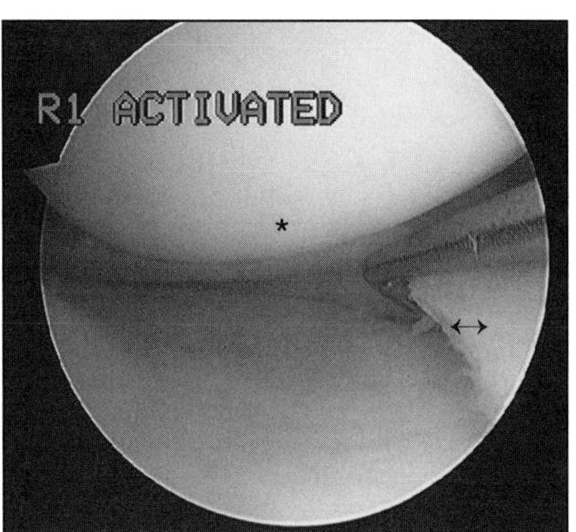

FIGURE 1.1 Normal cartilage of the femur (above probe, *) and a normal meniscus (under probe ↔).

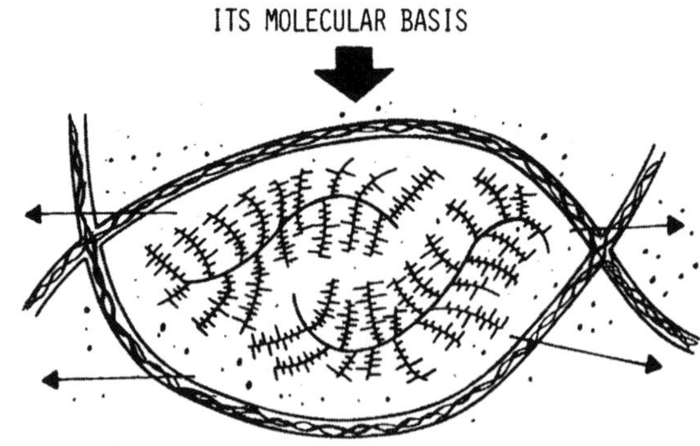

FIGURE 1.2 The viscoelastic properties of articular cartilage.

Reprinted, by permission, from J. Albright and R. Brand, 1987, *The scientific basis of orthopaedics* (New York: McGraw-Hill Companies), 358. © The McGraw-Hill Companies, Inc..

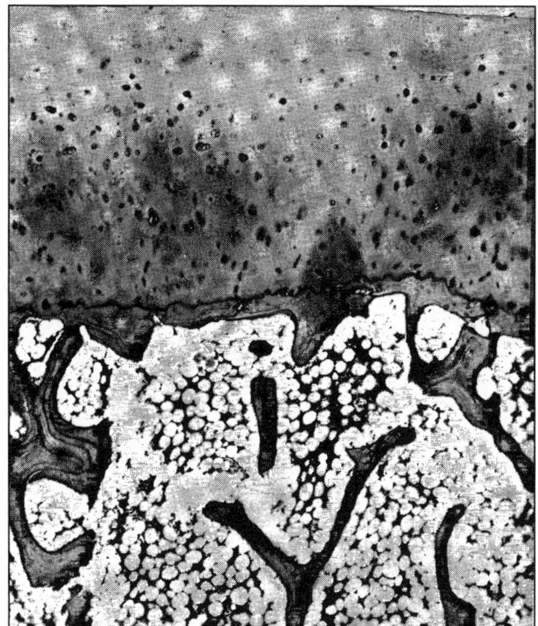

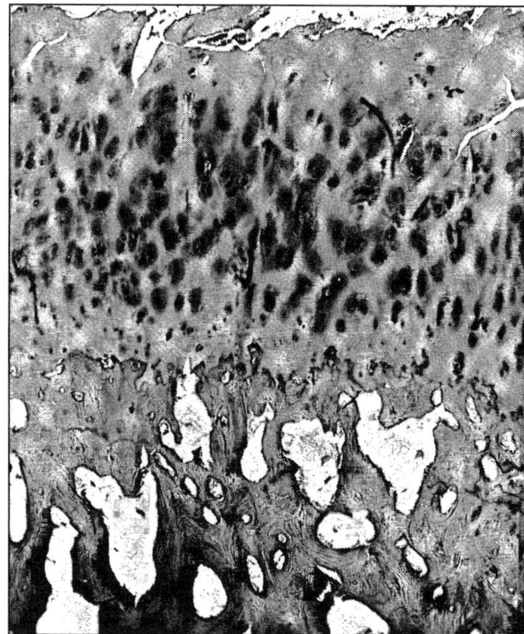

FIGURE 1.3 *(a)* Normal articular cartilage of an elderly patient; *(b)* a degenerating cartilage of an elderly patient.
Reprinted, by permission, from J. Albright and R. Brand, 1987, *The scientific basis of orthopaedics* (New York: McGraw-Hill Companies), 359. © The McGraw-Hill Companies, Inc..

the added stress by increasing metabolic activity. These pathways, which have been extensively studied at the cellular level, cause early OA chondrocytes to undergo transient proliferation and produce amplified quantities of various enzymes and growth factors. The resulting imbalance between the degradation and synthesis of the cartilage matrix catalyzes osteoarthritic changes. Ultimately, the proteoglycan moiety is split, disrupting the viscoelastic properties and exposing the collagen framework to increased stress, fatiguing the cellular structure and inducing its failure. Both chemical and collagen debris are released, passing to the synovial membrane and causing synovitis. Only at this point does OA become an inflammatory process.

Cartilage of any joint is subjected to high stresses in younger individuals, especially athletes. The interstitial fluid trapped in the ECM helps to absorb this kind of energy imparted to the cartilage during activities. As already described, although energy absorption is not the only function of cartilage, it is the main function. The overall level of activity decreases because both the quantity and quality of the structure of cartilage change. Thus, with decrease in the number of collagen fibrils and chondrocytes, less forces are dissipated and absorbed by the cartilage and more forces are imparted to the underlying subchondral bone. This is the reason patients with OA complain of pain and crepitus. Pain occurs because the underlying subchondral bone, unlike the articular cartilage, is well supplied with nerves.

Senescent Changes

With age, joint cartilage undergoes significant changes in its thickness, cell function and matrix properties, composition, and molecular organization. The already tenuous vascular supply undergoes further deterioration since the synovial fluid in the joint decreases in both quality and quantity. The cartilage matrix loses proteoglycan content (Buckwalter et al. 1993). This leads to decreased water content and an increase in the load on the cartilage since there is an accompanying decrease in the fluid flux. (Fluid flux refers to movement of fluid into and out of the cartilage matrix as it experiences loads in different conditions; cartilage cells use this fluid flux to equalize and balance pressures within the matrix.) The tensile properties, which are mainly dependent on the collagen, may or may not change as significantly. The overall activity of the cartilage decreases, affecting the general cellular response to mechanical loads, pressure changes, nutrients, and cytokines. The response to growth hormone (insulin-like growth hormone) decreases, leading to a higher susceptibility to injury and arthritis formation. Chondrocytes producing this growth hormone decrease in number as well, further decreasing its response in older persons (Buckwalter et al. 1993). The matrix catabolism increases and this brings about an imbalance of cartilage metabolism, in turn leading to arthritis formation (Buckwalter et al. 1993). The deformation of the cartilage changes the mechanical, electrical, and physiochemical signals and thus has a further role in progressive arthritis.

Injury to cartilage, more likely to occur in older than in younger people, can be microscopic, macroscopic, or a combination of the two. Cartilage injury can lead to chondrocyte damage, proteoglycan structure disruption, and increased collagen concentration, making the cartilage stiffer (Buckwalter et al. 1993). With skeletal maturity, superficial fibrillation of articular surfaces of the joint occurs. These changes may reach an irreversible stage more easily in older individuals. Fibrillations up to a certain point may be considered normal, but beyond this point they are indications of injury to the underlying cartilage. Superficial fibrillations of the cartilage are seen mainly during arthroscopy of the joints, and depending on how deep and how extensive they are, are given different grades (I to IV). Grade I is minimal involvement or a softening of the cartilage; grade II is fibrillation (figure 1.4);

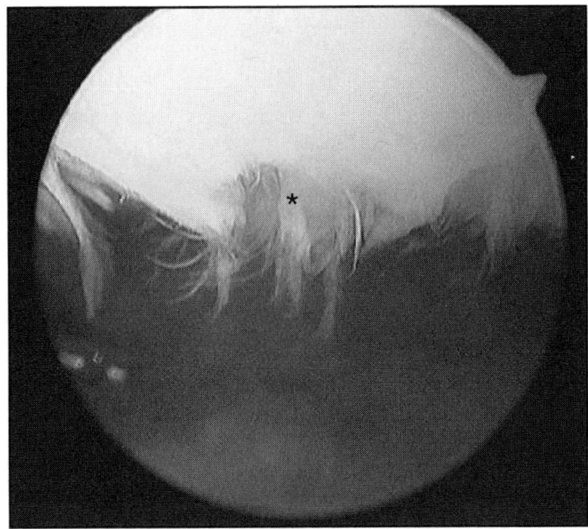

FIGURE 1.4 Grade II articular injury (patellar chondral lesion, *).

Cartilage

	Young	Old (OA)
Absorption		
Water	65-76%	Increased in early stage of OA Decreased in later stages
Proteoglycan	5-10%	Increased in early stage Decreased in later stage
Collagen	10-20%	Increased in percentage
Non-collagenous protein	5-10%	Increased
Minerals	1-2%	Increased
Fibronectin	Minimal	Increased
Type X collagen	Small amount	Increased with age
Type III collagen	None (absent)	Present in increasing quantity with age
IL-1	Decreased amount	Increased
Nitric oxide	Decreased (%)	Increased (%)
Free radicals	Decreased	Increased
Extracellular matrix	Increased	Increase in breakdown of structure
Fluid flux	Smooth	Decreased fluid flux
Response to growth hormone	Good	Decreased
Chondrocytes	Increased amount	Decreased

grade III is fissuring of the cartilage; and grade IV is cartilage loss with exposure of the underlying bone.

The healing of articular injury is compromised due to the lack of blood supply in the joint. An area of injured cartilage may result in increased loads on the surrounding "normal" cartilage, leading to propagation of the injury. Because tissue damaged by injury may be replaced by other types of collagen (not type II), which can lead to a decrease in the functional quality of the cartilage, the accumulated effects of small (or large) injuries over the decades can cause serious problems in the older active person.

JOINT STRUCTURES

It is well understood that structures composing the joint undergo a gradual decrease in blood supply with aging. This can bring about arthritic changes (decrease in space, osteophyte formation, etc.) with an effect on the joint's function and motion. This section deals with the meniscus, labrum, and capsule and ligaments.

Meniscus

Our understanding of meniscus comes mainly from studies in the knee joint. Although some other joints in the body contain meniscus (acromioclavicular, sternoclavicular, or triangular fibrocartilage complex in the wrist), most joints do not have meniscus. Wherever menisci are present, their main role is to distribute joint forces within the meniscus itself and to act as a shock absorber for the joint.

Menisci have different shapes and sizes depending on their joint locations. For example, in the knee joint they are semilunar pieces of fibrocartilage that extend the tibial articulation of the knee. In fact, menisci in the knee render the articulation between the femur and tibia congruous in addition to assisting with its load-bearing function. This explains why injury to the meniscus (whether traumatic or degenerative) tends to cause incongruity in the articulation of the bones of the knee and to lead to increased forces on the femur and the tibia with loads on the joint. The presence of menisci in the knee joint also increases the effective surface area of contact and helps in equal distribution of forces to the underlying cartilage; consequently, with meniscus loss (or injury), the load is taken up by the surrounding articular cartilage along with the bone, and arthritis tends to set in at a much faster pace.

Structure and Function

The fibrocartilaginous, viscoelastic tissue known as the meniscus consists of an ECM, a complex interlocking array of collagen fibers with proteoglycan and water. In addition to serving as a "shock absorber" for the joint, the meniscus lubricates the joint to aid in smooth motion and helps with load transmission. The main collagen in the meniscus is type I (more than 90%). The orientation of collagen fibers in the various meniscus zones, along with the water content, helps with load-bearing and -sharing properties (Mow et al. 1992). Recently the function of the meniscus has become much better understood at both the macroscopic and microscopic levels.

The meniscus has been divided into three different zones according to the amount of blood supply: the red–red zone (peripheral 10-25% with best vasculature), the red–white zone (intermediate vasculature), and the white–white zone (outer half with poorest vasculature). The varying degrees of vascularity explain why healing after a meniscus tear is zone dependent.

The knee joint has two C-shaped menisci, the medial and the lateral. Each meniscus is composed of horns—anterior, middle, and posterior. Each meniscus has longitudinal fibers, horizontal fibers, and circumferential fibers, with an interwoven mixture of radial and oblique fibers (see figure 1.1). With trauma to the meniscus, fibers are torn in a similar distribution to the direction of the force causing the injury. In degenerative types of tears, the meniscus tears in a complex manner such that the various types of fiber orientations are affected, making it difficult to distinguish between longitudinal, radial, and circumferential tears. In the knee, most degenerative, complex tears are found in the outer two-thirds of the menisci. Consistent with their function of stabilizing the joint, in a knee with no anterior cruciate ligament (ACL) the menisci take up the role of a knee stabilizer. It is for this reason that some people continue to have stable knee joints in spite of ACL tears.

The role of the meniscus in proprioception of the knee joint is well documented. Often people who have had a meniscectomy or have sustained a meniscus injury complain about losing the proprioceptive sense of the knee joint (a sense of balance and of the ability to feel the knee joint). Many patients with a meniscus injury complain that the joint has lost its stability or "gives way." In fact the knee joint is not unstable from a traditional standpoint, as it is with a tear of the ACL, posterior cruciate ligament, or other ligaments. Rather the feeling of joint instability is attributable to the loss of function of proprioceptive fibers in the meniscus in situations of meniscus loss or tear.

Senescent Changes

Menisci respond to aging, physiological stresses, and immobilization. With senescence, the collagen as well as the non-collagenous contents of the meniscus

Meniscus

	Young	Old
Type I collagen	Main type	Decreased
Other types	Minimal	Increased with age
Aggrecan	Decreased	Increased
Cellularity	Highly cellular	Decreased
Dry collagen	Decreased	Increased
Tissue surface	Smooth	Fibrillation/erosion
Water	60-75% of total weight	Decreased
Proteoglycans	Increased	Decreased
Meniscal fibrochondrocytes	Increased	Decreased
Diffusion (outer one-third)	Increased diffusion	Compromised

increase with a decrease in cellularity and water content. With this accumulation of dry collagen, there is an increase in the degradative proteases and calcium pyrophosphate crystal levels. This has a detrimental effect on the mechanical and functional properties. As suggested earlier, the outer two-thirds of the meniscus has a decreased potential to heal; and since this is the meniscus most affected by senescence, the healing potential of the meniscus drops much further still. The declining vascular supply and nutrition give rise to complex tears involving both the circumferential and horizontal collagen fibers.

Labrum

The labrum is a fibrous structure surrounding the periphery of the glenoid (figure 1.5). It attaches to the glenoid cartilage through a fibrocartilaginous transition zone (Cooper et al. 1992).

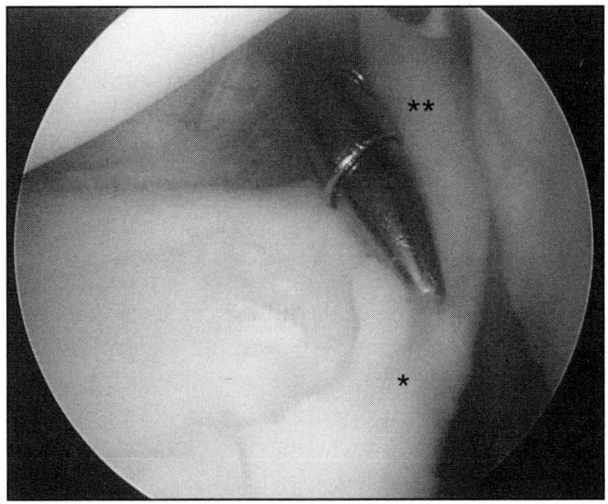

FIGURE 1.5 Trocar showing a normal superior labrum (*) and biceps tendon (**).

Normal Structure and Function

As with the meniscus of the knee joint, the labrum is triangular in cross section and contains proteoglycans and a very small amount of elastin. Its roles include load transmission, shock absorption, stabilization, articular cartilage nutrition, and probably proprioception (Cooper et al. 1992). It acts to increase the surface area of the glenoid and the joint surface, thus adding to the stability and load transmission across the shoulder joint (Cooper et al. 1992). The glenoid labrum acts as a static stabilizer of the G-H joint by deepening the glenoid socket by about 50%. In addition, it acts as a buttress to limit humeral head translation and serves as an attachment site for the G-H ligaments.

The labrum's unique biomechanical and physiological properties are attributed to its complex 3-D network of collagen fibers, proteoglycans, glycoproteins, and fibrochondrocytes. Unlike the meniscus, though, the labrum does not have areas of avascularity. Vessels are more numerous peripherally, however, and there is less vascularity at the fibrocartilaginous junction between the glenoid and the labrum.

Senescence

The elastin component in the labrum appears to increase with age. With increasing age, the labrum loses some of its ECM properties, which alters the pattern of joint loading. This may be a reason for accelerated articular cartilage degeneration with age. The depth of the labrum decreases with age due to its degeneration, forcing the cartilage to bear increasing forces across the joint.

Capsule and Ligaments

Capsule and ligaments are specialized, dense, fibrous musculoskeletal tissues. Their main role is to provide stability as well as mobility to the joints. Age-related injuries to these structures can cause the joint to become unstable or incapable of adequate movement. The capsule forms a complex structure that covers the joints and contains the synovial fluid. It is reinforced with distinct thickenings or ligaments—dense connective tissues that link bone to bone. The ligaments act to dynamically stabilize the joints during their motion (Gohlke, Essigkrug, and Schmitz 1994).

Normal Structure and Function

Under microscopic examination, the collagen fibers of the ligaments are relatively parallel and aligned along the axis of tension, but they have a more interwoven arrangement than in tendons. Characteristic sinusoidal patterns within the bundles are observed within the ligaments. Fibroblasts are responsible for producing and maintaining the extracellular components. In young persons, growth factors such as transforming growth factor-β (TGF-β), epidermal growth factor (EGF), and platelet-derived growth factor (PDGF) have been shown to stimulate fibroblast cell division and matrix synthesis.

The major biochemical component of ligaments is water, about 60% to 80%. Collagen constitutes approximately 70% to 80% of dry weight, with type I collagen accounting for about 90% of the collagen. Formation of cross-links between collagen fibers gives the ligaments their strength characteristics. The proteoglycans contain water molecules and affect the viscoelastic properties. Protein elastin helps the ligament to return to its original length after a load is removed.

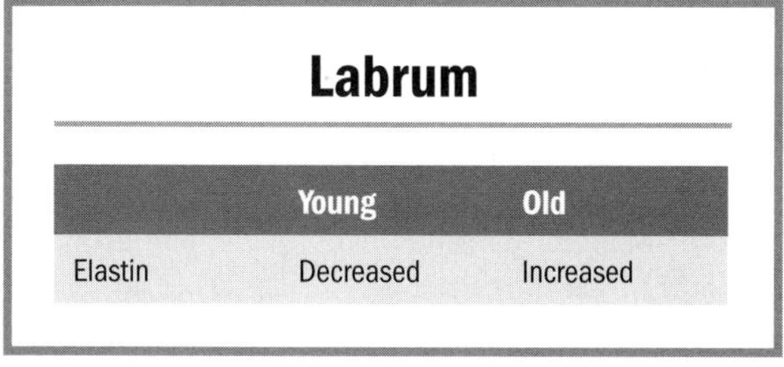

Labrum

	Young	Old
Elastin	Decreased	Increased

Senescent Changes

Age is a predominant factor in differences in the properties of the insertion sites of the ligaments (Buckwalter et al. 1993). In younger individuals, ligament injury is more predominant at insertion sites, whereas in older people, midsubstance tears are more common. As ligaments age, the structural and material properties change in response to loading conditions. For example, the load at failure of the ACL (which occurs along a continuum of ages, with 40 years being a fairly widely accepted average) is 33% to 50% of that seen with younger individuals (Buckwalter et al. 1993). The same has been reported in the shoulder, especially the inferior glenohumeral ligament (IGHL). Similar changes occur in most ligaments, placing increased stresses on the other structures within the joint.

Biochemical changes include a decrease in water and a relative increase in dry collagen content. Fibroblasts assume a more elongated shape and become less active metabolically. The cross-links increase in concentration to give the ligaments a stiffer, more stable form as compared to the immature, labile, more flexible form in younger individuals. Also, the effect of TGF-β, EGF, and PDGF on fibroblast proliferation diminishes with age. This leads to a detrimental effect on both the ligament substance and its insertion site such that the threshold to failure is lower because of decreased flexibility and ability to adapt to loads.

With aging, people tend to become less active, and this further leads to detrimental effects on the properties of ligaments. As already mentioned, the load at failure decreases with less activity or immobilization. Increased subperiosteal bone resorption along with increased osteoclastic activity at the ligament insertion site has been observed in older, less active individuals compared to older, more active counterparts or younger active people. Also, as noted previously, the recovery period after any kind of injury or immobilization is shorter in younger individuals. The quality of repair is also affected in senescence; the collagen alignment remains less organized after repair in older people. Additionally, the percentage of functional loss as compared to preinjury levels is more affected with senescence.

Intervertebral Disc

Intervertebral discs contribute greatly to normal spine function. These are cartilaginous structures that lie within two adjacent vertebral bodies, throughout the spine. While they function as load absorbers, their

Capsule and Ligaments

	Young	Old
Insertion	Strong	Weakened
Tears	Insertion	Midstructure
Load at failure	High	Low
Water	Increased content	Decreased
Dry collagen	Less in amount	Increased
Stiffness	Minimal	Increased
Cross-links	Decreased	High
Fibroblasts	Active	Less active
Density of fibroblasts	Increased	Decreased
Partial injury healing	Complete	Incomplete
Healing	Complete/ adequate	Compromised

contribution to the stability of the spine has also been proven. Movement would not be possible in the spine if the discs were not present. Senescent changes affect the disc also, as with any other musculoskeletal tissue, which is why we see disc degeneration and spine issues more in older age.

Structure

The disc is separated from vertebral bone by the hyaline cartilage endplate. This is present both superior and inferior to the disc. The outer portion of the disc is known as the **annulus fibrosis,** and the inner, softer structure is the **nucleus pulposus.** These two differ in the type of cartilage that predominates. While the annulus fibrosis is composed mainly of type I collagen, the nucleus pulposus is composed of type II collagen. A zone between the two makes for a smooth transition.

The matrix is formed from collagens, elastin, proteoglycans, and non-collagenous proteins. The collagens give the disc its form and strength. The concentration or dry weight of collagen progressively decreases from the outer annulus (60-70%) to the inner nucleus pulposus (10-20%). Proteoglycans, which give the disc its resiliency and stiffness to compression, decrease in concentration (10-20% of dry weight) from the periphery to the central nucleus (50% of dry weight). Elastin, whose role is unclear, is found in trace amounts in both the outer and inner layers of the disc. Non-collagenous proteins, which help to adhere the matrix cells to each other and organize and stabilize the matrix, are found in slightly higher amounts in the nucleus as compared to the annulus.

The blood supply of the inner central disc depends mainly on the diffusion of nutrients and metabolites through the matrix. This is because the small blood vessels lie mainly on the outer layer of the annulus, penetrating only into the outer part of the nucleus layer. The innervation setup seems to be similar, with free nerve endings on the outer layer of the annulus and no nerve endings on the inner layer of the nucleus.

The **annulus fibrosus** makes up the peripheral portion of disc structure, and, as already mentioned, is composed of fibrocartilage and type I collagen. These densely packed collagen fibers of annulus run obliquely between vertebrae and are arranged primarily in concentric layers. The outer concentric ring is highly organized, with all its fibers oriented in the same direction. The direction of the fibers in successive layers alternates, with one layer crossing another at angles of 30° to 60°. Some annular fibers extend past the periphery of the endplate. This probably offers added stability to the bone and the cartilage. The deeper fibers either insert into the cartilage at each end of the disc or blend with nucleus pulposus. Like other dense fibrous tissue, the annulus has about 60% to 70% water content. The connective tissue cells in this layer resemble fibroblasts in appearance. On the outer side of the annulus, these fibroblasts lie with their long axis parallel to the collagen fibrils, while in the inner region, more cells take on a rounded, spherical shape.

During development, there is a sharp demarcation between the annulus fibrosis and the nucleus pulposus. With growth, this boundary becomes less defined and is called the **transition zone.** As the name implies, this layer is a mixture of composition of the deeper gelatinous nucleus pulposus layer and the outer, more stout fibrocartilaginous annulus fibrosis.

The **nucleus pulposus** is a collection of delicate collagenous fibers in a mucoprotein gel rich in polysaccharide and is composed of mainly type II collagen. Since the nucleus has a high water content, it functions to resist compressive loads. It is here that the load distribution of the body takes place. The water content helps to distribute the forces, just as in the cartilage (discussed earlier in the chapter). The nucleus pulposus has a water content of about 90% at birth and about 70% in adults. The cells in this layer have an appearance resembling that of chondrocytes. These cells assume a more rounded shape as compared to the outer fibrocartilaginous annulus layer.

Senescent Changes

Like other musculoskeletal structures, the intervertebral disc undergoes alteration in its structure with maturation and aging. The nucleus pulposus undergoes the most change. The concentration of clear gelatinous nucleus, along with the notochordal tissue, decreases from birth to old age. As already noted, the transition zone forms with age; it is not found in the newborn. With the loss of gelatinous material during aging, the clear-appearing nucleus at birth gradually becomes opaque. Water content declines with advancing age and is reduced by pressure borne by the disc. This explains the loss in the height of a person during an active day.

Gradual loss of proteogylcan content explains the loss of water with aging. People in their 30s begin to show a gradual loss of fluid and concomitant fibrous replacement of the nucleus; by the sixth or seventh decade the nucleus becomes fibrocartilage. By this time it becomes difficult to separate the inner disc from the transition zone or the outer annular disc. Annulus also shows coarsened and hyalinized fibers and fissuring of the lamellae.

The percentage of necrotic cells in the disc increases from about 1% to 2% in a newborn to about 50% in adults, further increasing to about 80% in the elderly. The reason is probably compromise in the diffusion of nutrients with age. The diffusion likely decreases due to decreased water content, decrease in the number of viable notochordal cells, increase in the number of necrotic cells and cell metabolites, and increase in the opacity of the tissue. As explained earlier, the blood supply of the inner nucleus is already at a disadvantage since the blood vessel supply comes from the peripheral annulus. This also becomes an important factor in repair of the disc after injury. Because of all these factors, the potential to heal any kind of tear or injury to the disc decreases with increasing age.

Intervertebral Disc

	Young	Old
Gelatinous nucleus	High content	Low content
Notochordal cells	Higher amount	Decreased
Transitional zone	Absent	Present
Water content (%)	Increased	Decreased
Fibrocartilage (%)	Decreased	Increased
Dry collagen (%)	Increased	Decreased
Proteoglycan (%)	Increased	Decreased
Lamellae	Smooth	Coarsened, fissured
Necrotic cells	1-2%	50-80%
Diffusion	Good	Compromised
Cell metabolites	Low	High

MUSCULOTENDINOUS STRUCTURES

This section deals with tendon and skeletal muscle. Most skeletal muscles in the human body exert their effects (contraction or relaxation) through their insertion endpoints onto bone, which are generally tendons. It is the skeletal muscle contraction that stabilizes the joint against resistance and imparts motion to the joint. Muscle turns into tendon prior to insertion on the bone, so the interaction between these two (albeit they are continuous structures) is paramount to function of the joint involved. Tendons (like ligaments) have the ability to resist large tensile loads with minimal deformation. On the other hand, muscles have the ability to generate different loads under different demands; and as compared to tendons, muscles are more changeable in their lengths. The junction between the two structures is called the musculotendinous junction. It is here that energy generated by the bigger muscle is most effectively transferred to the smaller tendon.

Tendon

It is through the tendon—the insertional point of muscle into bone—that the muscle exerts forces onto the bone. As muscle turns into tendon, the fibrous structure becomes more organized. This leads to a decrease in the amount of space it occupies. This smaller area of tendon can then insert onto bone. If muscles did not decrease in size to become tendons prior to their insertion, our arms and forearms, and legs and thighs, would be the same size from proximal to distal. This would be highly energy consuming since the surface area would not decrease as the muscle inserted onto bone.

Normal Structure and Function

Most understanding of intra-articular function of the tendons comes from the shoulder rotator cuff tendons (Clark and Harryman 1992), which help to stabilize the glenohumeral joint by imparting direct compression of the humeral head to the glenoid. Tendons stabilize the joints both statically and dynamically. Statically, the presence of tendons in or around the joint makes the joint stable whether it is moving or not; that is, tendons act as checkreins. In dynamic stabilization, when the joint is moving, the tendons by virtue of their contraction or tightening add stability to the joint. This is one of the reasons joints do not dislocate with daily movement activities.

Orientation of the tendinous fiber strands and the interwoven fiber patterns varies. This explains differences in biomechanical properties of different tendons, in the response to different loads, and in intratendinous tears.

Tendons are dense, primarily collagenous tissues that link muscle to bone. They have highly organized parallel-oriented bundles of collagen. This orientation helps transmit the load generated by muscle to bone. Like ligaments and capsule, tendons are composed of both non-collagenous and collagenous tissue. The non-collagenous component, even though it contributes less in weight than the collagenous tissue, plays an important role in the structural makeup of tendon. Fibronectin, for example, occurs in all dense fibrous tissue. Its functions and real structural contribution are still being defined. The collagen content is primarily type I collagen (95%).

Proteoglycans, though in a small concentration, support the function of collagenous tissue (Spindler and Wright 2002). Depending on the type of demand on the tendon, different regions within the tendon have different concentrations of glycosaminoglycan, aggrecan, and biglycan content. Aggrecan is the shortened name of the large aggregating chondroitin sulfate proteoglycan and is the most abundant of the proteoglycans. Many different aggrecan molecules (about 100) combine to form the aggregate. Transforming growth factor-β stimulates the production of aggrecan and biglycan (Spindler and Wright 2002). Tendons undergoing tensile loads have a smaller concentration of proteoglycans than those undergoing primarily compressive loads. Proteoglycans are water-carrying molecules and more proteoglycan means more water. Therefore, compressive loads are easier to handle with increased proteoglycan since water makes the force distribute evenly. Similarly, tensile loads are more like "stretching" loads and water does not play much of a role since the distribution of water is not required.

Senescence

Structural and degenerative changes have been reported in tendons with age. The overall diameter of the tendon decreases. The total cell count, amount of crimp (sinusoidal patterns), and mean fibril diameter decrease. The metabolic activity of the fibroblasts in tendons also decreases. The dry weight of both the collagen and its cross-links, which hold the tendon's **collagen fibers** together, increases. This is important because the nerves and blood vessels that supply the tendon lie between these fibers. When the tendon terminates into bone, the collagen bundles (or fibers) become smaller and more intertwined with each other. This intertwining increases the surface area of the insertion and leads to a strong fixation onto the bone. Along with the increase in collagen and its cross-links is a decrease in the amount of glycosaminoglycans. Biomechanically, all these changes contribute to tendons becoming drier and stiffer in older individuals as compared to young persons, as well as to their lower failure threshold (figure 1.6).

The typical progression in older people of decreases in activity leading to reduced demands on the body, resulting in lowered muscle strength, causes diminished biomechanical tendon properties as well. The exact histological changes have yet to be completely defined. These changes may be harder to reverse in an older patient who starts exercising later in life. The

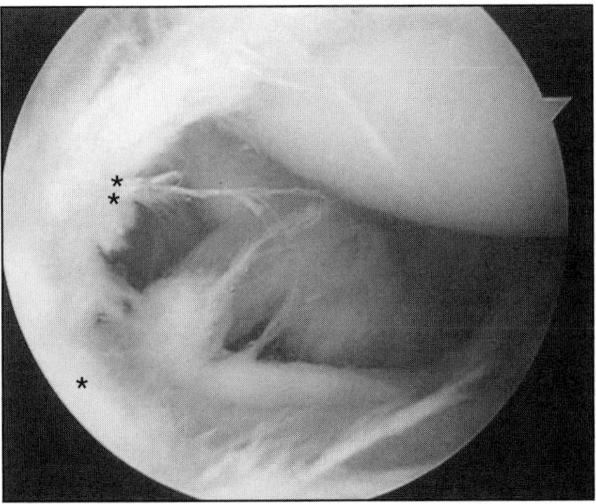

FIGURE 1.6 Partially torn biceps tendon (**) and labrum (*).

potential for healing in the degenerative age-related nontraumatic tear is also limited (figure 1.7).

Skeletal Muscle

Skeletal muscle is one of the best examples of a biological structure–function relationship. At both macro- and microscopic levels, the primary function of skeletal muscle is for movement and generation of force. The myotendinous junction is a highly specialized region for taking up the force generated by the skeletal muscles.

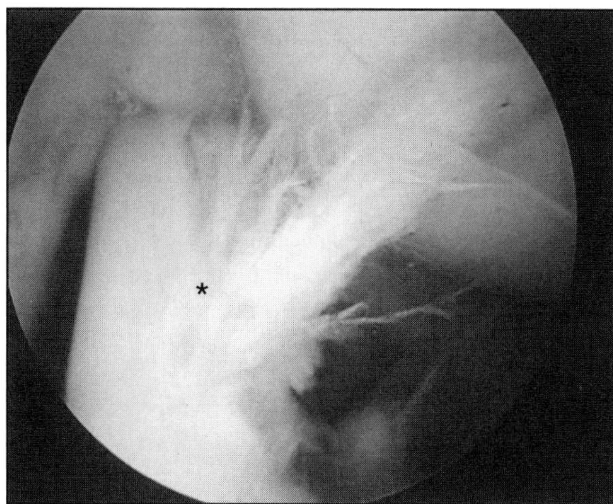

FIGURE 1.7 Biceps pathology (*).

Structure and Function

A muscle acts on bone and joint motion by acting through the myotendinous junction and eventually through the tendon. Muscles do not act in isolation. Synergistic and antagonistic muscles in the same limb carry out different motions, in coordination with each other. The best example can be seen in the shoulder muscle.

Seventeen muscles act in or around the shoulder girdle. Electromyographic (EMG) studies have indicated a complex array of activity of these muscles, even to do a simple task. The fact that EMG activities can be reproduced with a particular joint motion suggests that various muscles work in complete harmony with each other. When a particular muscle or group of muscles is injured, the other muscles adjust and adapt to the given function and take up increased activity and load.

The two types of muscle fibers, type I and II (Garrett and Best 1994), are generally present in equal amounts in the body. Type I, slow-twitch oxidative fatigue-resistant fibers, are used for endurance aerobic-type activities. These also have a slow rate of contraction. Type II are fast-twitch anaerobic fibers

Tendon

	Young	Old
Fibril diameter	Thick	Narrow
Cell count	High	Low
Crimp	High	Low
Glycosaminoglycans	High content	Low content
Stiffness	Decreased	Increased
Energy to tear/rupture	High	Low
Tensile strength	High	Low
Fibroblast	Rounded/plump	Flattened/elongated
Rough endoplasmic reticulum (%)	High	Low
Water (%)	High	Low
Vascularity	Good	Compromised

with a high strength of contraction. Growth hormone has a positive effect on both types of muscle fibers in younger individuals (Terjung et al. 2000). Response to activity is better in young muscles. Motor units are single peripheral motor neurons innervating a group of skeletal muscle fibers. In young, healthy athletes, the number of motor units is high and shows a high response to exercise and activity.

Senescent Changes

Muscle mass decreases slowly between 25 and 50 years of age. After this, the rate of muscle atrophy increases. This leads to a natural decrease in muscle strength, and muscle stiffness increases. The muscle diameter decreases also, significantly in the type II fibers (Luff 1998). Decreased average activity associated with aging is further detrimental to muscle strength and the ability to absorb energy before failure. Moreover, if disuse and immobilization are encouraged (e.g., when a shoulder is in a sling or a knee in an immobilizer for too long), the muscles involved in that joint manifest a loss of endurance and strength and an increase in stiffness. Loss of strength in any muscle group can mean that the other muscles around the joint may have to take up an increased load related to activity, thus becoming exposed to risk of failure. Decreased muscle strength also has a deleterious effect on the bone and motor endplates (Luff 1998). That is, muscle insertion into bone through the tendon brings additional blood supply to the bone; with aging, as the muscle is affected, so is the bone (decrease in quantity and quality of bone cells). (This can lead to much easier avulsion of muscle from bone since the area has a compromised blood supply. Avulsions, though, are not commonly seen in older individuals mainly because the force generated by the muscle undergoes a decrease at the same time.)

The response of the muscle fiber to growth hormone also decreases during aging. The number of motor units is diminished, with loss of fast motor units first. There is a reorganization of the other motor units, which may explain the reduction of reaction times and voluntary motor movements in elderly persons.

Muscle

	Young	Old
Mass	High	Gradually decreases
Diameter	Thick	Narrow
Strength	High	Low
Muscle cells	High amount	Low
Contracture against loads	High	Low
Hormonal levels (growth hormone, testosterone, thyroxin)	High	Low
Healing	Brisk	Slower
Cross-sectional area	Bigger	Smaller
Contractile proteins (%)	High	Low
Oxidative capacity	High	Low
Macrophage activity	High	Low
Repair/injury from regenerating myotubules	Good repair potential	Compromised
Mechanism of healing	Regenerating muscle	Replacement with scar
Blood supply	High/good	Compromised

All these factors in senescence make it even more important for joints not to be immobilized for too long in older persons. Loss of muscle strength and endurance also means early fatigue, and fatigued muscles have been shown to have an earlier and higher failure rate. This may be one reason it is more common to see an increase in both partial and complete muscle tears in the elderly as compared to young patients. Shoulder rotator cuff tears in the elderly are a good example. Muscles in older persons also have a decreased ability to heal after any kind of insult. This leads to longer-duration, more time-consuming rehabilitation after injury or surgery in muscles.

SUMMARY

The musculoskeletal system undergoes numerous senescent changes in its physiology as an individual ages. Given all these changes, it becomes crucial to help maintain the structure and functions of the musculoskeletal system through patient education, physical therapy, rehabilitation, exercise, and early treatment of certain conditions. Muscle strengthening exercises and prevention of motion loss may be the most important means by which therapists and athletic trainers can contribute to the health and function of aging joints. Immobilization for long periods, unless strictly indicated, should be avoided. A specific training program should be based on the older patient's social needs, reason for participation, and baseline functional level. This should not be like the training program for a younger population. Modifying the intensity factors, duration, and frequency of training may be especially crucial.

An overall conservative attitude after any musculoskeletal pathology on the part of patients, their families, and their physicians unfortunately results in decreased activity and further overall decline in function. Therapists and trainers must be prepared to counter this conservative attitude, realizing that a proper physical therapy program can largely reduce the decline in joint function with age. An early referral to an orthopedic surgeon or physical therapist following a musculoskeletal system injury or in situations of pathology may avoid many effects of disuse and senescence. An orthopedic surgeon can evaluate the musculoskeletal problem and triage it toward the right program and for the best results for that particular patient, whether or not it requires surgery.

CHAPTER

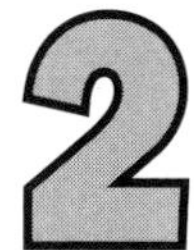

Exercise Testing and Prescription

Rafael F. Escamilla, PhD, PT, CSCS

Currently one in five Americans is 55 years or older (U.S. Department of Commerce 2000). The United States Census Bureau has projected that by the year 2010, one in four Americans will be 55 years or older (U.S. Department of Commerce 2000). With people living longer and staying active, it is important to understand the benefits of various forms of exercise. Associated with aerobic and anaerobic fitness are numerous physiological changes that occur with aging (Galloway and Jokl 2000; Mazzeo et al. 1998). The following statistics are based on many different populations, and the changes listed typically begin to some degree after age 25, regardless of nutritional, exercise, educational, ethnic, or social status.

- An increase in blood pressure (BP) and total peripheral resistance (Stratton et al. 1994)
- A decrease in maximum heart rate (HRmax), stroke volume, cardiac output, left ventricular diastolic filling rate and contractility, arterial–venous oxygen difference (a-$\bar{v}O_2$ difference), and ejection fraction, leading to a 5% to 20% decrease in maximum oxygen consumption ($\dot{V}O_2$max) per decade after age 25 (Mazzeo et al. 1998; Miller et al. 1986)
- A decrease in pulmonary function (Brischetto et al. 1984)
- A decrease in plasma volume, red blood cells, and total blood volume (Davy and Seals 1994)
- An increase in glucose intolerance and insulin resistance (Shimokata et al. 1991)
- A decrease in bone mineral density (especially in postmenopausal women) of approximately 1% per year (Burger et al. 1994)
- A decrease in basal metabolic rate (Shimokata and Kuzuya 1993)
- A 3% to 5% per decade increase in body fat (Kyle et al. 2001; Mazzeo et al. 1998)
- A 3% to 5% per decade decrease in the size and number of muscle fibers (sarcopenia) and motor units, especially fast glycolytic motor units (Type IIb) (Booth, Weeden, and Tseng 1994)
- A decrease in muscular strength and endurance of approximately 15% between ages 50 and 70, and approximately 30% per decade after age 70 (Mazzeo et al. 1998)
- An increase in motor neuron atrophy and denervation, and a decrease in nerve conduction velocity (Booth, Weeden, and Tseng 1994)
- A decrease in joint flexibility, an increase in crystallinity of collagen, and a decrease in tissue extensibility (Bell and Hoshizaki 1981; Kuhlman 1993)

These physiologic changes that occur with aging can lead to cardiovascular and musculoskeletal dysfunctions and are exacerbated by physical inactivity. A recent report of the Surgeon General indicated that over 60% of adults in the United States do not engage in regular activity; 25% of adults are not active at all, and less than 20% of adults obtain enough exercise for discernable health and exercise benefits (U.S. Department of Health and Human Services 1996). The Surgeon General's report also provided two important conclusions:

- Significant health benefits can be obtained by including moderate amounts of physical activity (e.g., 30 min of brisk walking or raking leaves, 15 min of running, or 45 min playing volleyball) on most, if not all, days of the week. Through a modest increase in daily activity, most Americans can improve their health and quality of life.

- Additional health benefits can be gained through greater amounts of physical activity. People who can maintain a regular regimen of activity that is of longer duration and of more vigorous activity are likely to derive greater benefit.

Employing aerobic exercise (exercise continuous in nature that elicits an increased sustained heart rate for a prolonged period of time) and anaerobic exercise (exercise intermittent in nature, such as strength training, in which a short period of exercise is followed by a short period of rest) can attenuate, and in some cases reverse, most physiologic changes associated with aging (Schilke 1991). This chapter focuses on three areas related to aerobic and anaerobic exercise in the active healthy individual over 50 years of age:

- Current research findings on the effects of aerobic and anaerobic exercise
- Aerobic and anaerobic exercise testing
- Aerobic and anaerobic exercise prescription

EFFECTS OF STRENGTH TRAINING IN THE AGING

Studies of the effects of low- and high-intensity strength training on muscle strength and hypertrophy in the aging population are shown in table 2.1. These data show clearly that strength training increases both muscle strength and muscle mass. Numerous studies (the table presents a small sample) involving both males and females over a wide range of ages (40-90 years old) have shown that strength training (higher-intensity strength training appears more effective than low-intensity strength training) produces numerous efficacious effects that aid in minimizing injuries, maximizing performance, enhancing rehabilitation, improving function, and decreasing the risk of coronary heart disease (CHD):

- An increase in muscle strength (Fiatarone et al. 1990; Pyka et al. 1994)
- An increase in muscle hypertrophy (Frontera et al. 1988; Taaffe et al. 1996)
- An increase in neuromuscular function (Hakkinen et al. 2000; Taaffe et al. 1999)
- An increase in bone strength and density and a decrease in osteoporosis (Layne and Nelson 1999; Nelson et al. 1994)
- A positive effect on pain or disability in individuals with osteoarthritis (Baker and McAlindon 2000)
- An increase in ligament and tendon strength (Hakkinen et al. 2000; Taaffe et al. 1999) and thickness (Kannus et al. 1997)
- An increase in balance and decrease in risk of falling and subsequent injury (Buchner et al. 1997; Gregg, Pereira, and Caspersen 2000)
- An increase in gait stability, mobility, and walking speed and efficiency (Judge, Underwood, and Gennosa 1993; Schlicht, Camaione, and Owen 2001)
- An increase in stair climbing and chair rising ability (Brill et al. 1998)
- An increase in hormonal adaptations (Kraemer et al. 1999)
- A decrease in glucose intolerance and insulin resistance and a decrease in the risk factors associated with type II diabetes (Eriksson et al. 1997; Honkola, Forsen, and Eriksson 1997)
- A decrease in BP (Martel et al. 1999)
- A decrease in body fat (Campbell et al. 1994; Toth, Beckett, and Poehlman 1999)
- An increase in basal metabolic rate (Campbell et al. 1994; Lemmer et al. 2001)
- An increase in protein requirements from 0.60 to 0.80 g/kg body weight to 1 to 1.6 g/kg body weight (Campbell et al. 1994; Lemon 1998)
- An increase in positive mood and a decrease in anxiety and tension (Tsutsumi et al. 1998)
- A reduction in the risk of CHD (Tanasescu et al. 2002)

STRENGTH TESTING FOR THE AGING INDIVIDUAL

Before strength testing of the aging active individual, a medical examination should take place and a health questionnaire should be completed to determine any contraindications to exercise. An orthopedic examination may also be warranted prior to strength testing to ensure that there are no musculoskeletal impairments that could be exacerbated with strength testing. The subject should have sufficient time to acclimate to the test exercises and should be able to properly perform each exercise. It is important that the patient perform proper stretching and progressive warm-up before testing. For example, a warm-up prior to lower extremity testing may consist of 5 min of stretching exercises for the hamstrings, quadriceps, and gluteus

TABLE 2.1 Sample of Studies Representing the Effects of High- and Low-Intensity Resistance Training on Muscle Strength and Hypertrophy in the Aging

Reference	Bemben et al. 2000	Fiatarone et al. 1990	Frontera et al. 1988	Nelson et al. 1994	Pyka et al. 1994	Taaffe et al. 1996
Strength training protocol	Machine upper and lower body exercises for high-intensity (80% 1RM) and low-intensity (40% 1RM) groups	Lower extremity machine resistance exercises	"Thigh-knee" Universal machine	Hip extension, knee extension, lat pulldown, back extension, abdominal flexion	12 Nautilus and Universal machine lower and upper body exercises	Leg press, knee extension, and knee flexion for high-intensity (80% 1RM) and low-intensity (40% 1RM) groups
Sex (M, F)	F	M, F	M	F	M, F	M, F
Number of subjects	17	10	12	20	11	13 M, 12 F
Age (years)	41-60	90 ± 1	60-72	50-70	61-78	69-79
Frequency (days/week)	3	3	3	3	3	3
Duration (weeks)	26	8	12	52	52	52
Training sets × repetition maximum (RM)	3 × 8 reps (80% 1RM) for high-intensity group; 3 × 16 reps (40% 1RM) for low-intensity group	3 × 8 reps (80% 1RM)	3 × 8 reps	3 × 8 reps (80% 1RM)	3 × 8 reps	3 × 7 reps (80% 1RM) for high-intensity group; 3 × 14 reps (40% 1RM) for low-intensity group
Strength testing protocol	1RM machine upper and lower body exercises	1RM machine knee extension	1RM "thigh-knee" Universal machine	1RM for hip extension, knee extension, and lat pulldown	1RM for each of the 12 strength training exercises	1RM for leg press, knee extension, and knee flexion
Mean significant increase in muscle strength	30% increase in high-intensity group; 27% increase in low-intensity group	174 ± 31% increase	112% increase in knee extensors; 227% increase in knee flexors	12% increase (average of the three strength testing exercises)	64 ± 11% increase (average of the 12 strength testing exercises)	59 ± 8% increase in high-intensity group; 42 ± 8% increase in low-intensity group
Mean significant increase in muscle hypertrophy	20% increase in rectus femoris (both high- and low-intensity groups); 33% increase in biceps brachii (high-intensity group only)	12 ± 5% increase in quadriceps, hamstrings, and adductors	11% increase in quadriceps; 34% increase in type I fibers; 27% increase in type II fibers	Total body muscle mass increased 1.2 ± 0.4 kg	48% increase in type I fibers; 62% increase in type II fibers	28 ± 9% and 22 ± 9% increase, respectively, in type I and II fibers (high-intensity group); 10 ± 3% and 18 ± 9% increase, respectively, in type I and II fibers (low-intensity group)

maximus and 5 min of walking or cycling. Finally, one should thoroughly explain the testing procedures to the subject and obtain informed consent.

The gold standard for strength testing is the 1-repetition maximum (i.e., 1RM, the heaviest weight that can be lifted for one repetition), usually performed using a weight training machine or free weight exercises. However, when a 1RM is not practical or is potentially dangerous, a 4- to 8RM (i.e., the heaviest weight that can be lifted for four to eight consecutive repetitions) may be used instead. It is also important to make sure that subjects do not hold their breath during a lifting test, thus performing the Valsalva maneuver, which increases BP and impedes blood flow back to the heart. The Valsalva maneuver is more likely to occur during maximal exertion compared to submaximal exertion.

Manual muscle tests (MMT) can also be used to assess muscle strength. These tests are performed by health professionals and are typically assigned a numerical score between 0 and 5 depending on whether a muscle's strength is qualitatively assessed as zero activity (0/5), trace activity (1/5), poor (2/5), fair (3/5), good (4/5), or normal (5/5).

Tests other than the 1RM and MMT can also be used to assess muscle strength, as explained in the following subsections. Some of these tests assess muscular endurance and power in addition to muscular strength and provide age-related norms for comparison and fitness classification.

Lower Body Strength Tests

Common exercises employed to test lower extremity strength include the 1RM barbell squat and machine leg press. The barbell squat is typically used by people competing in sport or activity to test lower extremity strength, since it is more sport specific than other tests. The machine leg press is more commonly used by nonathletes and older individuals, since it is easier and safer to perform. Age-related lower extremity strength norms for the Universal leg press machine are shown in table 2.2.

A combination of lower extremity strength and power can be tested during the sit-to-stand. Sitting on the front edge of a rigid chair (44.5 cm high) with knees even with the tips of toes and with feet approximately shoulder-width apart, the subject stands up straight with the knees and hips fully extended, and in a continuous motion returns back to the sitting position until the buttocks just make contact with the chair. The subject continues to perform this standing and sitting movement as fast as possible for 10 consecutive repetitions.

It is important to maintain good form and technique throughout the test, keeping the arms straight and at the side, trunk slightly inclined forward at the bottom position, head up and looking straight ahead, and without bouncing up from the chair. The subject should wear low-heel shoes or be tested barefooted.

TABLE 2.2 Age-Related Lower Extremity Strength Norms for the Universal Leg Press Machine*

			AGE					
Classification	Percentile	Group	<20	20-29	30-39	40-49	50-59	60+
Superior	99	Male	>2.82	>2.40	>2.20	>2.02	>1.90	>1.80
		Female	>1.88	>1.98	>1.68	>1.57	>1.43	>1.43
Excellent	80	Male	2.28	2.13	1.93	1.82	1.71	1.62
		Female	1.71	1.68	1.47	1.37	1.25	1.18
Good	60	Male	2.04	1.97	1.77	1.68	1.58	1.49
		Female	1.59	1.50	1.33	1.23	1.10	1.04
Fair	40	Male	1.90	1.83	1.65	1.57	1.46	1.38
		Female	1.38	1.37	1.21	1.13	0.99	0.93
Poor	20	Male	1.70	1.63	1.52	1.44	1.32	1.25
		Female	1.22	1.22	1.09	1.02	0.88	0.85
Number of subjects (n)		Male	60	424	1,909	2,089	1,286	347
		Female	20	192	281	337	192	44

* Values listed for each age group are from the 99th percentile (excellent) down to the 20th percentile (poor), and are expressed as the ratio of the 1-repetition maximum weight lifted to body weight.

The *Physical Fitness Specialist Certification Manual*. The Cooper Institute, Dallas, Texas, revised 2003, reprinted with permission.

Age-related equations for men and women have been developed to predict the normal amount of time needed to perform 10 consecutive repetitions during the sit-to-stand (Csuka and McCarty 1985): These equations are as follows:

Women: time (s) = 7.6 + 0.17 * age (yr); r = .71

Men: time (s) = 4.9 + 0.19 * age (yr); r = .88

Age-related performance norms for the time needed to complete 10 consecutive sit-to-stand repetitions as quickly as possible are shown in table 2.3.

Upper Body Tests

Common exercises employed to test upper extremity strength include the 1RM barbell or machine bench press. The barbell bench press is typically used by persons competing in sport or activity to test upper extremity strength, since it is relatively sport specific. The machine bench press is more commonly used by nonathletes and older persons, since it is easier and safer to perform. Age-related upper extremity strength norms for the Universal bench press machine are shown in table 2.4.

The body weight push-up can also be used to test both upper extremity muscular strength and endurance. The starting position for men is with the hands shoulder-width apart, elbows fully extended, back straight, feet supported on toes, and head up. From this position the subject descends until he touches the tester's fist (placed on the floor under subject's chest), and in a continuous motion ascends until the elbows are fully extended. The subject performs as many push-ups as possible without pausing. The modified push-up, which is used for females, is performed in the same way except that both knees are on the ground and flexed 90°. Age-related upper extremity strength and endurance norms for the push-up are given in table 2.5.

TABLE 2.3 Age-Related Lower Extremity Sit-to-Stand Strength and Power Norms (n = 139) for Mean and Upper Limit Times Needed to Complete 10 Consecutive Sit-to-Stand Repetitions As Quickly As Possible

	FEMALE		MALE	
Age (years)	Mean time (s)	Upper limit*	Mean time (s)	Upper limit*
20	10.9	16.0	8.8	12.3
25	11.8	16.8	9.8	13.3
30	12.6	17.6	10.8	14.2
35	13.4	18.5	11.7	15.2
40	14.3	19.3	12.7	16.2
45	15.1	20.1	13.7	17.2
50	15.9	20.9	14.7	18.1
55	16.8	21.8	15.6	19.1
60	17.6	22.6	16.6	20.1
65	18.4	23.5	17.6	21.1
70	19.3	24.3	18.5	22.0
75	20.1	25.2	19.5	23.0
80	20.9	26.1	20.5	24.0
85	21.8	27.0	21.5	25.0

*The upper limit time values demarcate the breakpoint separating normal from abnormal performance.

Reprinted from *American Journal of Medicine*, Vol. 78(1), M. Csuka and D.J. McCarty, Simple method for measurement of lower extremity muscle strength, pp. 77-81, copyright 1985, with permission from Excerpta Medica, Inc.

TABLE 2.4 Age-Related Upper Extremity Strength Norms for the Universal Bench Press Machine*

		Group	AGE					
Classification	**Percentile**		**<20**	**20-29**	**30-39**	**40-49**	**50-59**	**60+**
Superior	99	Male Female	>1.76 >0.88	>1.63 >1.01	>1.53 >0.82	>1.20 >0.77	>1.05 >0.68	>0.94 >0.72
Excellent	80	Male Female	1.34 0.77	1.32 0.80	1.12 0.70	1.00 0.62	0.90 0.55	0.82 0.54
Good	60	Male Female	1.19 0.65	1.14 0.70	0.98 0.60	0.88 0.54	0.79 0.48	0.72 0.47
Fair	40	Male Female	1.06 0.58	0.99 0.59	0.88 0.53	0.80 0.50	0.71 0.44	0.66 0.43
Poor	20	Male Female	0.89 0.53	0.88 0.51	0.78 0.47	0.72 0.43	0.63 0.39	0.57 0.38
	Number of subjects	Male Female	60 20	425 191	1,909 379	2,090 333	1,279 189	343 42

*Values listed for each age group are from the 99th percentile (excellent) down to the 20th percentile (poor), and are expressed as the ratio of the 1RM weight lifted to body weight.

The *Physical Fitness Specialist Certification Manual*. The Cooper Institute, Dallas, Texas, revised 2003, reprinted with permission.

TABLE 2.5 Age-Related Upper Extremity Strength and Endurance Norms for the Body Weight Push-Up (Men) and Modified Push-Up (Women) Exercises*

			AGE				
Classification	**Percentile**	**Group**	**20-29**	**30-39**	**40-49**	**50-59**	**60+**
Superior	99	Male Female	100 70	86 56	64 60	51 31	39 20
Excellent	80	Male Female	47 36	39 31	30 24	25 21	23 15
Good	60	Male Female	37 30	30 24	24 18	19 17	18 12
Fair	40	Male Female	29 23	24 19	18 13	13 12	10 5
Poor	20	Male Female	22 17	17 11	11 6	9 6	6 2
	Number of subjects	Male Female	1,045 579	790 411	364 246	172 105	26 12

*Values listed for each age group represent the total number of push-ups performed without pausing from the 99th percentile (excellent) down to the 20th percentile (poor).

The *Physical Fitness Specialist Certification Manual*. The Cooper Institute, Dallas, Texas, revised 2003, reprinted with permission.

Abdominal Strength Tests

Abdominal strength and endurance is commonly tested with the partial curl-up. Unlike the sit-up, the partial curl-up involves trunk (spinal) flexion without hip flexion, thus activating and isolating abdominal musculature without activating the hip flexors. Therefore the partial curl-up is more appropriate than the sit-up for those with low back problems, since during the sit-up the active hip flexors attempt to anteriorly tilt the pelvis and exert a force on the lumbar spine as they contract to flex the hips.

Before the start of the partial curl-up, two pieces of masking tape are placed on the ground parallel with each other and 10 cm apart. The partial curl-up begins with the subject supine, knees flexed approximately 90°, the feet flat and not anchored, the arms straight and parallel with the trunk, and the palms of the hands in contact with the floor with both middle fingers touching the piece of tape referenced as the zero mark line. Keeping the arms straight and feet flat, the subject lifts the head and scapulae off the ground by flexing the trunk until the hands move toward the feet 10 cm and touch the second piece of tape. In a continuous motion the subject returns to the starting position until both the head and scapulae make contact with the ground. For a 1-min duration the subject performs as many consecutive curl-ups as possible, without resting, at a constant cadence of 25 curl-ups per minute. A metronome is set at a cadence rate of 50 beats/min, so for each beat the subject will either curl up or return to the starting position. It is important that the subject maintain the rate established by the metronome throughout the 1-min duration; when the subject is unable to do so, the test is terminated and the number of partial curl-ups completed is recorded. Abdominal strength and endurance norms for the 1-min partial curl-up exercises are shown in table 2.6.

STRENGTH TRAINING PRESCRIPTION IN THE AGING

Once strength testing is complete and the person's goals have been established, a strength training program can be prescribed. This section deals with strength training prescription and covers principles for strength training, types of strength training, and common systems of strength training.

Training Principles for Strength Training

To properly prescribe different types and systems of strength training, one must understand several training principles. These include progressive overload, intensity, volume, rest intervals, duration, frequency, mode, periodization, specificity, reversibility, fitness level, and recovery.

Progressive Overload

The basic premise of **progressive overload** is to progressively increase the load on the musculoskeletal system. Once muscles, tendons, ligaments, and bones adapt to a given stimulus, additional loads must be placed on these structures over time for further adaptation to occur. For strength training, progressive overload typically involves increasing the weight and decreasing the repetitions, as well as increasing the number of sets performed (e.g., 100 kg × 10 reps × 2 sets for weeks 1-4; 120 kg × 8 reps × 3 sets for weeks 5-8; 140 kg × 6 reps × 4 sets for weeks 9-12). Another way of doing this is through small increases in load over time with the same number of repetitions (e.g., 100 kg × 8 reps for weeks 1-4; 110 kg × 8 reps for weeks 5-8).

Intensity

Training intensity is synonymous with the amount of weight, load, or resistance being lifted. The greater the load lifted, the greater the training intensity. Intensity

TABLE 2.6 Age-Related Abdominal Strength and Endurance Norms for the 1-Min Partial Curl-Up Exercise*

		AGE					
Classification	Group	15-19	20-29	30-39	40-49	50-59	60-69
Excellent	Male	25	25	25	25	25	25
	Female	25	25	25	25	25	>18
Very good	Male	23-24	23-24	23-24	22-24	19-24	16-24
	Female	23-24	23-24	23-24	21-24	16-24	11-17
Good	Male	21-22	21-22	21-22	16-21	14-19	10-15
	Female	21-22	19-22	16-21	13-20	9-15	6-10
Fair	Male	16-20	13-20	13-20	11-15	9-13	4-9
	Female	16-20	13-18	11-15	6-12	4-8	2-5
Needs improvement	Male	<15	<12	<12	<10	<8	<3
	Female	<15	<12	<10	<5	<3	<1

*Values listed for each age group represent the total number of partial curl-ups performed in 1 min.

Reprinted with permission from the Canadian Society for Exercise Physiology, *The Canadian Physical Activity, Fitness & Lifestyle Appraisal: CSEP's Plan for Healthy Active Living*, Ottawa, Ontario, 1996.

is most commonly expressed in terms of a percentage of an individual's 1RM. Training studies have shown that strength is maximized through high-intensity training between approximately 80% and 95% of an individual's 1RM, which equates to training with the heaviest resistance that can be performed between approximately 3 and 8 repetitions (i.e., between a 3RM and an 8RM) (Stone, O'Bryant, and Garhammer 1981; Taaffe et al. 1996). As shown in table 2.1, performing 3 sets of 8 repetitions, which equates to a training intensity of approximately 80% 1RM, has been shown to be very effective in increasing both strength and hypertrophy in aging persons. The risks associated with training at intensities greater than 80% 1RM may be greater than the benefits for muscle strength and hypertrophy, since higher-intensity training increases the risk factors associated with musculoskeletal injuries.

With the use of free weights or machine weight as resistance, the number of repetitions that relate to a given percentage of 1RM is highly variable depending on the exercise employed, the muscle group being worked (smaller muscles produce fewer repetitions for a given percentage of 1RM, and larger muscles produce higher repetitions for a given percentage of 1RM), and the training level (trained or untrained) of the individual (Hoeger et al. 1990). Nevertheless, for trained individuals the relationship between performing repetitions to failure and a percentage of one's 1RM can be estimated as follows (Mayhew, Ware, and Prinster 1993):

10RM ≈ 74% to 76% 1RM

9RM ≈ 76% to 78% 1RM

8RM ≈ 79% to 81% 1RM

7RM ≈ 81% to 83% 1RM

6RM ≈ 84% to 86% 1RM

5RM ≈ 86% to 88% 1RM

4RM ≈ 89% to 91% 1RM

3RM ≈ 92% to 94% 1RM

2RM ≈ 94% to 96% 1RM

In addition, one can estimate a person's 1RM by dividing the load employed during performance of a given number of repetitions to failure by the corresponding percentage of the 1RM the person is training at. For example, consider someone who can bench press 100 kg for a total of eight repetitions. Since the corresponding intensity for an 8RM is between ≈79% and 81% 1RM (upper and lower limits), the individual's estimated 1RM is calculated as follows:

estimated 1RM = load / repetitions = 100 kg / 0.81
= 123 kg for the lower limit

estimated 1RM = 100 kg / 0.79
= 127 kg for the upper limit

Therefore, the person's 1RM for the bench press is estimated to be between 123 and 127 kg.

Volume and Duration

Training volume for any given exercise is determined by multiplying together the total number of sets, repetitions, and the load (or resistance). For example, 3 sets of 8 repetitions of bench press with 100 kg has an exercise volume of (3)(8)(100 kg) = 2400 kg. Typically, volume increases as intensity decreases, and volume decreases as intensity increases. For example, consider an individual who has a 150-kg 1RM bench press. Performing high-intensity training for 4 sets of 4 repetitions at 90% of the 1RM would yield an exercise volume of (4)(4)(0.90)(150 kg) = 2160 kg. If that same athlete performed 4 sets of 8 repetitions at a lower intensity, 80% of the 1RM, the exercise volume would be (4)(8)(0.80)(150 kg) = 3840 kg. In this example the lower training intensity of 80% 1RM produced 78% greater volume than the higher training intensity of 90% 1RM. Higher-volume training is reserved for the competitive individual, since it enhances muscle strength and size.

Training duration, the total quantity of time needed during resistance training, varies depending on the type of strength training. As the number of exercises, repetitions, sets, and rest intervals increases during a session, training duration will also increase. A typical strength training session lasts between 20 and 60 min. Training duration also refers to the number of weeks or months a given strength training program is adhered to. A strength training program typically lasts 4 to 12 weeks before intensity, duration, frequency, or mode is modified, which is in accordance with periodization concepts.

Rest Intervals and Recovery

Rest intervals refers to the total rest time between repetitions, sets, and exercises for a given muscle group. In training a given muscle group, a 2- to 3-min rest interval between sets is common in strength training, often increasing with increasing intensities (e.g., 4- to 5-min rest interval for >90% 1RM training intensities) and decreasing with decreasing intensities (e.g., 1- to 2-min rest interval for 70-80% 1RM training intensities; 30- to 60-s rest interval for 40-60% 1RM training intensity). The increase in rest intervals with higher-intensity training compared to lower-intensity training is necessary in part because of the greater number of motor units recruited and a larger accumulation of lactate, as well as to allow complete **recovery** in training with near-maximal loads. Also, multi-muscle, multi-joint exercises (e.g., squat, power cleans, bench press), which require large energy expenditures, require longer rest times than single-muscle, single-joint exercises (e.g., leg extensions, leg curls, arm curls), which have much lower energy expenditures.

Rest intervals are also needed between exercise sessions in order to allow time for muscle and connective tissue to repair and regenerate from training. Compared to low-intensity training, high-intensity training (e.g., training with >80% 1RM, performing plyometric exercises or eccentric muscle contractions) causes more muscle and connective tissue damage and requires greater time to repair and regenerate. In general, 48 to 72 h is needed between training sessions for a group of muscles and connective tissue to adequately recover, with increasing amounts of recovery time needed as an individual ages. Adequate rest and protein intake are two of the most common factors for muscle regeneration. An increase in protein requirements from 0.60 to 0.80 g/kg body weight to 1 to 1.6 g/kg body weight is important for aging persons in order to prevent muscle atrophy, as well as maintain and gain muscle mass due to high-intensity strength training (Campbell et al. 1994; Lemon 1998).

Frequency

Training frequency refers to how often you engage in a strength training program. It is often expressed as total number of training sessions per week. A typical strength training frequency is once per day and two to five times per week. Although strength training once per week has been shown to both build and maintain strength (McLester, Bishop, and Guilliams 2000; Taaffe et al. 1999), other studies have shown that strength gains are maximized when strength training occurs two to three sessions per week as compared to one session per week (McLester, Bishop, and Guilliams 2000), or three sessions per week as compared to two (Braith et al. 1989). Interestingly, even when volume and intensity were kept constant between one day per week (3 × 3-10 repetitions) and three days per week (1 × 3-10 repetitions) during a 12-week strength training program, strength gains were significantly greater with the three-day per week protocol (McLester, Bishop, and Guilliams 2000).

The majority of the 40 to 50 strength training studies in the literature involving the aging that reported strength gains typically employed three or more training sessions per week consisting of three sets of approximately eight repetitions. Therefore these data suggest that performing multiple strength training sessions per week is superior in producing strength gains compared to performing a single strength training session per week. However, several studies have shown that strength gains can be maintained with as little as one strength training session per week (Taaffe et al. 1999), or one training session every two to four weeks (Tucci et al. 1992), as long as the training is of higher intensity. From these data one can deduce that the intensity of training is more important than duration or frequency of training in maintaining strength gains, and one training session per week may be preferred by individuals who have time constraints and whose goals are not to maximize strength gains but simply maintain strength.

For either higher-fit individuals or those who are deconditioned, it may be appropriate to split a longer training session involving several muscle groups into multiple shorter training sessions throughout the week that involve only one or two muscle groups. For example, a high-fit individual may train chest and shoulders one day, back and biceps the next day, hips and thighs the next day, and so on. This is referred to as split routine training. A long training session may also be split into multiple shorter training sessions throughout the day. For example, instead of training chest and shoulders together during a training session, one can train the chest in the morning and the shoulders in the evening.

An advantage to splitting a longer training session into multiple shorter sessions is that the effects of physiological and psychological fatigue are more pronounced during long sessions; this implies that if the shoulders are trained last within a session they may not receive as effective a workout as they would if trained at the beginning of the session when the person is mentally and physically fresh. A split routine allows an individual to devote full effort and intensity to each muscle group. The same is true for a deconditioned person who is training the entire body by performing three sets of eight exercises three times per week. This person may elect to perform four upper body exercises in the morning and four lower body exercises in the evening, or perform four upper body exercises one day and four lower body exercises the following day.

Mode

The most common **modes** of strength training include resistance machines, free weights, body weight resistance, and resistance from elastic bands. Numerous types of machines are now on the market, such as commonly used variable resistance machines (VRM), which often employ a cam to vary the lever arm throughout the range of motion. There are also several types of isokinetic machines, which maintain a relatively constant speed of movement regardless of how much effort an individual employs.

An excellent paper addressing the advantages and disadvantages of free weights and machines was recently published (Haff 2000). Some advantages of resistance training with machines include the following:

- It is safe.
- The machines are easy to use.
- Little knowledge of proper exercise form and technique is required.
- A spotter is not required for safety.
- Little time is required to set up and change the weight.
- Muscle isolation is excellent.

For example, it can be difficult to isolate knee flexion using free weights; but with machines, knee flexion can be isolated in multiple positions, such prone, sitting, and standing. Each of these positions works the hamstrings differently due to the varying length–tension relationship of muscle that occurs in each position.

A potential advantage of the VRM is that it is designed to match muscle torques generated throughout a range of motion. For example, the muscle torque generated by the elbow flexor muscles during an arm curl exercise initially is small at full elbow extension (small muscle moment arms), progressively increases to maximum at 90° elbow flexion (large muscle moment arms), and then progressively decreases as the elbow continues to flex. The VRM is designed to match these curves by means of asymmetrically shaped cams in which the resistance moment arm varies throughout the range of motion. During the arm curl exercise, the resistance torque would start out small at full elbow extension to match the small muscle torque produced at this position, would progressively increase and peak at 90° elbow flexion to match the large muscle torque at this position, and would then decrease throughout the remaining range of motion. In effect, less resistance is offered at weaker joint positions and greater resistance is offered at stronger joint positions. However, it has been shown that some VRM do not effectively match muscle torque curves of the body throughout a given range of motion (Johnson, Colodny, and Jackson 1990). Some disadvantages of machines are that they

- can be expensive,
- often are heavy and bulky,
- lack specificity to most movements that occur in sport due to largely single-plane motion,
- do not require balancing the weight during lifting through a range of motion,
- do not allow for explosive training since many machines hinder acceleration (e.g., VRM), and
- may not offer an eccentric phase of the lift (e.g., some isokinetic machines).

Free weights, including both barbells and dumbbells, are also very common in strength training. Some advantages of free weights are that they

- are relatively easy to use;
- offer numerous multi-joint, multi-muscle exercises;
- are inexpensive;
- take up little space (especially dumbbells);
- are more sport specific than machines since they allow the weight to accelerate and move in multiple planes;
- require more muscle activity from synergists and stabilizers in order to balance the weight, and have a large energy expenditure compared to machines;
- allow both concentric and eccentric muscle movements;
- allow countermovements similar to those in sport activities (e.g., the squat has a movement similar to jumping);
- provide range of motions and muscle activation patterns similar to those in sport;
- provide endless exercise variations; and
- elicit greater proprioception and coordination development compared to machines.

Some disadvantages of free weights are that they

- require a greater knowledge of proper exercise form and technique,
- require more time to set up and change weight,
- are not as safe as machines, and
- may require a spotter for safety.

Body weight resistance and elastic tubing can also be used effectively in strength training. Common body weight exercises include push-ups and pull-ups for upper body development, squats and lunges for lower body development, and back extensions and partial curl-ups for trunk development. Some body weight exercises, such as sit-to-stand and wall squat exercises, are appropriate during rehabilitation and strengthening, especially for persons who are elderly.

Elastic tubing is very inexpensive, takes up little room, and can be used to develop all the major muscle groups. One disadvantage of using elastic tubing is that the resistance may not be great enough for maximal strength development in the larger, more powerful muscles of the body, such as the thighs, hips, chest, and back.

Periodization

When muscles and connective tissues are given the same stimuli for a prolonged period of time, the strength gains exhibited in these tissues begin diminishing. To continue to stimulate muscles and connective tissues, training intensities, volumes, and exercises must periodically be changed (Stone 1990). This is referred to as **periodization.** Periodization is also important in preventing psychological staleness that results from performing the same program for a prolonged period of time.

Periodization is a system of training that varies training intensities and volumes throughout a yearlong training cycle referred to as a macrocycle (Stone 1990; Stone, O'Bryant, and Garhammer 1981). Periodization training has been shown to produce superior strength and power gains compared to single-set or multi-set training with a constant repetition scheme (Kraemer et al. 2000; Kraemer et al. 1997), even when the training effort is submaximal (Kraemer et al. 1997). In addition, periodization training has been shown to increase physical performance abilities in athletes (Kraemer et al. 2000). Therefore, periodization may be appropriate for the aging athlete who has a desire to compete in sport or other activities.

A typical macrocycle is broken down into three to four mesocycles, each three to four months in duration; and each mesocycle can in turn be broken down into three to four microcycles, each three to four weeks in duration. A common periodization pattern for the strength athlete involves beginning a training microcycle with higher volume and lower intensities and progressively increasing intensity and decreasing volume (Stone, O'Bryant, and Garhammer 1981). For example, consider a four-month mesocycle composed of four microcycles of four weeks each.

The initial four-week microcycle could involve a higher training volume of 4 sets of 12 to 14 repetitions and a lower training intensity of 60% to 70% of 1RM. This higher-volume–lower-intensity training microcycle, referred to as the **preparatory phase** (Stone, O'Bryant, and Garhammer 1981), will gradually allow the muscles and connective tissue to adapt to new stress. Also, the first microcycle allows people to adapt to performing new exercises that they may not be familiar with, with an emphasis on proper lifting form and technique. The strength gains during this initial microcycle will primarily be due to neural factors, with strength gains from muscle hypertrophy usually occurring after four to eight weeks of training.

The second four-week microcycle, referred to as the **hypertrophy phase** (Stone, O'Bryant, and Garhammer 1981), could involve 70% to 80% 1RM intensity and a training volume of 4 sets of 8 repetitions. The emphasis of this cycle is muscle hypertrophy, which research has shown to be effective with a moderate to high volume using multiple sets and a training intensity between approximately 8- and 12RM, equivalent to approximately 70% to 80% 1RM. As muscles increase in size, their potential for strength also increases, since the force a muscle can generate is directly proportional to that muscle's physiological cross-sectional area (Brand, Pedersen, and Friederich 1986). Compared to what happens in younger individuals beyond puberty, muscle hypertrophy occurs to a lesser extent in the elderly, who instead experience a greater period of strength gains due to neural factors (Welle, Totterman, and Thornton 1996).

The third four-week microcycle, referred to as the **strength phase** (Stone, O'Bryant, and Garhammer 1981), could involve training at 85% to 90% 1RM intensity and decreasing the training volume to 4 sets of 4 to 6 repetitions. The emphasis of this cycle is on muscle strength. However, as previously mentioned, intensities higher than approximately 80% 1RM increase the risk of musculoskeletal injuries, so these intensity levels should be reserved only for those who are trying to maximize their strength gains or those who compete in sports or activities that require a high level of strength.

The final four-week microcycle, referred to as the **power phase** (Stone, O'Bryant, and Garhammer 1981), involves training at the highest intensity levels (approximately 90-95% 1RM) and decreasing the training volume to 3 to 5 sets of 2 to 3 repetitions. The emphasis of this cycle is muscle power, which research has shown to be maximized in select explosive exercises (i.e., clean and jerk, power cleans, snatch) employing maximal or near-maximal loads (Garhammer 1993; Garhammer and McLaughlin 1980). This high level of intensity training is not appropriate for most aging individuals due to the higher risk of musculoskeletal injuries; rather it is reserved only for those involved in high-intensity training for sport, such as senior or masters level (over 40 years of age) weightlifting or powerlifting competition.

Specificity, Reversibility, and Fitness Principles

• The **specificity principle** states that muscles and connective tissue adapt specifically to the demands placed on them. This is known as the SAID principle (Specific Adaptation to Imposed Demands). For example, for muscles to hypertrophy, they have to be trained at an optimal intensity for that specific adaptation, which as previously mentioned is approximately 70% to 80% 1RM (8-12RM). Similarly, for muscles to maximally adapt to becoming stronger, a higher intensity should be employed (approximately 80-95% 1RM); for bones to increase in density and become stronger, weight-bearing exercises should be employed. In addition to muscle and connective tissues, the SAID principle also applies to exercise selections for sport-specific movements. For example, the squat movement is sport specific to jumping in basketball and may be preferred over the machine leg press in the aging athlete who participates in recreational basketball. In addition, the squat develops the largest and most powerful muscles of the body (i.e., gluteals, quadriceps, hamstrings, and erector spinae), which are important in both running and jumping, and there is a high energy cost associated with performing the squat.

• The **reversibility principle** states that strength gains are transient and are reversible with disuse. Furthermore, losses in strength due to disuse occur at a greater rate than gains in strength due to training. However, as previously mentioned, strength gains can be maintained with as little as one strength training session per week (Taaffe et al. 1999) as long as the training is of high intensity.

• The **fitness principle** states that unfit people achieve strength gains at a faster rate than trained individuals, but also lose strength due to disuse at a faster rate. As previously mentioned, the initial strength gains experienced by unfit persons are largely due to neural factors, such as increased neuromuscular coordination between muscles and decreased sensitivity in the Golgi tendon organs. Over time, strength gains gradually begin to plateau as each individual approaches his or her "genetic ceiling" for strength.

Types of Strength Training

Several types of training can be used for muscle strengthening, including isometric, dynamic, eccentric, and isokinetic training:

• **Isometric training** occurs when tension develops in the muscle without a change in muscle length. Isometric training reached its peak popularity in the 1950s and 1960s largely due to the work of two Germans, Hettinger and Muller (Hettinger and Muller 1953). Studies 3 to 15 weeks in length have shown moderate strength gains from multiple maximum isometric contractions 3 to 10 s in duration (Garfinkel and Cafarelli 1992; Komi et al. 1978). While isometric training is appropriate in rehabilitation settings in which joint movements are contraindicated, they are not as effective a form of strength training for athletes or higher-level individuals because of the static nature of the exercise, since dynamic strength training through a range of motion is more sport specific. In addition, the strength gained through isometric training is very specific to the angle in which the exercises are performed. For example, performing isometric shoulder abduction at a 30° angle will build strength specific to 30° shoulder abduction and does not transfer to smaller or greater angles of shoulder abduction.

• **Dynamic training** involves both concentric (muscle shortening) and eccentric (muscle lengthening) muscle contractions in which joint motion occurs throughout a range of motion. Common modes of dynamic training are free weights, machines, body weight exercises, and tubing exercises, which have all been previously discussed.

• **Eccentric training,** often referred to as negative training, involves eccentric muscle contractions only. A greater amount of weight can be lowered at a given rate compared to the amount of weight that can be raised at that same rate. This allows an individual to lower a weight in a controlled manner well in excess of that person's 1RM. Athletes commonly use spotters to help lift the weight up, with the athlete lowering the weight eccentrically. This entire process is then repeated for multiple repetitions and sets. Research has shown that eccentric training results in strength gains similar to those with isometric, concentric, and isokinetic training, and that it is most effective when used in combination with concentric contractions (Morrissey, Harman, and Johnson 1995). However, one undesirable effect of eccentric training is an excessive amount of muscle and connective tissue damage, which results in increased muscle soreness and an increased recovery period. Performing eccentric training exclusively is not a practical choice for most aging individuals, except perhaps for those in training for competition.

• **Isokinetic training** is performed on accommodating resistance machines that involve moving through a range of motion at a constant speed. The harder an individual pushes or pulls against the machine, the more the machine accommodates to this force by producing an equal but opposite reaction force (torque). This accommodation in resistance maintains a relatively constant speed according to the speed setting on the machine. Most isokinetic machines generate speeds up to 300° to 500°/s, allowing both concentric and eccentric contractions. However, since many movements in sport and other activities are performed at speeds well above isokinetic speeds, and since movement speeds are not controlled in sport and activity, isokinetic exercises are not very sport specific. Isokinetic training studies have shown significant strength increases in people performing approximately one to five sets of 5 to 15 repetitions between 60° and 120°/s for three days per week and 8 to 20 weeks (Mannion, Jakeman, and Willan 1992). Morrissey and colleagues (Morrissey, Harman, and Johnson 1995) provide an excellent review comparing the specificity and effectiveness of resistance training modes relative to different types of training (e.g., static vs. dynamic, concentric vs. eccentric, weight training vs. isokinetic).

Common Systems of Strength Training

Several different systems of training have been shown to be effective in building strength.

Single Sets Versus Multi-Sets

For a given exercise, **single-set systems** consist of performing a single set of repetitions to failure, while **multi-set systems** consist of performing multiple sets of repetitions to failure. No known studies involving a population greater than 50 years of age have compared strength gains between single-set and multi-set training. In people between approximately 18 and 50 years of age, however, numerous studies have shown that both single-set training and multi-set training produce strength gains, although multi-set training produced significantly greater strength gains (Borst et al. 2001; Kraemer et al. 1997). Moreover, multi-set training involving both a constant and a varied number of repetitions and sets has been shown to be superior to single-set training in maximizing strength and power gains, especially in athletes training for sport and employing periodization techniques (Kraemer et al. 2000). This is contrary to previous beliefs (Carpinelli and Otto 1998) that single-set training is just as effective as multi-set training in producing strength gains. This implies that individuals who desire to maximize strength gains should employ a multi-set system of training rather than a single-set system. However, since single-set systems are effective in maintaining or producing strength gains, single-set training systems are an effective alternative for those who have limited time for resistance training and whose goal is not to maximize strength gains but rather to remain active through maintaining a functional strength base to enhance their daily activities.

Systems Employing Varying Resistance Between Sets

- The **DeLorme system** of training is one in which the initial set is light and each subsequent set progressively adds greater resistance. The DeLorme system became popular in the 1950s and 1960s when DeLorme and colleagues reported significant strength gains during short-term training studies in which people performed three sets of 10 repetitions (DeLorme and Watkins 1948). In the original DeLorme system the resistance employed was equal to 50% of the lifter's 10RM for the first set, 66% of the 10RM for the second set, and 100% of the 10RM for the third set. One may employ variations of these training percentages when using the DeLorme system.
- In the **Oxford system** of training, after a warm-up the initial set is heavy and each subsequent set employs progressively smaller resistance. Like the DeLorme system, the Oxford system became popular in the 1950s and 1960s. Significant strength gains have been reported using the Oxford technique (Zinovieff 1951). The resistances with the Oxford technique are the same as in the DeLorme system but in reverse order: The resistance is equal to 100% of the lifter's 10RM for the first set, 66% of the 10RM for the second set, and 50% of the 10RM for the third set. With the Oxford system one may use variations of these training percentages.
- The **pyramid system** combines the light-to-heavy and heavy-to-light systems. A lifter can progress from light to heavy resistance on the way up the pyramid and from heavy to light resistance on the way down the pyramid. Conversely, in an inverse pyramid a lifter can progress from heavy to light resistance on the way up the pyramid and from light to heavy resistance on the way down. An typical example employing a pyramid system for strength training is as follows:

Set 1: 10RM
Set 2: 8RM
Set 3: 5RM
Set 4: 3RM
Set 5: 5RM
Set 6: 8RM
Set 7: 10RM

The Superset System

The **superset system** is typically performed in one of two ways. One type of superset consists of one set of two to four exercises that work the same muscle group, with little or no rest. For example, in the supine position, the exerciser first performs the dumbbell incline bench press, then dumbbell flys (butterflys), and finally dumbbell pullovers. These three exercises emphasize development of the upper, middle, and lower portions of the pectoralis major, respectively. Supersetting with three exercises as in this example is referred to as the tri-set system of training.

A different type of superset system involves performing, with little or no rest, one set of two to four exercises that work muscle groups with opposite muscle actions. Pairs of agonist–antagonist exercises are most common in this type of superset, which allows the agonist muscle group to rest while the antagonist muscle group works (and vice versa). For example, the biceps curl exercise may immediately follow the triceps push-down exercise, or the leg extension exercise may immediately follow the leg curl exercise. Superset systems are common in bodybuilding, and muscle hypertrophy is believed to occur from such training. Due to the large number of repetitions performed and the high exercise volume, this type of training also produces a higher level of muscular endurance and has a high energy expenditure.

The Circuit System

The **circuit system** of training consists of multiple exercises (typically 8-12) using higher repetitions (typically 12-20 repetitions 30 to 45 s in duration) and lower intensities (40-60% or 1RM), with minimal rest intervals between exercises or sets (10-30 s). This type of training is most beneficial for people whose primary aim is to increase their cardiovascular fitness and muscular endurance (Beckham and Earnest 2000), such as persons who are deconditioned, have excess body fat and need to lose weight, or have cardiovascular issues (e.g., hypertension, cardiovascular disease). In addition, studies have shown that strength increases also occur with circuit training, especially for the deconditioned (Wilmore et al. 1978). Circuit training is effective for those who need a supervised structured program and have limited time to work out.

The circuit is commonly set up so an individual moves from one exercise to another in a timed sequence (e.g., an audiotape specifies when to start and stop an exercise and when to rotate and set up for the next exercise), such as a 30-s exercise period followed by a 15-s period to move to and prepare for the next exercise. For example, after people perform 30 s on the bench press, they quickly rotate to and set up for the leg press during the 15-s rest interval, perform 30 s on the leg press, rotate and set up for the next exercise, and so forth. Following this format, a 12-exercise circuit would take approximately 10 min to perform. The circuit could be performed two to three times, thereby allowing two to three sets of each exercise in 20 to 30 min, which makes the circuit time efficient.

A circuit is often set up to use alternating upper and lower body exercises or to alternate muscle groups (e.g., [1] bench press, [2] leg press, [3] lat pulldowns, [4] leg extensions), thus allowing one muscle group to rest and recover while another muscle group is being worked. Also, multi-joint, multi-muscle exercises should compose most of the exercises in the circuit since these have a greater energy expenditure and develop overall muscular strength and endurance to a greater extent than single-joint, single-muscle exercises. A circuit commonly consists of resistance machines rather than free weights since they are safer and easier to learn how to use, and since changing resistance takes minimal time.

EFFECTS OF AEROBIC EXERCISE IN THE AGING

It is important that health care professionals recognize and emphasize to their patients or clients how exercise will enhance their overall well-being, both physically and mentally. Research involving both males and females over a wide range of ages between 40 and 90 years old has shown that aerobic training produces numerous efficacious cardiovascular effects in the aging individual:

- A decrease in all-cause mortality (Blair et al. 1989; Lee, Hsieh, and Paffenbarger 1995)
- A decrease in cardiovascular diseases (CVD), such as CHD and stroke (Blair et al. 1989; Paffenbarger et al. 1986)
- An increase in $\dot{V}O_2$max due to central and peripheral adaptations (Kohrt et al. 1991; Stratton et al. 1994)
- An increase in stroke volume, end-diastolic volume, left ventricular volume, cardiac output, and a-$\bar{v}O_2$ difference (Seals et al. 1994; Stratton et al. 1994)
- An increase in plasma blood volume (Convertino and Ludwig 2000)
- An increase in capillary and mitochondria density, myoglobin, and oxidative enzymes in skeletal muscles (Hepple et al. 1997)
- A decrease in heart rate (HR) at rest and at a given submaximal exercise workload (Stratton et al. 1994; Woolf-May et al. 1998)

- A decrease in minute ventilation and pulmonary function (Etnier et al. 1999)
- A decrease in systolic blood pressure (SBP) and diastolic blood pressure (DBP) at rest and at a given submaximal exercise workload, and a decrease in left ventricular mass (Halbert et al. 1997; Kelley and Sharpe Kelley 2001)
- An increase in high-density lipoproteins (HDL), a decrease in low-density lipoproteins, and a decrease in the ratio of total cholesterol to HDL cholesterol (Motoyama et al. 1995; Sunami et al. 1999)
- A decrease in plasma triglycerides (Schuit et al. 1998)
- A decrease in overall body fat and intra-abdominal fat (Bunyard et al. 1998; Toth, Beckett, and Poehlman 1999)
- An increase in glucose tolerance and insulin sensitivity, and a decrease in the risk factors associated with type II diabetes (Dengel et al. 1998; DiPietro et al. 1998)
- An increase in basal metabolic rate (Poehlman et al. 1990; Withers et al. 1998)
- A decrease in colon or prostatic cancer (Blair et al. 1989)
- An increase in bone mineral density and a decrease in osteoporosis with weight-bearing exercise (Chien et al. 2000)
- A positive effect on pain, function, or disability in individuals with osteoarthritis (Baker and McAlindon 2000; Ettinger and Afable 1994)
- An increase in balance and postural stability, with a decrease in risk of falling and subsequent injury (Buchner et al. 1997; Messier et al. 2000)
- An increase in gait mobility and walking speed and efficiency (Binder et al. 1999; Silver et al. 2000)
- An increase in the function of chair rising and stair climbing (Binder et al. 1999)
- An enhanced immune system (Woods et al. 1999)
- A decrease in anxiety, tension, and depression and enhanced feelings of well-being (Altchiler and Motta 1994; Moore and Blumenthal 1998)

AEROBIC (CARDIORESPIRATORY) EXERCISE TESTING FOR THE AGING

Testing cardiorespiratory fitness (aerobic power) is important because such fitness is inversely related to CVD and premature death and provides numerous other benefits associated with health and well-being, as shown in the preceding list. Cardiorespiratory fitness reflects the ability of the circulatory and respiratory systems to deliver oxygen to the working muscles, as well as the overall functional capacity of the heart. Both the cardiorespiratory and musculoskeletal systems must function adequately in order to maximize VO_2 measurements.

The best indicator of cardiorespiratory fitness is $\dot{V}O_2max$, which is the maximum rate (per minute) at which O_2 can be taken up, distributed, and utilized by the working muscles during maximal exercise. Since $\dot{V}O_2max$ is the product of cardiac output and a-$\bar{v}O_2$ difference, and since cardiac output affects VO_2 to a much larger degree than a-$\bar{v}O_2$ difference, $\dot{V}O_2max$ is largely determined by the functional capacity of the heart.

$\dot{V}O_2max$ can be expressed in absolute terms ($L \cdot min^{-1}$), or more commonly absolute VO_2max is normalized by body weight and expressed in relative terms of $ml \cdot kg^{-1} \cdot min^{-1}$. One limitation of normalized $\dot{V}O_2max$ ($ml \cdot kg^{-1} \cdot min^{-1}$) is that it may underestimate $\dot{V}O_2max$ in people with high levels of body fat. Consequently, for persons who are obese it may be helpful to express $\dot{V}O_2max$ relative to fat-free mass.

Age- and gender-related normalized $\dot{V}O_2max$ fitness norms and classifications have been reported previously (Åstrand 1960; Balady et al. 2000; Nieman 1999), and one set of such norms is shown in table 2.7. The average predicted $\dot{V}O_2max$ values for healthy sedentary females are approximately 6 to 12 $ml \cdot kg^{-1} \cdot min^{-1}$ lower than for males, largely because women have a smaller heart volume, less blood volume (4-5 L compared to 5-6 L in men), and less hemoglobin to carry O_2 (12-16 g/dL for females compared to 14-18 g/dL for men).

$\dot{V}O_2max$ can also be expressed in terms of METs (metabolic equivalents). One MET represents an absolute energy requirement at rest, which is approximately 3.5 $ml \cdot kg^{-1} \cdot min^{-1}$ for an average healthy individual. For example, one can convert a $\dot{V}O_2max$ of 40 $ml \cdot kg^{-1} \cdot min^{-1}$ to METs by dividing by 3.5 $ml \cdot kg^{-1} \cdot min^{-1}$:

$$\dot{V}O_2max = (40\ ml \cdot kg^{-1} \cdot min^{-1}) / (3.5\ ml \cdot kg^{-1} \cdot min^{-1}) = 11.4\ METs$$

which is approximately the energy needed to run at a 7 mile/h pace (8.5 min/mile) (Balady et al. 2000). MET values for common activities and workloads are provided in various sources (Balady et al. 2000; Nieman 1999) and are helpful for prescribing the proper dose of exercise to a client.

$\dot{V}O_2max$ can be either measured directly during maximum exercise tests using indirect open-circuit spirometry (the gold standard for measuring $\dot{V}O_2max$) or estimated with regression equations when a person

TABLE 2.7 Cardiorespiratory $\dot{V}O_2max$ (ml · kg^{-1} · min^{-1}) Fitness Norms and Classifications

Fitness classification	Low	Fair	Average	Good	High	Athletic	Olympic
Male Age group							
20-29	<38	39-43	44-51	52-56	57-62	63-69	>70
30-39	<34	35-39	40-47	48-51	52-57	58-64	>65
40-49	<30	31-35	36-43	44-47	48-53	54-60	>61
50-59	<25	26-31	32-39	40-43	44-48	44-49	>56
60-69	<21	22-26	27-35	36-39	40-44	45-49	>50
Women Age group							
20-29	<28	29-34	35-43	44-48	49-53	54-59	>60
30-39	<27	28-33	34-41	42-47	48-52	53-58	>59
40-49	<25	26-31	32-40	41-45	46-50	51-56	>57
50-65	<21	22-28	29-36	37-41	42-45	46-49	>50

Reprinted, by permission, from I. Åstrand, 1960, "Aerobic work capacity in men and women with special reference to age," *Acta Physiologica Scandinavica* 49 (Suppl 169): 1-92; and reprinted, by permission, D.C. Nieman, 1999, *Exercise testing and prescription: A health-related approach* (New York: McGraw-Hill Companies).

is performing submaximal or maximal exercise tests. It is important to remember that regression equations developed to predict $\dot{V}O_2max$ are either population specific or generalized. Population-specific regression equations are developed from a homogeneous group of individuals, such as a group of college-age males. In contrast, generalized multiple regression equations (i.e., several variables in the equation) are developed from a nonhomogenous group of individuals that vary in age, weight, gender, and fitness level, such as a large sample of sedentary and active men and women between 20 and 70 years old with a mass between 50 and 100 kg.

The exercise specialist needs to know what exercise tests are most appropriate for testing a particular client and how the equations used for a given test were developed. For example, a multiple regression equation developed using healthy well-trained college-age males should not be used to predict $\dot{V}O_2max$ for sedentary elderly women. However, it has been shown that fitness level, rather than gender or age, is the most important component of population specificity (Balady et al. 2000). If a test is conducted properly and the assumptions in the following list are met, estimating $\dot{V}O_2max$ using regression equations during submaximal or maximal exercise tests is typically accurate within 10% of an individual's actual $\dot{V}O_2max$ determined by open-circuit spirometry.

When a maximal exercise test is not possible or practical, one can substitute a submaximal test, but several assumptions must be made. If these assumptions are not met, a 10% to 20% error in predicting $\dot{V}O_2max$ can result:

- A steady state HR is achieved for each exercise work rate.
- A linear relationship exists between HR, O_2 uptake, and work rate.
- Maximum HR (HRmax) is uniform for a given age, typically estimated by 220 – age.
- Mechanical efficiency, determined by measuring VO_2 for a given work rate, is constant for everyone.

Aerobic exercise testing should be valid (i.e., should measure what it purports to measure), reliable (i.e., showing repeatable and consistent results from one day to the next), relatively inexpensive, practical, and easily administered. All the submaximal and maximal tests discussed in this chapter that use regression equations to estimate $\dot{V}O_2max$ have been shown to have high test reliability and validity and are both practical and easy to administer.

Test validity can also be adversely affected if the mode of exercise for testing is unfamiliar to the subject. For example, the validity of testing on a cycle ergometer is diminished if the subject has never been on a cycle before. Often a walking test is more appropriate, since more people walk during their normal activities.

To assess reliability, a test may be repeated on consecutive days and the results compared. To be reliable, estimated $\dot{V}O_2max$ results for a given test performed on two consecutive days should be within 5% of each other. It is important to establish both intratester (same tester) and intertester (different tester) reliability when testing individuals. For example, a low intertester reliability may occur when one tester is very experienced and another tester has relatively little experience.

Test reliability also affects test validity. Unreliable tests result in invalid tests, since test scores cannot be trusted if they are not consistent. However, it is possible to have highly reliable test scores (r >.90) but poor validity, because consistent scores from one day to the next do not establish that you are actually measuring what you purport to be measuring. For example, using a test developed specifically for highly trained college-age female cyclists with sedentary elderly men (with limited experience on a bike) may result in very reliable test–retest scores, but will have very poor validity since the test is population specific for highly trained college-age female cyclists.

Health screening, risk assessment, and pretest evaluation should take place prior to testing. According to American College of Sports Medicine (ACSM) guidelines (Balady et al. 2000), symptomatic and apparently healthy men (<45 years old) and women (<55 years old) with no more than one CVD risk factor are considered at low risk of cardiac complications during exercise and can safely participate in submaximal or maximal-effort exercise without a medical evaluation by a physician. Major CVD risk factors include the following:

- Family history—sudden death related to CVD in father, brother, or son prior to 55 years or age or in mother, sister, or daughter prior to 65 years of age
- Current cigarette smoking, especially in those who smoke more than two to three packs per day
- Hypertension, with SBP >140 mmHg and DBP >90 mmHg
- A total serum cholesterol >200 mg/dL or HDL cholesterol <35 mg/dL
- Impaired fasting glucose, with fasting blood glucose >110 mg/dL
- Obesity, with a body mass index (BMI) >30 kg/m^2 or a waist girth >100 cm
- Sedentary lifestyle, defined as that of an individual who does not exercise regularly, or does not meet the minimal threshold of activity recommendations of 30 min or more of moderate physical activity on most days of the week (Balady et al. 2000)

In addition, older persons (men ≥45 and women ≥55 years old) or those with two or more CVD risk factors are considered at moderate risk of cardiac complications during exercise. These people can participate in submaximal exercise (i.e., moderate-intensity exercise that elevates heart rate between 60% and 80% HRmax) without a medical evaluation by a physician, but a medical evaluation by a physician is recommended in order for these individuals to participate in a maximal-effort exercise. Individuals classified as at high risk of cardiac complications during exercise have one or more signs or symptoms indicative of cardiovascular and pulmonary disease (e.g., pectoralis angina, shortness of breath at rest or with mild exertion, dizziness, ankle edema, tachycardia) or have known cardiovascular, pulmonary, or metabolic disease. ACSM guidelines recommend that high-risk individuals have a medical evaluation by a physician before participating in submaximal or maximal-effort exercise.

The Physical Activity Readiness Questionnaire (PAR-Q) or a similar form is recommended as a minimal pre-exercise health screening standard prior to exercise. A medical history questionnaire should also be given in order to classify the individual as low, moderate, or high risk of cardiac complications during exercise. The PAR-Q and medical history questionnaire provide the exercise professional information on health-related factors such as diseases, family history, medications, obesity, eating disorders, diet and nutrition, past and present exercise history, alcohol and other substance abuse, and cigarette smoking. Once an individual is cleared for exercise by a physician or by virtue of the PAR-Q and medical history questionnaire, exercise testing and subsequent training can commence.

There are several absolute contraindications for exercise, such as an abnormal electrocardiogram (ECG); unstable angina; uncontrolled cardiac arrhythmias; severe symptomatic aortic stenosis or heart failure; and acute pulmonary embolus, myocarditis, or pericarditis (Balady et al. 2000). Exercise testing should not be performed for subjects with absolute contraindications until their signs and symptoms are treated and have stabilized. Common relative contraindications for exercise include coronary stenosis, SBP >200 mmHg and DBP >110 mmHg at rest, tachyarrhythmias or bradyarrhythmias, hypertrophic cardiomyopathy, uncontrolled metabolic diseases (e.g., diabetes), and neuromuscular or musculoskeletal disorders that are exacerbated by exercise (Balady et al. 2000). Subjects with relative contraindications should be tested only after careful evaluation of the risk/benefit ratio of exercise testing.

When both aerobic and anaerobic testing occur during the same testing session, aerobic testing should precede anaerobic testing, since the elevated HR resulting from anaerobic testing may produce erroneous results during aerobic testing, which is typically dependent on HR. On the day of testing the subject should be well rested and in a relaxed state of mind; should be in a proper exercise environment (e.g., comfortable room temperature, since high temperatures and humid conditions increase HR); should be properly hydrated; should wear comfortable clothing; should not have eaten or had any alcohol, tobacco, or caffeine for at least 3 h prior to testing (since these increase HR); and should avoid any exercise. The subject should have sufficient time to acclimate to the exercises that will be used for testing and should be able to employ proper exercise form and technique. It is important that proper stretching and progressive warm-up occur before testing. Finally, the testing procedures should be thoroughly explained to the subject, informed consent should be obtained prior to testing, and appropriate equipment and certified medical personnel should be available throughout the testing period.

During exercise testing, BP and ECG monitoring is recommended for all high-risk CVD subjects, with a physician present, while the apparently healthy person or someone with low risk for CVD normally does not require such monitoring. The normal BP response to progressive exercise is a corresponding increase in SBP, typically 10 ± 2 mmHg/MET for inactive individuals (5-10 mmHg/MET increase in the active), with a possible plateau at maximal exercise (Balady et al. 2000). The normal response in DBP to progressive exercise is no change or a slight decrease, while an increase in DBP >15 mmHg suggests severe coronary artery disease (Balady et al. 2000).

Systolic BP and diastolic BP during maximal treadmill exercise generally increase with age, with mean SBP values for ages 18 to 79 ranging between 182 and 195 mmHg for males and between 155 and 196 mmHg for females, and mean DBP values for ages 18 to 79 ranging between 69 and 83 mmHg for males and between 67 and 83 mmHg for females (Balady et al. 2000). An SBP <140 mmHg is a poor prognosis during performance of maximal exercise (Balady et al. 2000), suggesting myocardial dysfunction. Similar to BP changes with exercise, the normal HR response to progressive exercise is a relatively linear increase of 10 ± 2 beats/MET for inactive subjects (5-10 beats/MET increase in the active) (Balady et al. 2000).

There are several absolute indications for terminating exercise testing (Balady et al. 2000):

- SBP >250 mmHg or DBP >115 mmHg
- Increase in DBP approaching 15 mmHg
- Moderate to severe angina, ataxia, dizziness, or syncope
- Signs of poor perfusion
- Subject's desire to stop
- Sustained ventricular tachycardia
- ST elevation (≥1.0 mm) in leads without diagnostic Q-waves
- Technical difficulties in monitoring ECG or SBP

There are also several relative indications for terminating exercise testing (Balady et al. 2000):

- Drop in SBP ≥10 mmHg from baseline BP despite increase in workload, in the absence of evidence of myocardial ischemia
- Increase of >15 mmHg in DBP—may suggest severe CHD
- SBP approaching 250 mmHg and DBP approaching 115 mmHg
- Fatigue, shortness of breath, wheezing, leg cramps, or claudication
- Increasing chest pains
- Arrhythmias other than sustained ventricular tachycardia
- ST or QRS changes such as excessive ST depression (>2.0-mm horizontal or downsloping ST segment depression)

For individuals with pulmonary disease, arterial O_2 saturation (S_aO_2) levels should be assessed throughout the exercise period. Normal resting S_aO_2 levels are 97% to 100%, with a decrease of 4% or more during exercise considered abnormal, especially if S_aO_2 is initially below normal resting values (e.g., a decrease in S_aO_2 from 91% to 87% is more problematic than a decrease in S_aO_2 from 97% to 93%) (Balady et al. 2000). Generally, an individual with S_aO_2 <90% will require supplemental O_2.

Prior to testing, resting measurements such as BP, HR, S_aO_2, height, weight, and body composition should be obtained. When $\dot{V}O_2$max is estimated by submaximal or maximal tests, more than one test may be performed and the estimated $\dot{V}O_2$max values averaged. A sample of common and easy-to-perform tests used to determine $\dot{V}O_2$max is discussed next. These include field tests, which require submaximal or maximal efforts during walking or running; submaximal or maximal treadmill or cycle ergometer tests; and submaximal step tests. Since many people are not as accustomed to cycling as to walking or running, maximal graded cycle protocols may produce 5% to 15% lower $\dot{V}O_2max$ values compared to maximal graded treadmill protocols.

Rockport 1-Mile Walk Submaximal Field Tests for Estimating $\dot{V}O_2max$

To test a subject using the Rockport 1-mile walk protocol (Kline et al. 1987), instruct the subject to walk as fast as possible for 1 mile on a track (or treadmill) while maintaining a normal walking motion (not racewalking). With use of a treadmill, one can determine the total walking time (in minutes) for a 1-mile distance by dividing 60 by the walking speed in miles/h (e.g., for a 4 mile/h walking speed, 60/4 = 15 min).

Immediately at the completion of the 1-mile walk, both time and end-of-test HR (from a heart rate monitor or a 15-s HR count, multiplied by four to convert HR to beats/min) are recorded. It is important that HR be taken immediately after exercise, since HR begins to decrease 10 to 15 s after the completion of exercise.

$\dot{V}O_2max$ in $ml \cdot kg^{-1} \cdot min^{-1}$ can be estimated using the following multiple regression equation:

$$\dot{V}O_2max\ (ml \cdot kg^{-1} \cdot min^{-1}) = 132.853 - 0.0769 * weight\ (lb) - 0.3877 * age\ (yr) + 6.315 * gender\ (0\ for\ females\ and\ 1\ for\ males) - 3.2649 * time\ (min) - 0.1565 * HR\ (beats/min)$$

Alternatively, $\dot{V}O_2max$ can be expressed in $L \cdot min^{-1}$ with use of the following multiple regression equation:

$$\dot{V}O_2max\ (L \cdot min^{-1}) = 6.9652 + 0.0091 * weight\ (lb) - 0.0257 * age\ (yr) + 0.5955 * gender\ (0\ for\ females\ and\ 1\ for\ males) - 0.2240 * time\ (min) - 0.0115 * HR\ (beats/min)$$

For example, a 50-year-old 180-lb male completing the 1-mile walk in 15.5 min with an ending HR of 128 beats/min would have the following estimated normalized and absolute $\dot{V}O_2max$:

$$\dot{V}O_2max = 132.853 - .0769 * 180 - .3877 * 50 + 6.315 * 1 - 3.2649 * 15.5 - .1565 * 128 = 35.3\ ml \cdot kg^{-1} \cdot min^{-1}$$

$$\dot{V}O_2max = 6.9652 + 0.0091 * 180 - 0.0257 * 50 + 0.5955 * 1 - 0.2240 * 15.5 - 0.0115 * 128 = 3.0\ L \cdot min^{-1}$$

Selected Submaximal Laboratory Tests for Estimating $\dot{V}O_2max$

A number of submaximal VO_2 tests for the laboratory are available. This section presents some of the most frequently used.

Single-Stage Treadmill Walking Test (Ebbeling et al. 1991)

To test a subject using the single-stage treadmill protocol, instruct the subject to walk at a brisk pace between 2 and 4.5 miles/h for a 4-min warm-up at 0% grade, which should elicit a HR between 50% and 70% of HRmax (note: if HR is not between 50% and 70% of HRmax, instruct the subject to increase walking speed). The subject then walks for another 4 min at the same speed as during the warm-up, but now at a 5% grade. At the end of this 4-min stage, HR is immediately recorded from an electronic HR monitor or from a 15-s HR count and multiplied by four to convert HR to beats/min. $\dot{V}O_2max$ is estimated using the following multiple regression equation:

$$\dot{V}O_2max\ (ml \cdot kg^{-1} \cdot min^{-1}) = 15.1 + 21.8 * speed\ (miles/h) - 0.327 * HR\ (beats/min) - 0.263 * speed * age\ (yr) + 0.00504 * HR * age + 5.98 * gender\ (0\ for\ females\ and\ 1\ for\ males)$$

Åstrand-Ryhming 6-Minute Step Test

The Åstrand-Ryhming 6-min step test (Åstrand and Ryhming 1954) has a stepping cadence of 90 steps/min (metronome set at 90 beats/min) and uses a 40-cm (15.75-in.) single step height for men and 33 cm (13 in.) for women. After 6 min of stepping, end-of-test HR is recorded (beats/min). $\dot{V}O_2max$ ($L \cdot min^{-1}$) can be estimated with use of the nomogram shown in figure 2.1. A line is connected on the nomogram from the subject's weight (kg) to the end-of-test HR, using the appropriate male or female column, and $\dot{V}O_2max$ is recorded where the line crosses the $\dot{V}O_2max$ line (see figure 2.1 for further explanation). Alternatively, $\dot{V}O_2max$ ($L \cdot min^{-1}$) can be estimated using the following regression equations (Marley and Linnerud 1976) instead of the nomogram:

$$Men: \dot{V}O_2max\ (L \cdot min^{-1}) = 3.7444 * [(weight\ (kg) + 5) / (HR\ (beats/min) - 62)]$$

$$Women: \dot{V}O_2max\ (L \cdot min^{-1}) = 3.750 * [(weight\ (kg) - 3) / (HR\ (beats/min) - 65)]$$

Because the nomogram in figure 2.1 was developed using subjects between 20 and 30 years old (Åstrand and Ryhming 1954), and because HR progressively decreases with age, an age-related HRmax correction factor was developed (Åstrand 1960), as shown in figure 2.1. For example, a $\dot{V}O_2max$ of 5.8 $L \cdot min^{-1}$ from the nomogram or regression equation would be corrected to 4.8 $L \cdot min^{-1}$ [(5.8 $L \cdot min^{-1}$) * 0.83 = 4.8 $L \cdot min^{-1}$] for a 40-year-old individual, or 4.0 $L \cdot min^{-1}$ with a known HRmax of 160 beats/min [(5.8 $L \cdot min^{-1}$) * 0.69 = 4.0 $L \cdot min^{-1}$]. To convert $\dot{V}O_2max$ from $L \cdot min^{-1}$ to $ml \cdot kg^{-1} \cdot min^{-1}$, use the following equation:

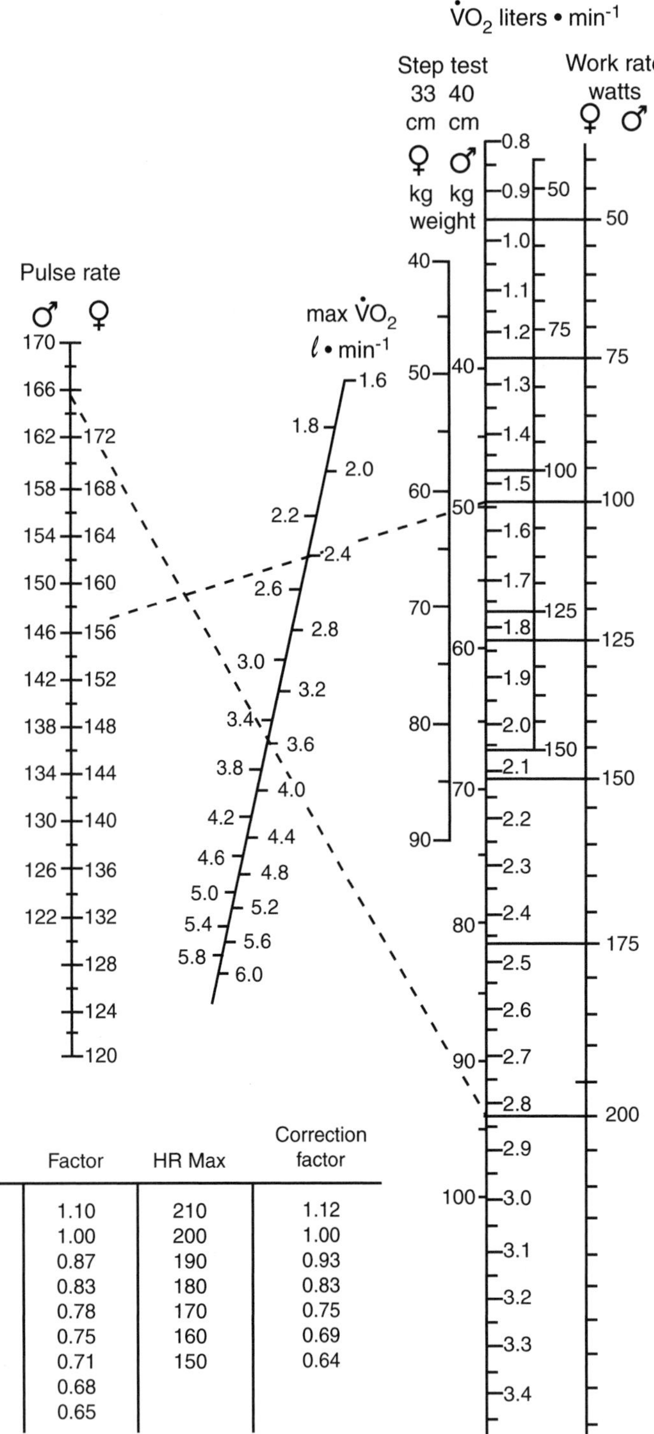

Age	Factor	HR Max	Correction factor
15	1.10	210	1.12
25	1.00	200	1.00
35	0.87	190	0.93
40	0.83	180	0.83
45	0.78	170	0.75
50	0.75	160	0.69
55	0.71	150	0.64
60	0.68		
65	0.65		

FIGURE 2.1 Nomogram (Åstrand and Ryhming 1954; Powers and Howley 1997) for estimating $\dot{V}O_2$max from HR values during 6 min of exercise at a single work rate in watts (W) involving a submaximal cycle ergometer test (50 rev/min cadence) or a 40-cm (men)- or 33-cm (women)-high step test (90 steps/min cadence). Examples of how to estimate $\dot{V}O_2$max for the cycle ergometer and step tests are shown by the two dashed lines on the nomogram. The first example shows a $\dot{V}O_2$max of 3.6 L · min^{-1} for a male during a cycle test for a 200-W work rate and an end-of-test HR of 166 beats/min. The second example shows a $\dot{V}O_2$max of 2.4 L · min^{-1} during a step test for either a 48-kg male with an end-of-test HR of 145 beats/min, or a 61-kg female with an end-of-test HR of 156 beats/min. Once $\dot{V}O_2$max is determined by the nomogram, multiply this value by the age correction factor shown at the bottom. For example, a 50-year-old individual with a $\dot{V}O_2$max of 3.6 L · min^{-1} from the nomogram would have an age-corrected $\dot{V}O_2$max of 2.7 L · min^{-1} (3.6 L · min^{-1} * 0.75). If HRmax is measured directly from a maximal exercise test, then use the HRmax correction factor instead of the age correction factor. For example, a 50-year-old individual with an actual HRmax of 160 beats/min and a $\dot{V}O_2$max of 3.6 L · min^{-1} from the nomogram would have a HRmax-corrected $\dot{V}O_2$max of 2.48 L · min^{-1} (3.6 L · min^{-1} * 0.69).

From P.O. Åstrand and I. Ryhming, 1954, "A nomogram for calculation of aerobic capacity (physical fitness) from pulse rate during submaximal work," *Journal of Applied Physiology* 7: 218-221; and from S.K. Powers and E.T. Howley, 1997, *Exercise physiology: Theory and application in fitness and performance* (New York: McGraw-Hill Companies), 280, with permission of The McGraw-Hill Companies.

$$\dot{V}O_2max\ (ml \cdot kg^{-1} \cdot min^{-1}) = \dot{V}O_2max\ (L \cdot min^{-1}) * (1{,}000\ ml \cdot L^{-1}) / weight\ (kg)$$

For example, an age-corrected $\dot{V}O_2max$ of 4.8 L · min^{-1} is equivalent to 60 ml · kg^{-1} · min^{-1} for an 80-kg individual [(4.8 L · min^{-1}) * (1,000 ml · L^{-1}) / 80 kg = 60 ml · kg^{-1} · min^{-1}].

Åstrand-Ryhming 6-Minute Cycle Test

The Åstrand-Ryhming cycle test (Åstrand and Ryhming 1954) consists of 6 min of cycling at a single work rate that is high enough to elicit a HR between 125 and 170 beats/min (approximately 70-85% HRmax or 50-70% $\dot{V}O_2max$) (Åstrand and Ryhming 1954). A recommended pedaling rate during the test is 50 rev/min, since mechanical efficiency is high at this rate. Recommended work rates include 50 W (1 kp or 300 kg · m · min^{-1}) or 100 W (2 kp or 600 kg · m · min^{-1}) for unconditioned males, 100 or 150 W (3 kp or 900 kg · m · min^{-1}) for conditioned males, 50 or 75 W (1.5 kp or 450 kg · m · min^{-1}) for unconditioned females, and 75 or 100 W for conditioned females (Balady et al. 2000).

$\dot{V}O_2max$ is estimated using the nomogram shown in figure 2.1. A line is connected on the nomogram (figure 2.1) from the subject's work rate (watts) to the end-of-test HR, using the appropriate male or female column, and $\dot{V}O_2max$ is recorded where the line crosses the $\dot{V}O_2max$ line. As previously explained, an age-related or HRmax correction factor (figure 2.1) is used to adjust $\dot{V}O_2max$ for age or known HRmax, and $\dot{V}O_2max$ can be converted from L · min^{-1} to ml · kg^{-1} · min^{-1}.

Maximal-Effort Exercise Testing

The graded exercise test to exhaustion, with $\dot{V}O_2max$ measured directly, is considered the gold standard for assessing cardiorespiratory fitness (Balady et al. 2000). It is typically performed on a treadmill but can also be performed on a cycle ergometer. Maximal-effort field tests, such as running, can also be used to estimate $\dot{V}O_2max$. However, since the equipment needed to measure $\dot{V}O_2max$ directly is costly and typically not available to the health and exercise professional, regression equations can be used to predict $\dot{V}O_2max$.

As with submaximal tests, $\dot{V}O_2max$ can be estimated relatively accurately (within 10% of actual values) with maximal tests through use of appropriate regression equations. Although $\dot{V}O_2max$ estimated with regression equations is not necessarily any more accurate with maximal tests compared to submaximal tests, maximal tests can help provide a more accurate HRmax (instead of estimating using 220 – age), which one can use when prescribing an aerobic exercise program and determining a HR training zone.

The most important factor in calculating an accurate $\dot{V}O_2max$ involves the subject's providing a true maximal effort during the graded exercise test. Verbal encouragement is helpful in motivating the subject, and practicing the test prior to testing can also be helpful in allowing the subject to become acclimated to running on a treadmill up a grade or pedaling a cycle ergometer. When a subject is truly "maxed out," the end-of-test HR will typically be within 10 to 15 beats/min of the person's age-predicted HRmax (220 – age), with the person showing definite signs of fatigue (e.g., staggering; unable to keep up with a given work rate), and will provide a rate of perceived exertion (RPE) near maximum (Balady et al. 2000). The RPE is discussed in greater detail later in the chapter.

The Bruce Treadmill Test

The Bruce protocol (Bruce, Kusumi, and Hosmer 1973) is by far the most common maximal graded exercise test. The conventional Bruce protocol involves performance of up to six 3-min stages (stages 1-6) with speeds, grades, and METs for each stage as shown in table 2.8. Typically, the conventional Bruce protocol is an uphill walking test for stages 1 to 3, becoming an uphill running test for stages 4 to 6. For subjects who have difficulty starting off with the 10% grade in stage 1 for the conventional Bruce protocol, a modified Bruce protocol can be used; the subject begins the test using either a 0% or 5% grade (table 2.8). When maximal exertion is achieved and the subject is unable to continue, the time completed in minutes is recorded.

Foster et al. (1984) developed the following generalized regression equation (r = .98; standard error of estimate [SEE] = 3.35 ml · kg^{-1} · min^{-1}) for the conventional Bruce protocol (stages 1-6) for estimating $\dot{V}O_2max$ for symptomatic and asymptomatic active and sedentary males:

$$\dot{V}O_2max\ (ml \cdot kg^{-1} \cdot min^{-1}) = 14.76 - 1.379 * time\ (min) + 0.451 * time^2 - 0.012 * time^3$$

Pollock et al. (1982) developed the following generalized regression equation (r = .91; SEE = 2.7 ml · kg^{-1} · min^{-1}) for the conventional Bruce protocol (stages 1-6) for estimating $\dot{V}O_2max$ for asymptomatic active and sedentary females:

$$\dot{V}O_2max\ (ml \cdot kg^{-1} \cdot min^{-1}) = 4.38 * time\ (min) - 3.9$$

To estimate $\dot{V}O_2max$ using the modified Bruce protocol, use the ACSM metabolic equation for walking (Balady et al. 2000):

$$\dot{V}O_2max\ (ml \cdot kg^{-1} \cdot min^{-1}) = 0.1 * speed\ (m \cdot min^{-1}) + 1.8 * speed\ (m \cdot min^{-1}) * fractional\ grade\ (\% / 100) + 3.5$$

TABLE 2.8 Conventional (Stages 1-6) and Modified (Stages 0-6) Bruce Maximal Treadmill Protocol

Stage	Time (min)	Speed (miles/h)	Grade (%)	METs
0	3	1.7	0	2-3
0.5	3	1.7	5	3-4
1	3	1.7	10	4-5
2	3	2.5	12	6-7
3	3	3.4	14	9-10
4	3	4.2	16	12-13
5	3	5.0	18	14-15
6	3	5.5	20	17-18

For example, if an individual reaches maximum exertion at the end of stage 2 (12% grade and 2.5 miles/h, which converts to 67 m · min^{-1}), $\dot{V}O_2max$ would be estimated as follows: $\dot{V}O_2max = 0.1 * (67\ m \cdot min^{-1}) + 1.8 * (67\ m \cdot min^{-1}) * (12 / 100) + 3.5 = 24.7\ ml \cdot kg^{-1} \cdot min^{-1}$ (approximately 7 METs).

The Balke Treadmill Test

The Balke maximal treadmill protocol (Balke and Ware 1959) is basically a graded uphill walking test employing a relatively normal cadence. It is less intense compared to the Bruce protocol, but one drawback is that it may take twice as long to complete. In the Balke protocol the subject walks as long as possible at a constant speed of 3.3 miles/h at a 0% grade for the first minute, a 2% grade for the second minute, and at a 1% increase in grade every minute thereafter until a 25% grade is obtained. At 25% grade the speed is increased 0.2 miles/h every minute while the grade is kept constant.

Using 51 asymptomatic active and sedentary male subjects (35-55 years old), Pollock et al. (1976) developed the following generalized regression equation (r = .92; SEE = 2.7 ml · kg^{-1} · min^{-1}) for the Balke protocol to order to estimate $\dot{V}O_2max$ for asymptomatic active and sedentary males:

$$\dot{V}O_2max\ (ml \cdot kg^{-1} \cdot min^{-1}) = 1.444 * time\ (min) + 14.99$$

Pollock et al. (1982) developed the following generalized regression equation (r = .94; SEE = 2.2 ml · kg^{-1} · min^{-1}) for the Balke protocol to estimate $\dot{V}O_2max$ for asymptomatic active and sedentary females:

$$\dot{V}O_2max\ (ml \cdot kg^{-1} \cdot min^{-1}) = 1.38 * time\ (min) + 5.22$$

Age-related time norms, $\dot{V}O_2max$ norms, and fitness classifications for the Balke maximal treadmill test are shown in table 2.9.

The Storer-Davis Cycle Test

To perform the Storer-Davis cycle test (Storer, Davis, and Caiozzo 1990), the subject initially cycles with no resistance (0 W) for a 4-min warm-up. A constant pedaling cadence of 60 rev/min is maintained throughout the test. After the warm-up is complete, the work rate is increased in 0.30 kp · min^{-1} (15 W · min^{-1}) increments until the subject is unable to continue or is unable to maintain the constant pedaling cadence of 60 rev/min. To predict $\dot{V}O_2max$, the final work rate in watts is recorded and used in the following multiple regression equations:

$$\text{Men: } \dot{V}O_2max\ (ml \cdot min^{-1}) = 10.51 * watts + 6.35 * weight\ (kg) - 10.49 * age\ (yr) + 519.3\ ml \cdot min^{-1};\ SEE = 212\ ml \cdot min^{-1}$$

$$\text{Women: } \dot{V}O_2max\ (ml \cdot min^{-1}) = 9.39 * watts + 7.7 * weight\ (kg) - 5.88 * age\ (yr) + 136.7\ ml \cdot min^{-1};\ SEE = 147\ ml \cdot min^{-1}$$

To convert ml · min^{-1} to ml · kg^{-1} · min^{-1} in these equations, divide ml · min^{-1} by the subject's weight (kg). These equations have been shown to predict $\dot{V}O_2max$ to within 10% of its actual value in 95% of individuals (Storer, Davis, and Caiozzo 1990).

TABLE 2.9 Age-Related Time Norms, $\dot{V}O_2$max Norms, and Fitness Classifications for the Balke Maximal Treadmill Test, the 12-Min Run, and the 1.5-Mile Run

				AGE				
Classification	**Percentile**	**Test protocol**	**Group**	**20-29**	**30-39**	**40-49**	**50-59**	**60+**
Superior	99	Balke treadmill (time in min:sec)	Male	30:20	29:00	28:00	26:00	24:29
			Female	26:21	23:22	22:00	18:44	20.25
		12-min run (miles)	Male	1.94	1.89	1.85	1.77	1.71
			Female	1.78	1.66	1.61	1.48	1.55
		1.5-mile run (time in min:sec)	Male	7:29	7:11	7:42	8:44	9:30
			Female	8:33	10:05	10:47	12:28	11:36
		$\dot{V}O_2$max (ml · kg^{-1} · min^{-1})	Male	58.79	58.86	55.42	52.53	50.39
			Female	53.03	48.73	46.75	42.04	44.47
Excellent	80	Balke treadmill (time in min:sec)	Male	23:00	22:00	20:10	18:00	16:00
			Female	18:00	16:20	14:45	12:00	11:15
		12-min run (miles)	Male	1.65	1.61	1.54	1.45	1.37
			Female	1.45	1.38	1.32	1.21	1.18
		1.5-mile run (time in min:sec)	Male	10:16	10:47	11:44	12:51	13:53
			Female	12:51	13:43	14:31	15:57	16:20
		$\dot{V}O_2$max (ml · kg^{-1} · min^{-1})	Male	48.20	46.75	44.11	40.98	38.09
			Female	40.98	38.57	36.28	32.31	31.23
Good	60	Balke treadmill (time in min:sec)	Male	20:15	19:00	17:15	15:00	12:53
			Female	15:00	13:35	12:00	10:00	8:28
		12-min run (miles)	Male	1.54	1.49	1.42	1.33	1.24
			Female	1.33	1.27	1.21	1.13	1.07
		1.5-mile run (time in min:sec)	Male	11:41	12:20	13:14	14:24	15:29
			Female	14:24	15:08	15:57	16:58	17:46
		$\dot{V}O_2$max (ml · kg^{-1} · min^{-1})	Male	44.23	42.42	39.89	36.65	33.59
			Female	36.65	34.60	32.31	29.43	27.21
Fair	40	Balke treadmill (time in min:sec)	Male	18:00	16:32	15:00	13:00	10:30
			Female	13:00	12:00	10:01	8:13	6:35
		12-min run (miles)	Male	1.45	1.39	1.33	1.25	1.15
			Female	1.25	1.21	1.13	1.06	0.99
		1.5-mile run (time in min:sec)	Male	12:51	13:36	14:29	15:26	16:43
			Female	15:26	15:57	16:58	17:55	18:44
		$\dot{V}O_2$max (ml · kg^{-1} · min^{-1})	Male	40.98	38.86	36.69	33.76	30.15
			Female	33.76	32.31	29.45	26.85	24.49
Poor	20	Balke treadmill (time in min:sec)	Male	15:20	14:06	12:30	10:30	8:00
			Female	10:50	9:30	8:00	6:25	5:24
		12-min run (miles)	Male	1.34	1.29	1.23	1.15	1.05
			Female	1.16	1.11	1.05	0.98	0.94
		1.5-mile run (time in min:sec)	Male	14:13	14:52	15:41	16:43	18:00
			Female	16:33	17:14	18:00	18:49	19:21
		$\dot{V}O_2$max (ml · kg^{-1} · min^{-1})	Male	37.13	35.35	33.04	30.15	26.54
			Female	30.63	28.70	26.54	24.25	22.78
		Number of subjects	Male	1,675	7,094	6,837	7,094	1,005
			Female	764	2,049	1,630	7,094	202

Values listed for each age group represent performance times for the Balke test and 1.5-mile run, number of miles completed for the 12-min run, and the $\dot{V}O_2$max that corresponds with the values listed for the Balke test, the 1.5-mile run, and the 12-min run. Values listed are from the 99th percentile (superior) down to the 20th percentile (poor).

The *Physical Fitness Specialist Certification Manual*. The Cooper Institute, Dallas, Texas, revised 2003, reprinted with permission.

Selecting Maximal Field Tests for Estimating $\dot{V}O_2max$

Here are two of the most practical maximal field tests:

- **12-min run.** For the 12-min run test, a subject runs as fast as possible for 12 min and records the distance traveled in meters or miles. Using 115 asymptomatic U.S. Air Force male officers with an age range between 17 and 52 years (mean = 22 years), Cooper (1968) developed the following generalized regression equations (r = .90) for the 12-min run protocol to estimate $\dot{V}O_2max$:

$$\dot{V}O_2max\ (ml \cdot kg^{-1} \cdot min^{-1}) = (distance\ (m) - 504.9) / 44.73 \text{ or } \dot{V}O_2max\ (ml \cdot kg^{-1} \cdot min^{-1}) = (distance\ (miles) - 0.3138) / 0.0278$$

Age-related time norms, $\dot{V}O_2max$ norms, and fitness classifications for the 12-min run are shown in table 2.9.

- **1.5-mile run.** A subject runs as fast as possible for 1.5 miles and the time at completion is recorded. $\dot{V}O_2max$ is estimated using the following ACSM running equation (Balady et al. 2000):

$$\dot{V}O_2max\ (ml \cdot kg^{-1} \cdot min^{-1}) = 3.5 + 483 / (time\ in\ min)$$

Age-related time norms, $\dot{V}O_2max$ norms, and fitness classifications for the 1.5-mile run are shown in table 2.9.

AEROBIC EXERCISE PRESCRIPTION FOR THE AGING

Previously discussed research indicates clearly that numerous beneficial physiological effects and adaptations occur due to aerobic exercise. However, to maximize these benefits it is important to have a proper understanding of exercise prescription. Exercise prescriptions should be individualized to enhance the health, fitness, and well-being of the individual, both physical and mental, and should be specific to an individual's needs and goals. From the submaximal and maximal exercise tests described, a subject's $\dot{V}O_2max$ and cardiorespiratory fitness level are initially determined. In addition, resting and exercise HR, BP, ECG, and RPE may be determined. These data are important to know prior to the start of an exercise program so that one can prescribe exercise properly.

The basic components of an aerobic training session are a warm-up, an aerobic (endurance) training phase, and a cool-down. A 5- to 10-min general and specific warm-up should precede the aerobic training phase, typically involving callisthenic-type and stretching exercises and other types of light exercise (e.g., walking or slow jogging). The warm-up prepares the body for the aerobic phase by facilitating the transition from rest to exercise; enhancing mechanical efficiency by increasing blood flow, body temperature, O_2 delivery to the working muscles, and metabolic rate; decreasing muscle viscosity; reducing the risk of musculoskeletal injury; increasing nerve impulse conduction speed; and enhancing muscular performance. Muscles and connective tissues perform better, are more extensible, and move more efficiently through a greater range of motion when they are warm. A warm-up also decreases the risk of cardiovascular injuries, and in higher-risk individuals may decrease occurrence of ischemic ST-segment depression, threatening ventricular arrhythmias, and transient global left ventricular dysfunction following sudden strenuous exercise (Balady et al. 2000).

The cool-down slowly and gradually decreases the cardiovascular response to exercise, thus minimizing trauma to the body compared to a sudden stop in exercise. The cool-down involves a gradual decrease in exercise intensity and permits appropriate circulatory adjustments and return of HR and BP to near resting values. The cool-down enhances venous return, thus reducing potential for postexercise hypotension and dizziness, facilitates dissipation of body heat, increases the removal of lactate, and decreases potential harmful effects of a postexercise rise in plasma catecholamines. Omission of a cool-down in the immediate postexercise period is associated with an increased incidence of cardiovascular complications (Balady et al. 2000). These complications may result in a transient decrease in venous return, possibly reducing coronary blood flow when HR and myocardial oxygen demands may still be high; may result in ischemic ST-segment depression (with or without angina symptoms); and may result in serious ventricular arrhythmias.

Both a proper warm-up and cool-down prior to exercise may also decrease muscle soreness, since warmer and more extensible muscles and connective tissue experience less trauma and minute tears. The aerobic phase of the training session is the most important component of the training session in terms of enhancing cardiorespiratory fitness.

Manipulating the Variables of the Aerobic Prescription

Exercise prescription for the aerobic phase involves modulations in several interrelated variables, such as exercise mode, intensity, duration, and frequency (Pollock et al. 1998). These variables are discussed next.

Definitions of Variables

- **Exercise mode** refers to the type of exercise employed during the training session. The mode should be based on an individual's functional capacity, interests, time and equipment availability, and personal goals and objectives. Common aerobic activities include walking, running, cycling, swimming, stair stepping, hiking, cross-country skiing, skating, rowing, circuit weight training, and aerobic dance classes. People may participate in various aerobic-type sport activities, such as tennis, racquetball, basketball, and soccer.
- **Exercise duration** simply is the total amount of time spent in the aerobic phase of training. This is typically 20 to 60 min, but shorter durations of at least 10 min may be performed multiple times per day to achieve similar effects (e.g., three 10-min sessions vs. one 30-min session), which is especially appropriate for those who are deconditioned or symptomatic (e.g., cardiopulmonary patients).
- **Exercise frequency** refers to the total number of exercise sessions per week and is typically two to six sessions per week.

A deconditioned person may improve with only two sessions per week, while a higher-fit person may need five or more sessions per week to see further improvements. Also, an individual able to perform only lower-intensity exercise may need longer durations and frequencies of exercise to achieve an adequate cardiorespiratory effect and energy expenditure, especially those who need to lose excess body fat. In general, lower-frequency and -duration training is associated with higher-intensity exercise, while higher-frequency and -duration training is associated with lower-intensity exercise. It is important to begin an exercise program with both lower intensities and durations and to gradually increase these variables as the individual progresses. It is also important to modify mode, intensity, duration, and frequency (e.g., periodization) throughout a yearlong training program. Ways of manipulating these variables and establishing an appropriate training progression are discussed in greater detail next as specific methods of determining exercise intensity are introduced.

- **Exercise intensity** refers to the overall exertion perceived by an individual (i.e., the difficulty level) during a training session. Several methods can be used to quantify intensity, such as %HRmax, %HR reserve, or RPE.

Exercise Intensity, Duration, and Frequency

Exercise intensity, duration, and frequency are all interrelated and collectively determine the total work and volume performed, as well as the efficacy of the training session.

The ACSM recommends that every adult accumulate 30 min or more of moderate-intensity physical activity on most, preferably all, days of the week (Balady et al. 2000). However, this general statement does not provide information regarding the dose of exercise needed to elicit a desired cardiorespiratory effect or energy expenditure. Both longer-duration, lower-intensity exercise (e.g., 60 min of brisk walking) and higher-intensity, shorter-duration exercise (e.g., 20-30 min of running) are effective in enhancing cardiorespiratory fitness and expending calories.

High Intensity Versus Low Intensity

An inverse relationship exists between exercise intensity and duration in terms of caloric expenditure. For example, an average-size person can expend approximately 300 kcal with slow walking (3 miles/h) for 60 min (low intensity–high duration), very brisk walking (4.5 miles/h) for 45 min (moderate intensity–moderate duration), or running at 6 miles/h for 20 min (high intensity–low duration). Therefore, someone unable to perform higher-intensity exercise can still improve cardiorespiratory fitness and energy expenditure by exercising for longer durations with lower intensities. However, it is important to note that even though the percentage of kilocalories expended from fat is higher during lower-intensity compared to higher-intensity training, low-intensity aerobic activity does not necessarily equate to a greater total caloric expenditure from fat. More importantly, the total caloric expenditure for a given period of time is much greater with high-intensity compared to low-intensity training. To illustrate, consider table 2.10, which illustrates the effects of low- and high-intensity exercise on estimating kilocalories used from fat and carbohydrates and total caloric expenditure.

From these data it is clear that for a given period of time, higher-intensity training is just as effective (and may be even more effective) in burning fat as lower-intensity training. More importantly, caloric expenditure for the 30-min duration was 60% greater for higher-intensity training compared to lower-intensity training.

Research has shown several advantages of high-intensity training over low-intensity training (Lee, Hsieh, and Paffenbarger 1995; Tanasescu, et al. 2002). For example, both total energy expenditure and energy expenditure from vigorous activity, but not nonvigorous activity, have been shown to relate inversely to

TABLE 2.10 The Effects of Low- and High-Intensity Exercise on Estimating Kcal Used

Exercise intensity (%$\dot{V}O_2$max)	Average VO_2 ($L \cdot min^{-1}$)	Average RER*	Carbs (% kcal)	Fat (% kcal)	Carbs (kcal for 30 min)	Fat (kcal for 30 min)	Total (kcal for 30 min)
Low—50%	1.7 $L \cdot min^{-1}$	0.83	50	50	125	125	250
High—80%	2.7 $L \cdot min^{-1}$	0.92	70	30	275	125	400

*RER = respiratory exchange ratio (the ratio of carbon dioxide produced to oxygen consumed).

mortality (Blair et al. 1989; Lee, Hsieh, and Paffenbarger 1995; Paffenbarger et al. 1986; Tanasescu et al. 2002). In addition, death rates decline steadily as the energy an individual expends during aerobic-type exercise increases from 500 to 3,500 kcal/week, with death rates 20% to 30% lower in active men who expended 2,000 kcal/week compared to less active men (Paffenbarger et al. 1986).

Tanasescu et al. (2002) tracked 44,452 men 40 to 75 years old over 13 years to assess the amount, type, and intensity of physical activity in relation to the risk of CHD. They reported that total physical activity, running, weight training, and walking were each associated with reduced CHD risk. Running, rowing, and walking more than 1 h per week were associated with a CHD risk reduction of 42%, 18%, and 18%, respectively, which implies that running was more effective than walking in reducing CHD risk. Also, an increased, higher-intensity walking pace was more important than total duration of walking in reducing CHD risk. High-intensity exercise (>6 METs) was more effective than moderate-intensity exercise (3-6 METs) in reducing CHD risk, and moderate-intensity exercise was more effective than low-intensity exercise (<3 METs) in reducing CHD risk. Exercise intensity was related to a CHD risk reduction of 4% for each 1-MET increase in exercise intensity, independent of total exercise volume. These data provide strong evidence for the value of aerobic exercise, especially higher-intensity aerobic exercise, in reducing the risk of CVD.

If the energy requirement of an activity is in METs, the following equation can be used to convert to kcal $\cdot$ min^{-1}: kcal $\cdot$ min^{-1} = METs * 0.0175 * weight (kg). For example, consider the 10.2 METs required to run at a moderate pace on a flat surface at 6 miles/h, which implies an energy cost approximately 10 times that of rest (the individual will burn 10 times as many kilocalories compared to at rest). If we assume the individual weighs 80 kg, the energy cost required to run at a constant 6 miles/h is 14.3 kcal $\cdot$ min^{-1}. At this 10 min/mile pace it will take the person 30 min to run 3 mi, and he or she will expend approximately 430 kcal (14.3 kcal $\cdot$ min^{-1} * 30) during this time. Now consider this 80-kg individual walking the same 3-mile distance at a slow to moderate 3 mile/h (3.3-MET) pace. The energy cost at this slower pace is only 4.6 kcal $\cdot$ min^{-1}. Since at 3 miles/h it will take 60 min to complete the 3-mile distance, the total energy expended is approximately 280 kcal.

Compared to running 3 miles, walking 3 miles took twice as long and expended nearly one-third fewer kilocalories. Therefore, compared to lower-intensity aerobic exercise, higher-intensity aerobic exercise is more beneficial both in enhancing cardiorespiratory fitness and in expending a greater number of kilocalories in a shorter period of time. In addition, habitual vigorous exercise is associated with an overall decreased risk of primary cardiac arrest (Siscovick et al. 1984). However, higher-intensity exercise has been associated with an increased risk of musculoskeletal injury and lower adherence to training compared to lower-intensity exercise (Pollock et al. 1998).

Excess Post Oxygen Consumption

In addition to the O_2 cost of exercise, an excess amount of O_2 (relative to resting O_2 consumption of 1 MET) is also consumed after exercise during the recovery period in order to restore homeostasis of the body. This excess oxygen is referred to as excess postoxygen consumption (EPOC), which stays above resting levels of O_2 consumption up to approximately 24 h after exercise, with most of the increase being seen during the first few hours after exercise. The EPOC is needed in order to reconvert lactate back to glycogen; oxidize lactate in energy metabolism; restore O_2 levels in the blood and muscle (e.g., myoglobin); resynthesize ATP and CP stores in the working muscles; and decrease HR, ventilation, body temperature, and blood catecholamines (epinephrine and norepinephrine) back to resting levels.

The effect of EPOC on exercise intensity and duration has been examined by Quinn and colleagues (1994). Having eight trained female subjects (mean age 30.2 ± 5.0 years) walk briskly during multiple sessions at a constant intensity of 70% $\dot{V}O_2$max for either 20 min, 40 min, or 60 min, the authors reported an EPOC after a 3-h recovery period (consisting of quiet sitting) of 8.6 L (43 kcal) in the subjects who walked for 20 min, 9.8 L (49 kcal) in the subjects who walked for 40 min, and 15.2 L (76 kcal) in the subjects who walked for 60 min. These data indicate that people's metabolic rate stays elevated above 1 MET for several hours after completion of exercise (thus they are expending more kilocalories than they would if they did not exercise) and that for a given exercise intensity, longer-duration exercise is more effective than shorter-duration exercise in increasing EPOC.

Quantifying Exercise Intensity

The proper dose of exercise intensity needed to elicit a cardiorespiratory response has been quantified by several methods as summarized in table 2.11. These methods are discussed next.

Direct Method

The direct method of quantifying exercise intensities involves first directly measuring or predicting an individual's $\dot{V}O_2$max during submaximal or maximal exercise testing as already described. Appropriate training intensities needed to achieve moderate to high improvements in cardiorespiratory fitness are between 40% and 85% of $\dot{V}O_2$max. However, improvements in cardiorespiratory fitness are maximized with exercise intensities between 60% $\dot{V}O_2$max (lower limit) and 85% $\dot{V}O_2$max (upper limit), although training intensities between 40% and 55% of $\dot{V}O_2$max may be more appropriate for deconditioned or symptomatic individuals.

For example, optimal training intensities (60-85% $\dot{V}O_2$max) for a healthy 50-year-old individual with a $\dot{V}O_2$max of 49 ml · kg^{-1} · min^{-1} (14 METs) would be between 29.4 ml · kg^{-1} · min^{-1} (8.4 METs) and 41.7 ml · kg^{-1} · min^{-1} (11.9 METs). This implies that this individual should participate in activities that require an energy expenditure between 8.4 and 11.9 METs, which could include running on a flat surface between 5 miles/h (approximately 8.6 METs) and 7 miles/h (approximately 11.7 METs). As shown in table 2.7, a $\dot{V}O_2$max of 49 ml · kg^{-1} · min^{-1} would classify a 50-year-old male as having an "athletic" cardiorespiratory fitness level. Now consider a deconditioned 50-year-old male with a $\dot{V}O_2$max of only 30 ml · kg^{-1} · min^{-1} (8.6 METs). From table 2.7, this individual would be classified as having a "fair," below-average cardiorespiratory fitness level. Since this person is deconditioned, training intensities between 40% and 55% $\dot{V}O_2$max may be more appropriate—between 12 ml · kg^{-1} · min^{-1} (3.4 METs) and 16.5 ml · kg^{-1} · min^{-1} (4.7 METs). An activity that requires an energy expenditure between 3.4 and 4.7 METs is slow to fast walking on a flat surface between 3 miles/h (approximately 3.3 METs) and 4.5 miles/h (approximately 4.5 METs).

TABLE 2.11 Classification of Physical Activity Intensity, Based on Physical Activity Lasting up to 60 Min

Endurance-type activity	Relative intensity[a]			Absolute intensity (METs) in healthy adults[b]			
Intensity	%VO_2R or %HRR	%HRmax	RPE	Young (20-39 years)	Middle-aged (40-64 years)	Old (65-79 years)	Very old (>80 years)
Very light	<20	<35	10	<2.4	<2.0	<1.6	<1.0
Light	20-39	35-54	10-11	2.4-4.7	2.0-3.9	1.6-3.1	1.1-1.9
Moderate	40-59	55-69	12-13	4.8-7.1	4.0-5.9	3.2-4.7	2.0-2.9
Hard	60-84	70-89	14-16	7.2-10.1	6.0-8.4	4.8-6.7	3.0-4.25
Very hard	>85	>90	17-19	>10.2	>8.5	>6.8	>4.25
Maximal[c]	100	100	20	12.0	10.0	8.0	5.0

[a]Relative intensity includes (1) %VO_2R (percent of maximum O_2 uptake reserve), which is expressed as %($\dot{V}O_2$max - VO_2rest) + VO_2rest; (2) %HRR (percent of maximum heart rate reserve), which is expressed as %(HRmax - HRrest) + HRrest; (3) %HRmax (percent of maximum HR), which is expressed as %(220 - age); and (4) RPE (rate of perceived exertion), with complete RPE scales shown in figure 2.2. See text for sample calculations and additional explanations.

[b]Absolute intensity (METs) values are approximate mean values for men. Mean values for women are approximately 1 to 2 METs lower than those for men.

[c]Maximal values are mean values achieved during maximal exercise for healthy adults.

Reprinted, by permission, from M.L. Pollock, G.A. Gaesser, J.D. Butcher, J.P. Despres, R.K. Dishman, B.A. Franklin, and C.E. Garber, 1998, "American College of Sports Medicine position stand: The recommended quantity and quality of exercise for developing and maintaining cardiorespiratory and muscular fitness, and flexibility in healthy adults," *Medicine and Science in Sports and Exercise* 30: 975-991.

The approximate gross energy costs of several common aerobic type activities are as follows:

- Walking
  - -Slow (2.5-3 miles/h): 3 METs
  - -Brisk (3.5-4 miles/h): 4 METs
- Level-ground running
  - -6 miles/h (10 min/mile): 10 METs
  - -8 miles/h (7.5 min/mile): 13.5 METs
  - -10 miles/h (6 min/mile): 16 METs
- Level-ground cycling or stationary cycling for 80-kg individual
  - -Slow and leisurely (10-12 miles/h or 100-125 W): 6 to 7 METs
  - -Moderate and leisurely (12-14 miles/h or 125-150 W): 7 to 8 METs
  - -Fast and leisurely, or racing (15-16 miles/h or 175-200 W): 9 to 10 METs
- Golf (walking while carrying bag or pulling cart): 4 to 7 METs
- Hiking: 3 to 7 METs
- Tennis and racquetball: 4 to 12 METs
- Swimming: 4 to 8 METs
- Walking upstairs: 8 METs
- Walking downstairs: 3 METs
- Weight training (light to moderate intensity): 3 to 6 METs

%HRmax Method

Due to the relatively linear relationship between HR and VO_2, HR can be used as a guide to determine exercise intensity. If an individual's HRmax has not been determined through a maximal-effort exercise to exhaustion, it can be estimated by (220 – age) ± 12 beats/min. However, the standard deviation of ± 12 beats/min implies that two-thirds of people could have an actual HRmax that is 12 beats/min higher or lower than the age-predicted HRmax of (220 – age). In an attempt to improve the accuracy in estimating HRmax, one research group developed the following gender-specific multiple regression equations to predict HRmax using 2,010 men and women who were 14 to 77 years of age (Whaley et al. 1992):

Men: HRmax = 203.9 – 0.813 * age (yr) + 0.276 (HRrest) – 0.084 * weight (kg) – 4.5 * smoking code (1 for a smoker and 0 for a nonsmoker)

Women: HRmax = 204.8 – 0.718 * age (yr) + 0.162 * HRrest (beats/min) – 0.105 * weight (kg) – 6.2 * smoking code (1 for a smoker and 0 for a nonsmoker)

These equations take into account that individuals with a higher HRrest also tend to have a higher HRmax (and conversely, individuals with a lower HRrest also tend to have a lower HRmax) and that smokers and overweight individuals tend to have a lower HRmax. In addition, the equation HRmax = 200 – 0.5 * age (yr) has been shown to be relatively accurate in estimating HRmax in individuals with >30% body fat (Miller, Wallace, and Eggert 1993).

Once HRmax has been determined, the %HRmax method may be used to set exercise intensity and establish an optimal HR training zone. Appropriate training intensities needed to achieve moderate to high improvements in cardiorespiratory fitness are between 50% and 90% HRmax. However, improvements in cardiorespiratory fitness are maximized with exercise intensities between 70% HRmax (lower limit) and 90% HRmax (upper limit), which corresponds to approximately 60% and 85% of $\dot{V}O_2$max (table 2.11).

For example, using the HRmax method, an optimal HR training zone (70-90% HRmax) for a 50-year-old healthy individual would be between 119 and 153 beats/min. For deconditioned or symptomatic individuals, training intensities between 50% and 65% HRmax may be more appropriate. For a 50-year-old deconditioned person, a more appropriate training zone would be between 85 and 110 beats/min. People can use an electronic HR monitor during training to more easily determine if they are employing an exercise intensity that is within their HR training zone.

% Heart Rate Reserve Method

In the % heart rate reserve (%HRR) method, developed in Scandinavia and published in 1957 by Karvonen and colleagues (Karvonen, Kentala, and Mustala 1957), one determines intensity by taking a percentage of the difference between an individual's HRmax and HRrest (table 2.11). Appropriate training intensities needed to achieve moderate to high improvements in cardiorespiratory fitness are between 40% and 85% HRR. However, improvements in cardiorespiratory fitness are maximized with exercise intensities between 60% HRR (lower limit) and 85% HRR (upper limit). Although 60% and 85% HRR have been shown to correspond to approximately 60% and 85% of $\dot{V}O_2$max in younger subjects (table 2.11), recent data have indicated that in older adults %HRmax is more closely related to %$\dot{V}O_2$max than %HRR (Panton et al. 1996).

Although an optimal HR training zone using the %HRR method is between 60% and 85% HRR for most healthy individuals (60-75% HRR for average fitness status and 75-85% HRR for excellent fitness status or athletes in training), training intensities between 40% and 55% HRR may be more appropriate for deconditioned, symptomatic, or low fitness status individuals. An individual's optimal HR training zone can be calculated using what is known as the Karvonen formula:

$$60\text{-}85\%\ \text{HRR} = (60\text{-}85\%) * (\text{HRmax} - \text{HRrest}) + \text{HRrest}$$

For example, with use of the %HRR method, the optimal training zone (60-85% HRR) for a 50-year-old individual with a HRrest of 75 beats/min would be between 132 and 156 beats/min for optimal cardiorespiratory fitness. An advantage of the %HRR method over the %HRmax method is that it takes an individual's HRrest into account, which often reflects a healthy individual's fitness level. A lower HRrest equates to an increased fitness level, as shown in table 2.12. Consider another 50-year-old with a HRrest of 50 beats/min. Using the %HRR method this person's optimal training zone (60-85% HRR) would be between 122 and 152 beats/min, which is considerably different from the 132 to 156 beats/min just mentioned. However, using the %HRmax method, these two individuals would have identical target HR zones. The relationship between the %HRR method and the %HRmax method at varying intensities is shown in table 2.11. A sample training progression using %HRR for improving and maintaining cardiorespiratory fitness is shown in table 2.13.

Rate of Perceived Exertion Method (Borg Scale)

Original and modified (category-ratio) RPE scales (figure 2.2a-b) have been shown to be an easy and relatively reliable method for quantifying intensity either in conjunction with the direct and HR methods (table 2.11) or when HR or direct methods are not appropriate (e.g., for a cardiac patient on beta blockers, which decrease both HRmax and HRrest, in which case the %HRmax and %HRR may not be appropriate). High correlations exist between RPE, HR, VO_2, and workload. The original 15-grade Borg scale has a range from 6 to 20 (figure 2.2a) (Borg 1970, 1982). Appropriate training intensities needed to achieve moderate to high improvements in cardiorespiratory fitness (e.g., 60-90% of HRmax) have an RPE between 12 and 16 (table 2.11), which is between "somewhat hard" and "hard" on the original RPE scale.

SUMMARY

In conclusion, this chapter provides a scientific basis for anaerobic and aerobic exercise testing and prescription in the active aging individual. It is clear that the aging individual obtains physiological and psychological benefits from aerobic and anaerobic exercise that are similar to those for younger people, although the magnitudes differ. It is also clear that aerobic and anaerobic exercise can attenuate or in some cases

TABLE 2.12 Norms for Resting Heart Rate (Beats/Min)

	CLASSIFICATION						
Gender/age	Very poor	Poor	Below average	Average	Above average	Good	Excellent
M 18-25	82-103	74-78	70-72	66-69	61-65	57-59	40-54
F 18-25	84-104	77-81	72-76	68-71	64-67	59-63	42-57
M 26-35	81-102	74-78	69-71	65-67	61-63	55-59	36-53
F 26-35	84-102	77-81	72-74	68-70	64-66	60-62	39-57
M 36-45	83-101	75-80	70-72	66-69	62-64	58-60	37-55
F 36-45	83-102	77-81	72-75	69-71	65-67	61-63	40-58
M 46-55	84-103	77-81	72-74	66-70	63-65	58-61	35-56
F 46-55	85-104	77-82	73-76	70-72	65-69	61-64	43-58
M 56-65	84-103	76-80	72-75	68-71	63-65	59-61	42-56
F 56-65	84-103	79-81	73-77	69-72	65-68	61-64	42-59
M >65	83-103	74-79	70-73	66-69	62-65	57-61	40-55
F >65	86-97	78-83	73-76	70-72	66-68	60-64	49-59

TABLE 2.13 Sample Training Progression for Improving and Maintaining Cardiorespiratory Fitness

Program stage	Week	Exercise frequency (sessions/week)	Exercise intensity (% heart rate reserve)	Exercise duration (min)
Preparatory	1	2-3	40-50	10-15
	2	2-3	40-50	15-20
	3-4	3-4	50-60	15-20
	5-6	3-4	50-60	20-25
Improvement	7-9	3-4	60-70	20-25
	10-12	3-4	60-70	25-30
	13-15	4-5	65-75	25-30
	16-18	4-5	65-75	30-35
	19-21	4-5	70-85	35-40
	22-24	4-5	70-85	40-45
Maintenance	24+	2-5	70-85	20-45

a

6	No exertion at all
7	Extremely light
8	
9	Very light
10	
11	Light
12	
13	Somewhat hard
14	
15	Hard (heavy)
16	
17	Very hard
18	
19	Extremely hard
20	Maximal exertion

Borg RPE scale
© Gunnar Borg, 1970, 1985, 1994, 1998

b

0	Nothing at all	"No P"
0.3		
0.5	Extremely weak	Just noticeable
1	Very weak	
1.5		
2	Weak	Light
2.5		
3	Moderate	
4		
5	Strong	Heavy
6		
7	Very strong	
8		
9		
10	Extremely strong	"Max P"
11		
●	Absolute maximum	Highest possible

Borg CR10 scale
© Gunnar Borg, 1981, 1982, 1998

FIGURE 2.2 *(a)* The Borg RPE scale and *(b)* the Borg CR10 scale.

Reprinted, by permission, from G. Borg, 1998, *Borg's perceived exertion and pain scales.* (Champaign, IL: Human Kinetics), 47, 50.

reverse most physiological adaptations that occur due to aging. Understanding scientific principles of aerobic and anaerobic training will help the trainer, therapist, physician, and other clinicians and exercise specialists properly test and prescribe exercise for the active aging individual.

CHAPTER

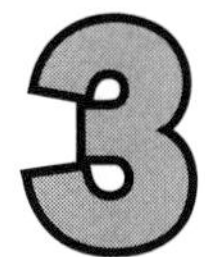

The Kinetic Chain

W. Ben Kibler, MD

The term "kinetic chain" refers to a particular conceptual framework for understanding the mechanisms by which athletes accomplish the complex tasks required for function in sport. Once these functional mechanisms are clear, the adaptations that occur as a result of athletic or recreational activity, and the maladaptations in flexibility and strength and clinical findings associated with athletic dysfunction due to injury, are more understandable. This knowledge can give the sports medicine clinician more tools to use in evaluation and treatment of athletes. This chapter describes the basics of the kinetic chain concept and illustrates its applicability and utility in treating older athletes.

DEFINING THE KINETIC CHAIN

The kinetic chain is a coordinated sequencing of activation, mobilization, and stabilization of body segments to produce an athletic activity (Putnam 1993). Body segments have been described according to the Hanavan model as a major bone and the joints on each end (figure 3.1). Kinetic chain activities have been grouped into open and closed chain (Kibler and Livingston 2001). Characteristics of open chains generally include free movement of the terminal segment, large terminal segment velocities, and relatively many degrees of freedom in the proximal segments. Characteristics of closed chains generally include fixed or minimal movement of the terminal segment, low terminal segment velocities, minimal degrees of freedom, and coupling of movements of the segments. Many kinetic chains exhibit both closed and open chain activity. Sequential force development throughout the segments in an overhead athlete is shown in figure 3.2.

The majority of force is developed in the legs and trunk in closed chain fashion (Kibler 1995), is funneled through the scapuloglenohumeral complex using closed chain biomechanics, and is transferred to the rapidly moving hand, which is acting in an open chain manner. The observational result in the tennis swing is shown in figure 3.3.

The feet are planted on the ground. Knee flexion/extension and trunk counter-rotation/rotation develop force from the ground that is sequentially transferred through the trunk to the shoulder. Arm rotation and forward motion are centered on a stabilized shoulder, and hand motion is transferred to the racket.

Kinetic chain sequencing serves three purposes:

- Efficient generation and transfer of kinetic energy and force to the distal segment (hand, foot) to move an object (ball, racket, body) (Putnam 1993), accomplished by using the "summation of speed" principle, in which the velocity and force developed in each segment are facilitated and augmented by the actions of proximal segments, similar to what occurs with a "cracking of the whip"
- Stabilization and positioning of the body segments and joints to regulate and absorb the developed forces at the joints, accomplished by creating anticipatory postural adjustments (APAs) that are integrated with the athletic activity pattern to maintain a stable base for activity (Cordo and Nashner 1982; Zattara and Bouisset 1988)
- Stabilization of body posture to counteract the eccentric loads and destabilizing effects of the athletic movements, accomplished by integrating proximal and distal muscle activation to spread loads over the entire extremity (Nieminen et al. 1995; Zhang, Bates, and Dufek 2000), by controlling eccentric and tension loads (Van Ingen Schenau, Bobbert, and Rozendahl 1987), and by

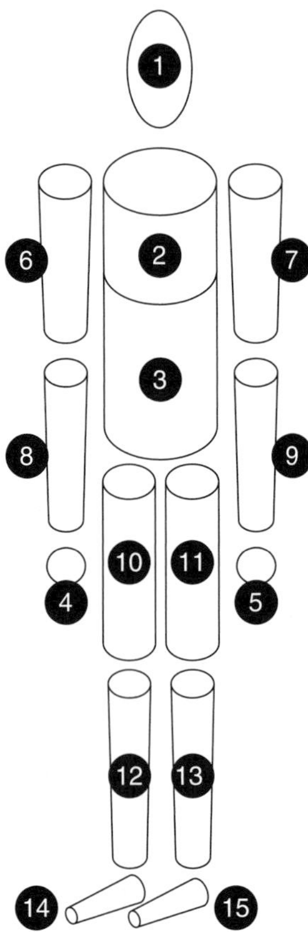

FIGURE 3.1 The Hanavan model of body segments.

From E.P. Hanavan, 1964, *Mathematical model of the human body* (Wright-Patterson Air force Base, Ohio) AMRL-TR-64-102.

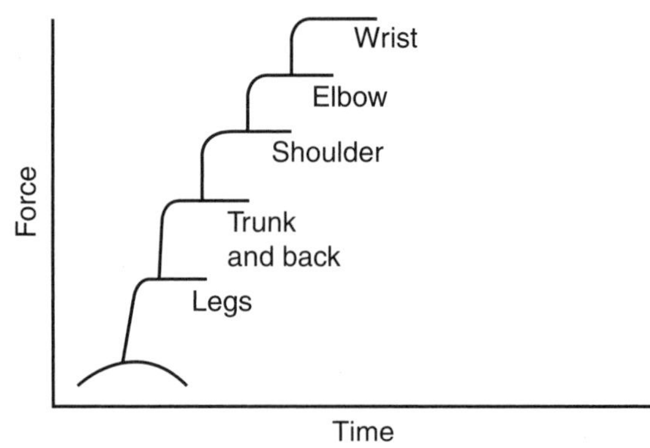

FIGURE 3.2 The kinetic chain of proximal-to-distal segment activation and force generation.

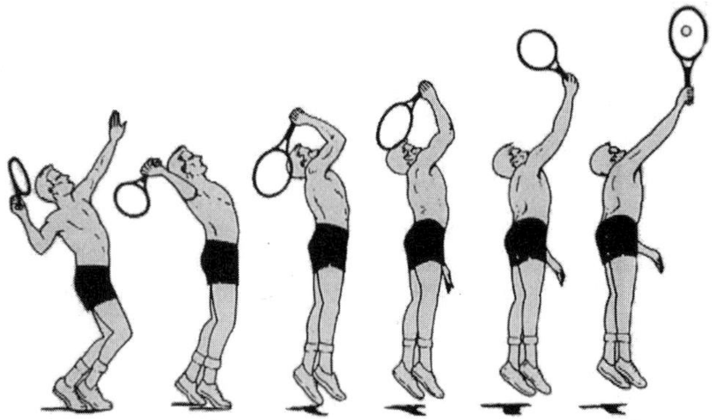

FIGURE 3.3 Sequential segment activation in the tennis serve. Note the ground reaction force creating trunk motion that then drives arm motion.

Copyright by W. Ben Kibler, MD.

placing joints in their most stable configuration in either the lower extremity (Bobbert and van Soest 2000) or upper extremity (Marshall and Elliott 2000)

Enhancing control of the kinetic chain can increase performance by improving performance parameters (strength, force, endurance) and decrease injury risk by diminishing risk factors (excessive loads in muscles or joints, decreased eccentric strength).

An effective kinetic chain must consist of three elements:

- The most basic element is **intact or functionally intact anatomy** of the joints, ligaments, bones, and muscles. "Functionally intact" means that the load-bearing capabilities, ranges of motions, and strength and power capabilities are adequate for the demands of the sport or activity.

- The second element is **appropriate physiological muscle activation**. This creates patterns of muscle activation to act upon the anatomy. These patterns generate force (Putnam 1993), harmonize the movements of several joints (Nichols 1994), and control loads and joint stiffness at individual joints. These activation patterns are task (throwing, jumping, catching, load absorbing) specific and allow the kinetic chains to be sport or activity specific. They are learned by repetition, are highly ordered, and are easily altered in injury or fatigue (Glousman et al. 1988).

- The third element is **appropriate biomechanical forces and motions** to result in the desired athletic function. This occurs when the physiological patterns activate functionally intact anatomy. The hand, foot, or body is then in the appropriate position, with the appropriate motion, to produce a desired effect. This sequential motion and position of the joints produces an "interactive" moment at a distal joint. The effect of the interactive moment is that distal segments do not have to independently develop the large forces seen in the distal segments (Bobbert and van Soest 2000; Putnam 1993). Also, the interactive moments create positions of the bones around a joint that allow the developed forces to "pass through" to the next segment. This minimizes loads on the joints and joint control structures, the ligaments and muscles. Most of the force development is from the proximal segments that have been the base of stability and larger mass (Elliott, Marshall, and Noffal 1995).

General descriptions of kinetic chains have been demonstrated for many sports and activities. The kinetic chains represent general patterns that appear to be reproducible for a specific activity with some variation between individuals doing the activity (Hirashima et al. 2002; Marshall and Elliott 2000).

KINETIC CHAIN IMPLICATIONS FOR INJURY, EVALUATION, AND TREATMENT

Kinetic chain integrity is vital for sport function. Alteration in the sequential activation, mobilization, and stabilization of the body segments occurs very commonly in association with sport dysfunction, either decreased performance or injury. This kinetic chain "breakage" has been demonstrated in both young and older athletes in many anatomical areas and as a result of repetitive, vigorous activities. It is usually acquired and can be created from many factors—remote injury, incompletely healed or rehabilitated injury, muscle weakness or imbalance, muscle inflexibility or joint stiffness, or improper mechanics. Kinetic chain breakage creates increased distal physiological or biomechanical requirements (increased muscle activation, or increased distal segment velocity, acceleration, or mass in order to "catch up" and develop the same kinetic energy or force at the distal segment) (Kibler 1995); changes the interactive moment at the distal joint (increasing the forces that must be absorbed at the joint) (Putnam 1993); or decreases the ultimate velocity or force at the distal segment (Toyoshima, Hoshikawa, and Miyashita 1974).

Examples of kinetic chain breakage include ankle inflexibility and gastrocnemius muscle weakness in plantar fasciitis (Kibler, Goldberg, and Chandler 1991), hamstring weakness in runners (Knapik et al. 1991), trunk muscle imbalance (Young, Herring, and Press 1996), scapular muscle weakness in shoulder impingement (McQuade, Dawson, and Smidt 1998), scapular dyskinesis in impingement and instability (Warner and Micheli 1992), and glenohumeral internal rotation deficit in shoulder injuries (Burkhart, Morgan, and Kibler 2000). Whether kinetic chain breakage is a primary cause of the injury or symptoms or is the result of the process of injury, exacerbating the symptoms, is not resolved. However, it is well established that kinetic chain breakages occur frequently. Some studies have shown these alterations in association with overt injury and clinical symptoms 49% to 100% of the time.

The frequent association of distant tissue alterations with clinical symptoms can lead to a "victims and culprits" approach to evaluation and treatment of sports medicine injuries, especially overload or chronic injuries (MacIntyre and Lloyd-Smith 1993). This approach allows a broad-based perspective on the pathophysiology underlying these injuries and an extensive clinical evaluation of all the physiological and biomechanical alterations that may be associated with the injury. The "victim" is the site of clinical symptoms, and the "culprits" are the distant alterations. For example, patellar tendinopathy may be associated with hip inflexibility or hip abductor weakness, and "tennis elbow" (lateral elbow tendinosis) may be associated with posterior deltoid weakness.

Any system of evaluation of injuries using the kinetic chain approach should take into account the broad scope of causative and contributing factors that may exist in addition to the clinical symptoms. These include joint flexibility, any intrinsic risk factors, and any biomechanical deficits that may be present. Our evaluation is based on a framework in which most of the factors are categorized into five main areas, called complexes (Kibler, Chandler, and Pace 1992). These complexes interact with each other in the causation of microtrauma injuries, can be present as a result of macrotrauma injuries, and are detectable on a clinical level. These complexes are the following:

- **Tissue injury complex:** that group of anatomic structures that have overt pathological change
- **Clinical symptom complex:** that group of overt symptoms and signs that clinically characterize the injury
- **Tissue overload complex:** that group of structures that have nonsymptomatic but clinically detectable changes
- **Functional biomechanical deficit complex:** alterations in biomechanics due to injury or overload
- **Subclinical adaptations:** substitute actions that the athlete uses to compensate for altered mechanics to maintain performance

These complexes interact in a negative feedback vicious cycle (Kibler, Chandler, and Pace 1992) to cause or maintain a soft tissue injury (figure 3.4). In microtrauma cases, an athlete may "cycle" as a "susceptible" athlete for some time before overt clinical symptoms appear. Most acute injuries exhibit fewer

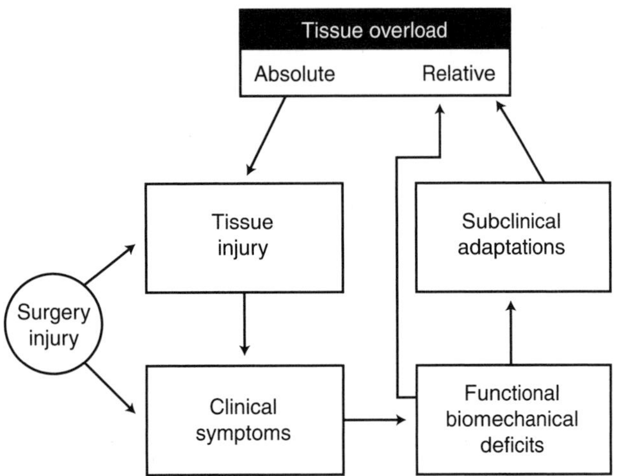

FIGURE 3.4 The negative feedback vicious cycle.

overloads and biomechanical deficits, but some of these may occur due to treatment, such as immobilization after Achilles tendon surgery. In this model, clinical symptoms are a relatively small part of the entire pathophysiologic picture. These obviously require treatment, but it is also important to emphasize restoration of function encompassing all of the physiological and biomechanical alterations, rather than only resolution of symptoms.

THE KINETIC CHAIN IN THE OLDER ATHLETE

There is minimal literature on kinetic chain function in older adults in normal athletic activities. However, observational analysis of kinetic chains of throwing, running, swimming, or golfing shows no differences in segment activation sequences between older and younger adults. Kinetic chain activations should be encouraged in older athletes as well because such activations will develop efficiencies in force development and joint protection. They will also create a proximal segment stability that can facilitate distant segment mobility, and will decrease the demands and loads on the distal segments.

Similarly, there is very little published research on distant tissue alterations or adaptations in older athletes, despite the high incidence of overload and chronic injuries in this age group. However, the factors known to be altered due to injury or maladaptation to sport in kinetic chain dysfunction in young athletes are known to also be altered in older athletes due to aging (Nichols, Medina, and Dean 2001). In addition, older athletes show decreased joint mobility due to arthrosis, bone spurs, or soft tissue stiffness. They exhibit decreased muscle flexibility and strength (Wilmore 1991). They have diminished capability for force and power development, as well as eccentric muscle activation for load absorption, and have decreased anaerobic endurance (Bosco and Komi 1980; Larsson 1978). These age-acquired alterations decrease the inherent capability of the muscles to protect themselves from injury and to protect joints from injury. Loss of flexibility is a key issue, because it can affect injury risk not only locally but also distantly, through creating kinetic chain breakage.

Moreover, there is no evidence that the kinetic chains for sport activities are different in older athletes. The mechanical and physiological requirements for the golf swing, the tennis strokes, and running and jumping, among other sport activities, are the same. The implications are that kinetic chain breakage would also present in overload or chronic injuries in older athletes and may play a major role in decreased performance, increased injury risk, and treatment and rehabilitation. Injury analysis should include negative feedback vicious cycle evaluation; rehabilitation should include kinetic chain rehabilitation; and preventive conditioning (prehabilitation) should include kinetic chain elements.

PRINCIPLES OF KINETIC CHAIN EVALUATION

The first principle to guide the evaluation is that kinetic chain maladaptations are very frequent in association with chronic musculotendinous injuries, so one should expect and look for them in the history and physical exam.

Second, the history should include questions about previous injury, either local to or distant from the present injury. Examples include previous ankle injury (present ankle injury or knee injury), previous hip injury or inflexibility (present knee pain, low back pain, or shoulder injury), previous back pain (present knee pain or shoulder injury), and previous shoulder injury (present shoulder injury or elbow injury). Also, one should ask questions about the exact nature of any treatment and rehabilitation of previous injury. In general, treatment based strictly on decreasing local symptoms (injections for tendinitis, brace for tendinitis, rest for any injury) and rehabilitation based on modalities (ultrasound, hot pack, electrical stimulation) will not address the kinetic chain alterations. Return to complete function may be more difficult and may lead to injuries in other parts of the kinetic chain.

Third, the physical exam should include some screening tests for distant parts of the kinetic chain to highlight deficits. Good screening tests include standing posture evaluation from front and back, the "one-leg stability series" of one-leg stance and one-leg squat (Kibler and Livingston 2001), sit and reach for lumbar flexibility, repetitive arm elevation/depression for scapular stability (Kibler and McMullen 2003), and glenohumeral rotation off a stabilized scapula (Burkhart, Morgan, and Kibler 2000). Further evaluation can take place if the screening exam shows alterations.

Fourth, rehabilitation can proceed up the kinetic chain, even when the injured area is still protected or healing. This can allow functional restoration of all areas; and when the injured area is capable of tolerating rehabilitation, all the other areas are capable of being integrated into the chain (Kibler, McMullen, and Uhl 2001).

This approach has been summarized in a rehabilitation book that provides more in-depth information (Kibler, Herring, and Press 1998).

EXAMPLES OF KINETIC CHAIN-BASED EVALUATION AND TREATMENT

This section gives examples of an approach for evaluation and treatment that may increase the completeness of the evaluation and the efficacy of rehabilitation techniques. Each condition is covered more extensively in other sections of the book.

Plantar Fasciitis

Plantar fasciitis is exacerbated by loss of dynamic protraction control of the foot and ankle. Several kinetic chain alterations may be present. Factors evident in the complexes include the following:

- **Clinical symptoms:** point tenderness over plantar fascial insertion into calcaneus, stiffness in the morning or upon standing after sitting
- **Tissue injury:** plantar fascia, short flexors
- **Possible additional tissues that may be overloaded:** gastrocnemius/soleus complex, Achilles tendon, gluteal muscles
- **Functional biomechanical deficits:** look for decreased active ankle dorsiflexion; decreased foot pronation/supination control or positive Trendelenburg sign with one-leg stance, or both; decreased strength in toe-off (figure 3.5).
- **Subclinical adaptations:** look for shorter stride on affected leg, look for leg external rotation with stance

Rehabilitation strategies that one should consider include increasing the flexibility of the plantar flexor muscles, increasing the eccentric strength of the plantar flexor muscles, and increasing hip abductor strength to control the pelvis over the planted leg to decrease pronation at the subtalar joint (figure 3.6).

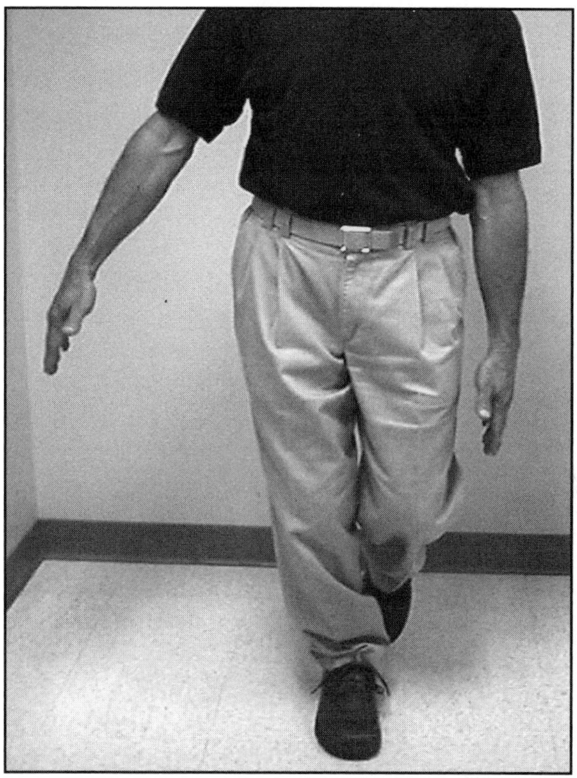

FIGURE 3.5 Positive Trendelenburg sign, with loss of hip control over the planted leg in one-leg stance.

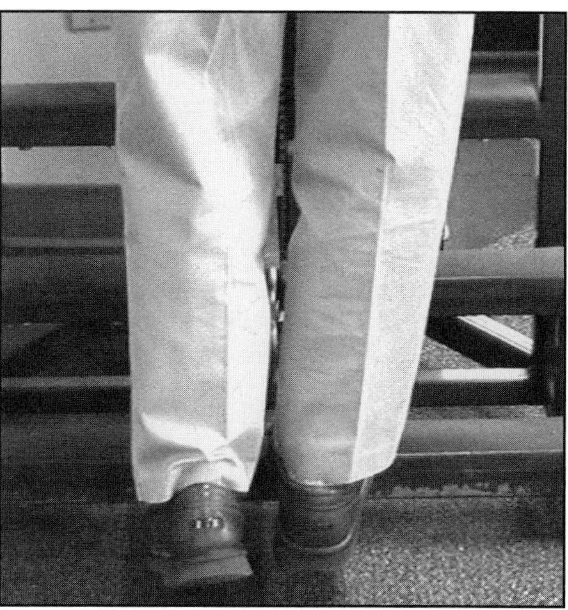

FIGURE 3.6 Plantar flexor eccentric exercise.

Achilles Tendinitis

Achilles tendinitis, like plantar fasciitis, may be exacerbated by kinetic chain alterations that decrease the control of heel movement in stance.

- **Clinical symptoms:** tenderness, ± swelling on Achilles tendon, ± palpable tender knot, pain on first activities diminishing with warm-up
- **Tissue injury:** Achilles tendon, in substance, calcaneal enthesis
- **Possible additional tissue overload:** gastrocnemius/soleus complex, hip abductors/rotators
- **Functional biomechanical deficits:** look for decreased active ankle dorsiflexion, decreased ankle inversion/eversion control and positive Trendelenburg sign upon single-leg stance
- **Subclinical adaptations:** look for decreased stride length, toe/heel landing pattern in stance
- **Rehabilitation considerations:** increase flexibility of plantar flexor muscles, increase hip abduction/rotation control to control pelvis over planted leg, introduce straight and diagonal lunges to increase eccentric muscle activation of entire leg (figure 3.7)

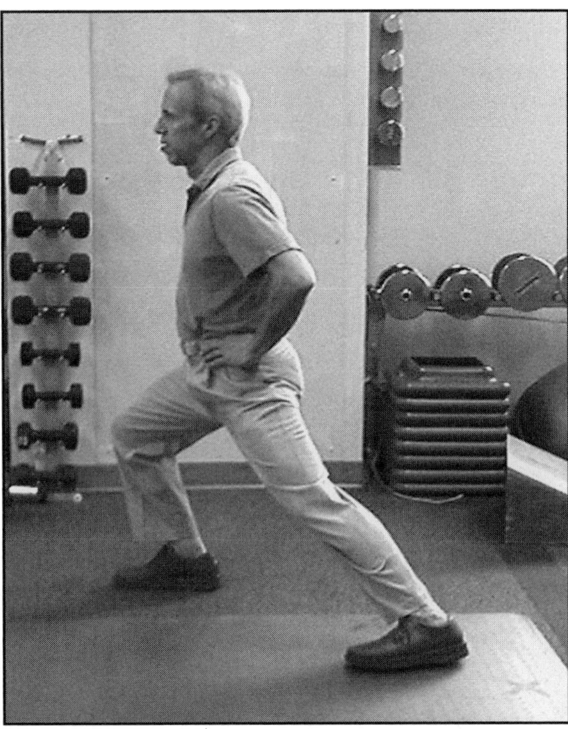

FIGURE 3.7 Diagonal lunges.

Anterior Medial Knee Pain

Anterior medial knee pain has local causes, including joint arthrosis, meniscal damage, plica, or patellofemoral problems, and may be exacerbated by kinetic chain alterations.

- **Clinical symptoms:** medial joint line tenderness, stiffness in the morning, patellofemoral crepitus, pain upon rotation, pain upon jumping, effusion after play
- **Tissue injury:** medial meniscus, medial articular cartilage, medial patellofemoral retinaculum
- **Possible additional tissue overload:** knee extensors, hip extensors/abductors
- **Functional biomechanical deficits:** look for quadriceps/iliotibial band inflexibility; hip rotation tightness; positive Trendelenburg sign with one-leg stance or squat; knee varus
- **Subclinical adaptations:** look for lack of knee extension with stance, hip/trunk flexion with walking or stair climbing
- **Rehabilitation considerations:** increase quadriceps and iliotibial band flexibility; increase patellar mobility; encourage coupled hip extension/knee extension (figure 3.8) muscle exercises, which maximize quadriceps activation and increase active knee motion; encourage half-lunges to increase eccentric control

Chronic Hamstring Muscle Strain

Chronic hamstring strain results from repeated episodes of reinjury. Each reinjury creates more deficits and adaptations.

- **Clinical symptoms:** point tender pain localized along the course of the muscle, either a defect (tear) or a palpable knot (scar), pain when running, stiffness at rest
- **Tissue injury:** hamstring at muscle–tendon junction
- **Tissue overload:** adductors, hip extensors
- **Functional biomechanical deficits:** look for hip flexion and knee flexion in stance or running, a positive Trendelenburg sign on one-leg stability testing
- **Subclinical adaptations:** shortened stride on injured leg, no pivoting on injured leg
- **Rehabilitation considerations:** hip stability exercises for strength and flexibility, stretching and mobilization for the shortened hamstrings,

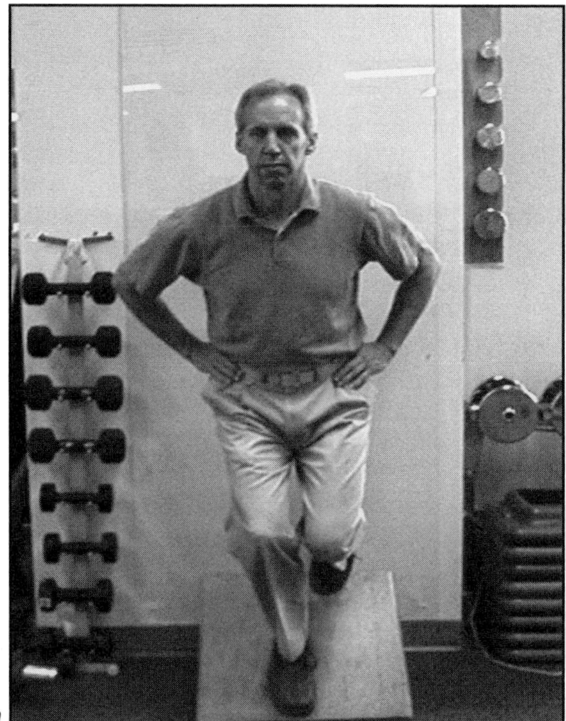

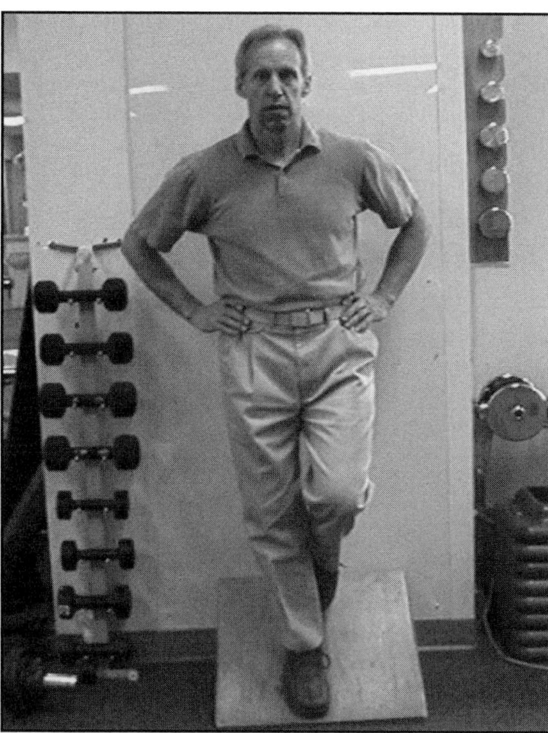

FIGURE 3.8 Coupled hip extension/knee extension to maximize quadriceps activation: *(a)* starting position and *(b)* ending position.

closed-chain exercises involving simultaneous hip extension and knee extension (return to play must be slow and guided due to tendency to recur)

Low Back Pain

Low back pain (LBP) is probably the most common musculoskeletal problem in older athletes. Much LBP is due to degenerative changes, but the exam should look for alterations that may benefit from rehabilitation.

- **Clinical symptoms:** low back pain in lumbosacral area, ± radiculopathy, stiffness in the morning, pain upon extension/flexion
- **Tissue injury:** depending on etiology, disc, nerve root, bone, joints
- **Tissue overload:** deep paraspinal muscles, joint capsules, hip rotators, hamstrings, psoas
- **Functional biomechanical deficits:** hip flexion tightness, hip rotation tightness, lumbar flexion/extension muscle imbalance
- **Subclinical adaptations:** hip flexion posture, lack of trunk extension
- **Rehabilitation considerations:** decrease pain, eliminate postural tightness, increase hip flexion/rotation flexibility, initiate core stability exercises

Rotator Cuff Tendinitis

Rotator cuff injury has obvious local causative factors (poor intrinsic blood supply, subacromial abrasion, direct or indirect trauma), but also may be associated with many kinetic chain alterations.

- **Clinical symptoms:** pain over anterior or lateral acromion; (+) impingement testing; pain and weakness with horizontal adduction, forward flexion, external rotation; pain at night.
- **Tissue injury:** rotator cuff tendon, partial or complete
- **Possible additional tissue overload:** shoulder capsule, scapular stabilizing muscles
- **Functional biomechanical deficits:** look for glenohumeral internal rotation deficit, scapular dyskinesis with lower trapezius weakness, upper trapezius hyperactivation, and acromial depression

- **Subclinical adaptations:** look for shoulder shrug with arm elevation, thoracic kyphosis, dropping the arm below shoulder elevation in throwing or serving
- **Rehabilitation considerations:** thoracic mobilization in extension; encourage coupled hip extension/trunk extension/scapular retraction; encourage scapular stabilization (elbows in back pockets) (figure 3.9); encourage early closed chain humeral head depression (figure 3.10); encourage coupled trunk movement/closed chain rotator cuff exercises (wall washes) (figure 3.11)

Lateral Elbow Tendinitis

Lateral elbow tendinitis (misnamed lateral epicondylitis, more properly named lateral elbow tendinosis) is common in older athletes and is commonly associated with mechanical kinetic chain deficits.

- **Clinical symptoms:** point tender pain over anterior epicondyle, over extensor carpi radialis brevis; pain with grip; pain with one-hand backhand tennis stroke
- **Tissue injury:** extensor carpi radialis brevis, occasionally extensor carpi radialis longus or joint capsule

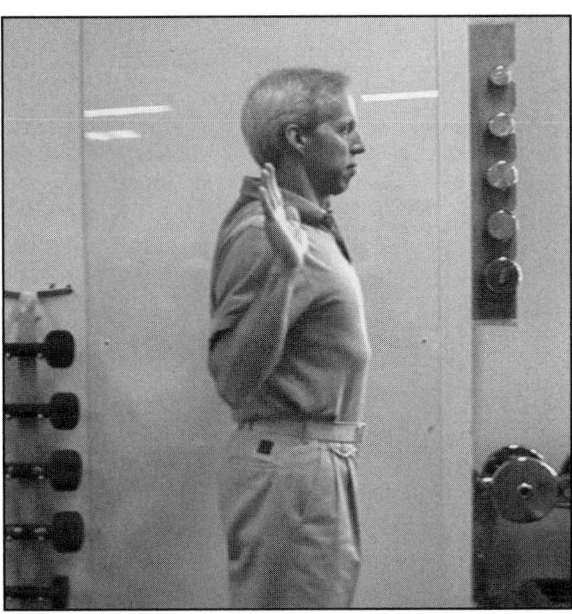

FIGURE 3.9 Scapular retraction exercises, ending with "elbows in back pockets."

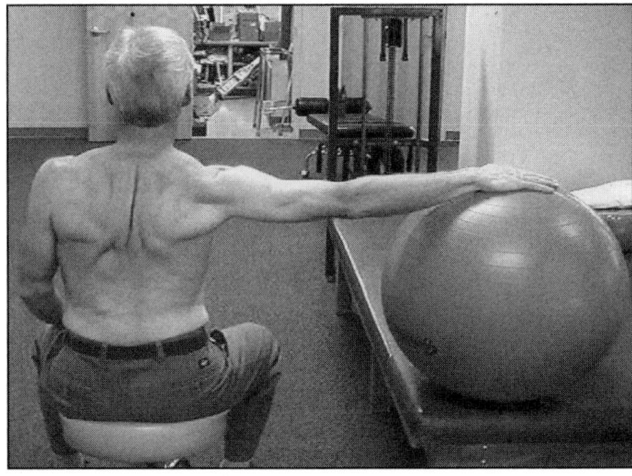

FIGURE 3.10 Closed chain humeral head depression, with hand on a ball to decrease shear on the rotator cuff and promote co-contractions.

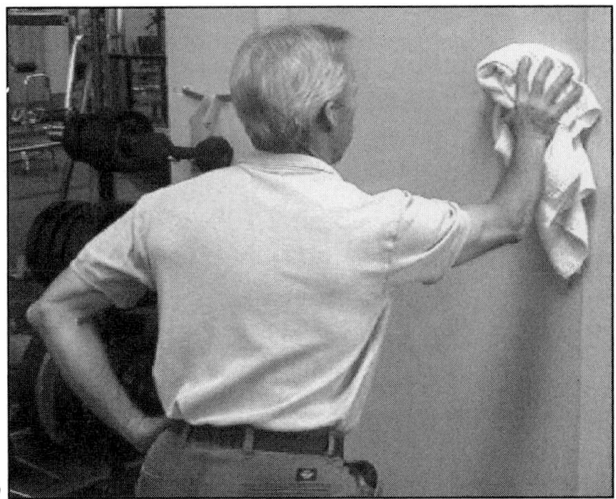

a

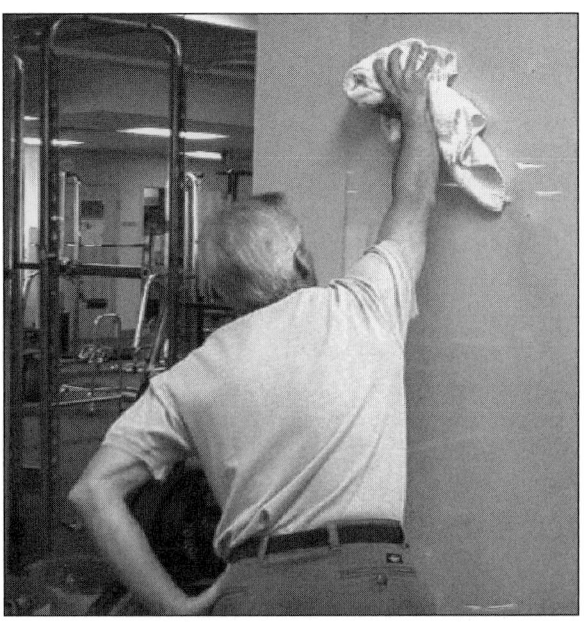

b

FIGURE 3.11 Coupled trunk movement/rotator cuff activation ("wall washes"): *(a)* starting position and *(b)* extended position (to complete exercise, return arm to starting position).

- **Possible additional tissue overload:** biceps, shoulder external rotators, lateral epicondyle
- **Functional biomechanical deficits:** look for scapular dyskinesis, alterations in scapular position and motion that alter scapular roles in activity, shoulder external rotation strength deficits
- **Subclinical adaptations:** look for alterations in hitting mechanics, including leading with the elbow, hitting the ball behind the body, or trying to swing the racket using the wrist extensors
- **Rehabilitation considerations:** correct mechanics; consider change to two-handed backhand; increase shoulder external rotation strength; increase wrist co-contraction strength

Wrist Tendinitis

The wrist, as the terminal segment, may be injured in throwing activities as a result of proximal kinetic chain deficits that create increased stress.

- **Clinical symptoms:** point tenderness over specific wrist tendons, ± crepitus and swelling
- **Tissue injury:** tendon, tendon sheath, or both
- **Tissue overload:** elbow flexor/extensors, biceps, deltoid
- **Functional biomechanical deficits:** elbow loss of motion, "short arming" (decreased range of motion at shoulder) the throwing motion
- **Subclinical adaptations:** excessive cocking/flexion of wrist in hitting motion
- **Rehabilitation considerations:** start rehabilitation at the shoulder, increasing range of motion and strength, and correct altered mechanics

SUMMARY

Kinetic chain activation allows efficient force development and load regulation to accomplish athletic functions. Athletic dysfunction is commonly associated with alterations in kinetic chain activations. In the older athlete, the alterations acquired through sport activities are added to alterations due to the aging process. Evaluation and treatment of athletic dysfunction and symptoms in the older athlete should include examination for distant kinetic chain alterations that may be causative or additive to the dysfunction.

CHAPTER

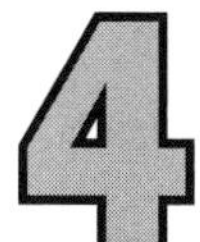

Soft Tissue Care: Flexibility, Stretching, and Massage

Carol C. Figuers, PT, EdD

In order to continue to successfully train and compete in sport and recreation, the mature patient needs to pay particular attention to achieving and maintaining soft tissue flexibility. Stretching, postural awareness, and massage are all avenues toward keeping an individual able to exercise, train for a sport, or even be competitive. These options are also conservative and noninvasive and allow a good deal of personal management and decision making. This chapter offers some general guidelines for using these approaches in both the prevention and treatment of soft tissue injury. In addition, special consideration is given to the age-related changes in soft tissues and how these may impact flexibility and function.

AGE-RELATED SOFT TISSUE CHANGES

Soft tissue, which can restrict mobility, includes muscles, fascia, tendons, ligaments, joint capsules, articular cartilage, intervertebral discs, and skin. All of these structures undergo biological and mechanical age-related changes. Older skeletal muscle is more prone to contraction-induced mechanical injury and has a decreased ability to regenerate injured tissue (Buckwalter et al. 1993). Fascia, tendons, and ligaments demonstrate excessive collagen cross-bridging with age, resulting in increased stiffness (Seto and Brewster 1991). All soft tissue suffers from a lack of hydration with age, particularly the intervertebral discs, often resulting in limited mobility and stiffness. Decreased water content in connective tissue and increased coarseness of elastin with aging reduce overall tissue plasticity (Menard and Stanish 1989).

If soft tissue in the joint area is less extensible, the muscular attachments must accommodate for this loss of range of motion. If the muscles themselves are inflexible, there is a greater potential for injury in the form of muscular strains or sprains. Soft tissue flexibility may also be impaired through disuse, injury, or a disease process such as osteoarthritis. In healthy, active soft tissue, new collagen involved in growth or healing is laid down in an organized pattern in response to applied stress. If motion is restricted, for example due to immobilization, the fiber orientation is more irregular, resulting in further limitation to movement (Seto and Brewster 1991).

Flexibility of soft tissue is therefore a major issue for the senior athlete or exercise enthusiast. If the athlete has been physically active for many years, this activity itself has helped to prevent much of the flexibility loss due to immobility. In fact, many young athletes are able to train and perform with minimal formal stretching of soft tissue. However, the mature and active patient must be aware of the physiological changes in soft tissue with aging and proactive in maintaining healthy soft tissue mobility. A new mind-set may be required, one that includes soft tissue stretching and mobilization.

POSTURE

Posture can be thought of as both static and dynamic. Static postures such as sitting and standing can reflect muscular imbalances and result in soft tissue tightness, inflexibility, and potential for injury. One example is standing or sitting with the head held forward, causing tightness in the cervical extensor musculature (figure 4.1*a*). "Forward head" is a posture often seen as people work at computers or drive a vehicle. Another area of tightness caused by a static posture is tight hamstring muscles consequent to sitting. Many people over age 50 who participate in sport or exercise are fairly sedentary when not training or competing and may spend a large amount of time either sitting at a desk or driving or riding in a car. These "inactivities" can enhance muscle tightness, which can influence soft tissue mobility needed during exercise.

Dynamic posture can be thought of as the body's alignment during movements, including sport or exercise. Certain sports require the body to be held in specific positions, such as forward flexion of the trunk and head during cycling. Swimming strokes (except for backstroke) involve mainly forward trunk and shoulder motions. These dynamic postures may result in decreased flexibility in the pectoral muscles and "forward head." Any forward or flexed posture can contribute to potential problems with decreasing bone density seen with aging. Although physical activity appears to counteract the process of demineralization, all mature patients should continue to be vigilant in avoiding excessive forward flexion and should attempt when possible to correct their postures to neutral in sport and other daily activities (figure 4.1*b*).

By identifying both static and dynamic postures that athletes utilize throughout their days, one may discover areas of soft tissue inflexibility and be able to recommend appropriate interventions.

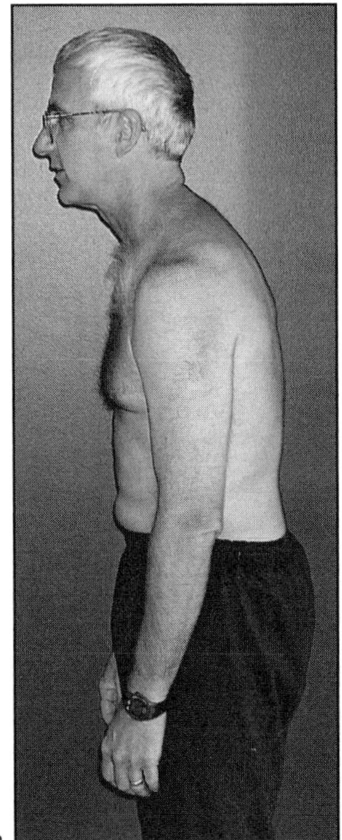

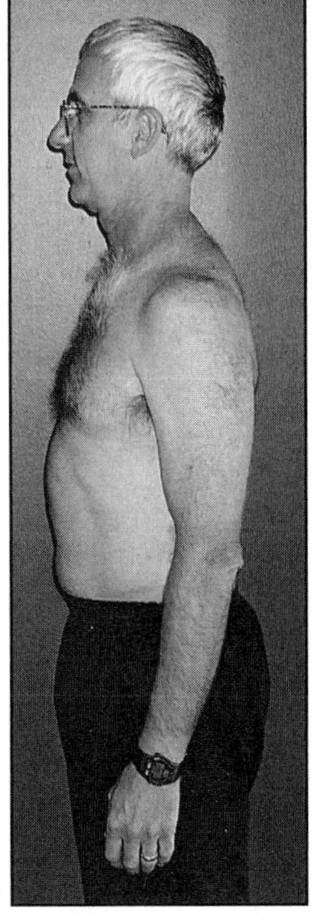

FIGURE 4.1 *(a)* Forward head posture and *(b)* healthy cervical posture.

SOFT TISSUE STRETCHING

In order to maintain flexibility for exercise, training, and competition, stretching should be routine for active seniors. Stretching as a warm-up prior to physical activity or sport should follow the guidelines and procedures outlined in this text. Particularly for the older individual, increased time and decreased speed with stretching are important. In order to make a significant change in muscle length or range of motion, the focus may be more specific to that location and will require a prolonged stretch. Stretching exercises can be performed in either passive or active modes. In passive stretching, one person applies a stretching technique directly to the soft tissue, for example a tight muscle group, of another individual. The patient is therefore receiving a passive stretch. A solid knowledge of anatomy and physiology is important for safe application of passive stretching techniques.

Individuals can also carry out active or self-stretching exercises. All stretching routines should be based upon the physical properties of connective tissue to maximize the stretching effort. In order to permanently lengthen tissue, plastic rather than elastic changes must occur. The optimum environment for creating soft tissue length change through stretching is comprised of three elements:

- Elevated temperature
- Low force
- Long duration

In other words, prior to a stretch, soft tissue should be warm, through either low-level physical activity or applied moist heat. A safety guideline is not to stretch cold muscles or soft tissue. The force of the stretch should be a feeling of mild stretch with no pain. The stretch should be slow and should be maintained for 20 to 30 s. Bandy and Irion (1994) reported that a 30-s hamstring muscle stretch was as effective as a 60-s stretch in subjects with a mean age of 26 years. In a recent study on the duration of stretching in subjects aged 65 years and older, Feland and colleagues (2001) suggest that a longer holding time (60 s) is more effective in an older population. They theorize that a longer-duration stretch in an older population may be beneficial to overcome the collagen deposition and muscle stiffness associated with aging. Based on the age-related soft tissue changes discussed earlier, low-intensity and long-duration stretching is extremely important in creating elastic changes in the mature active patient.

Each stretch should be repeated several times, with one extremity or muscle group stretched at a time. In

1990, Taylor and colleagues examined the elongation of the muscle–tendon unit following various stretching sets and determined that after approximately four stretches, additional improvement in length was minimal. In order to prevent soft tissue injury as well as maximize the flexibility available in soft tissue, patients should perform stretching exercises regularly, daily if possible. A stretch should never be performed in a ballistic or "bouncing" motion. This may activate a "stretch response," causing the muscle being stretched to actually shorten, thus leading to possible soft tissue damage. Anyone engaging in stretching should attempt to minimize potential muscular strain by keeping the back as straight as possible. This is particularly important for the older patient, who, as noted earlier, may be at some risk for osteoporosis and forward flexion of the spine.

Precautions for Stretching

Kisner and Colby (1996) recommend the following measures to avoid injury during stretching.

1. A joint should never be passively forced past its normal range of motion.
2. Avoid stretching in the area of a recent or newly united bony fracture.
3. Avoid excessive stretching of soft tissues that have been immobilized for a long period of time (e.g., in a cast or splint).
4. If joint or muscle soreness is present for more than 24 h following stretching, too much force may have resulted in inflammation. A temporary feeling of tenderness, however, may normally be experienced following stretching.
5. Avoid stretching tissue that is swollen, as this may result in further pain and swelling.
6. Avoid overstretching muscles that are weak, particularly postural muscles such as in the neck and back.

Active Stretching Program

This section provides a general set of stretching exercises for common areas of soft tissue tightness. Ideally, the patient's stretching program would be individualized based on a thorough musculoskeletal examination performed by a provider with appropriate training and expertise. The exercises described should be perceived as a mild stretch and should be discontinued if any pain or discomfort occurs. Stretches provided in this text focus on areas of the upper body, lower body, and trunk, which may become tight or inflexible through physical use and postural deviations.

Upper Body

Chin Tuck (for Cervical Extensors)

Slowly tuck your chin in, pulling head over body. Do not look down or up; look straight ahead.

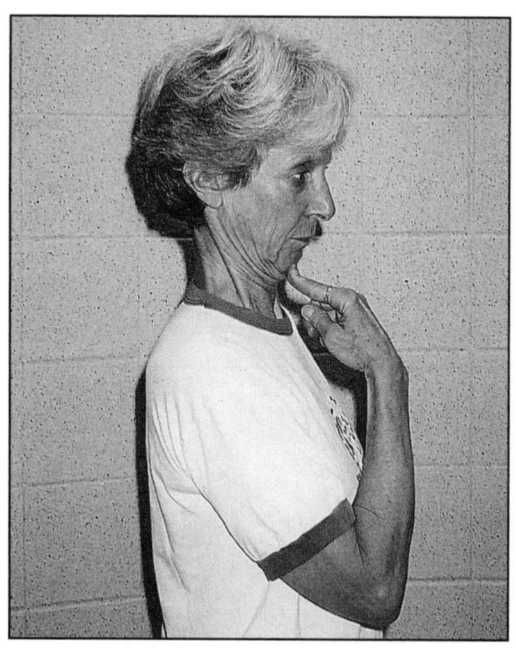

Pectoral Stretch (for Pectoral Muscles)

Standing in a corner or doorway, place hands on wall with arms out and elbows at 90°. Lean trunk forward until you feel a stretch across the front of your upper chest. You may vary the portion of pectoral muscle being stretched by slightly raising or lowering your hands on the wall.

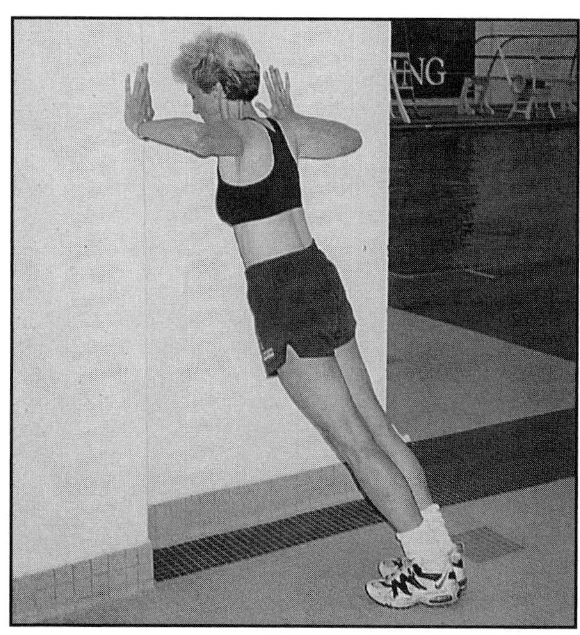

Inferior Capsule Stretch (for Latissimus and Infraspinatus)

Lift one arm up over your head with the elbow bent and pointing upward. Grasp that elbow with the opposite hand and slowly pull the elbow behind your head until you feel a stretch in your shoulder and upper arm.

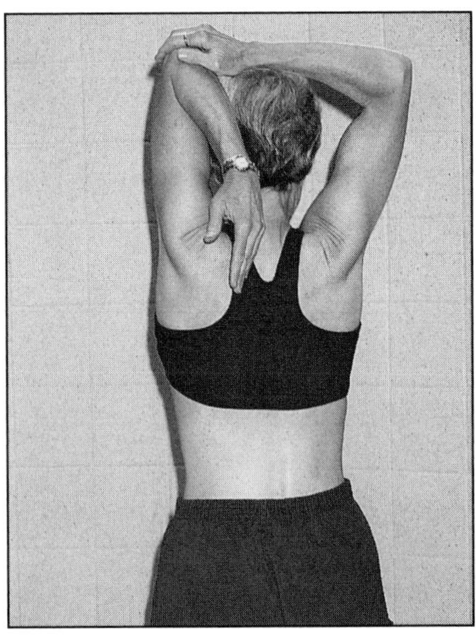

Posterior Capsule Stretch (for Rhomboids, Infraspinatus, and Middle Trapezius)

Raise one arm to shoulder height and grasp that arm right above the elbow. Slowly pull the elbow and arm across your chest, feeling a stretch in the back of that arm and shoulder.

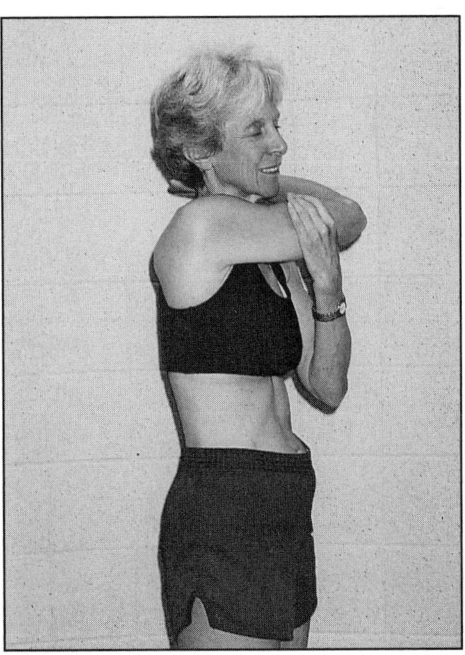

Lower Body

Hamstring Stretch

Sitting. Sit with one leg straight and the other knee bent. Place the bottom of the bent leg's foot against the inside of the straight leg. Turn your trunk and face the straight leg. Keep your back straight and slowly lean forward over the straight leg in the direction of the foot. A stretch should be felt along the back of the leg rather than in the low back.

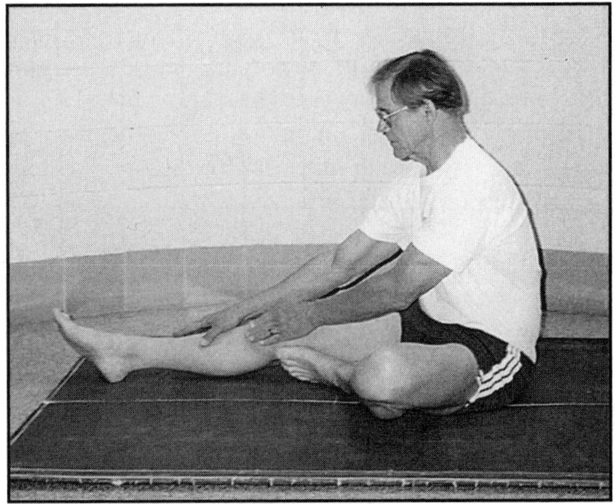

Standing. Place one leg on a bench or raised surface. With both feet pointing straight ahead, slowly lean forward at the hip in the direction of the propped leg. Keep your back and knees straight until you feel a stretch in the back of the propped thigh.

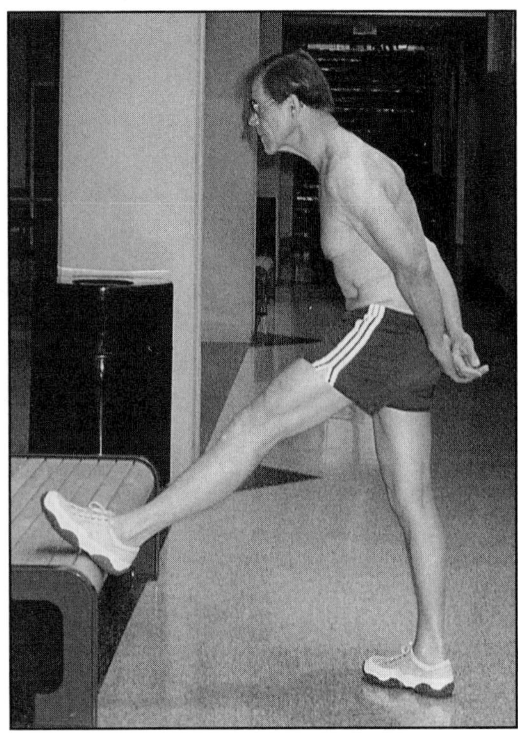

Alternative Hamstring Stretches Using Therapy Ball

Sit on therapy ball and extend one leg in front, keeping the other leg behind for balance. Slowly reach toward the forward leg, with back remaining straight, until a gentle stretch is felt.

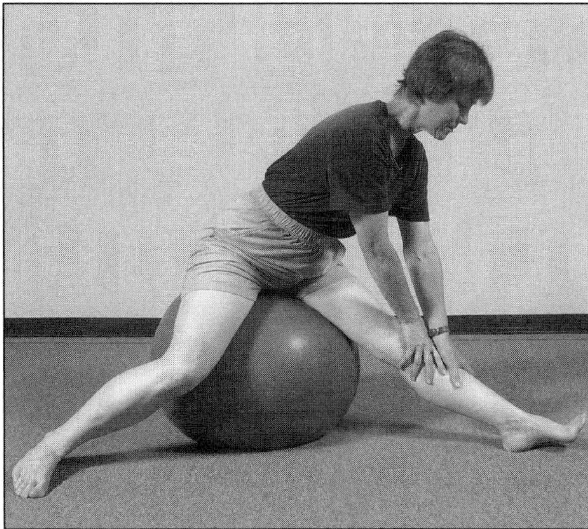

Lie on your back with both legs resting on therapy ball. Slowly straighten one leg, keeping knee and upper leg against ball. Hold a gentle stretch of the hamstrings on that leg.

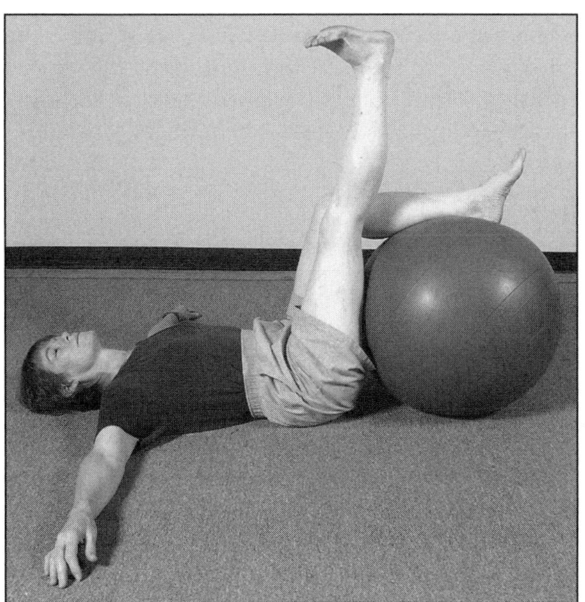

Quadriceps Stretch

Stand holding on to a fixed surface. Bend one knee behind you and grasp the ankle of that bent leg with the hand from the same side. With the knee pointed down, slowly bring the ankle back toward the buttocks, feeling a stretch across the front of the thigh. Keep the back straight and do not lean forward or back.

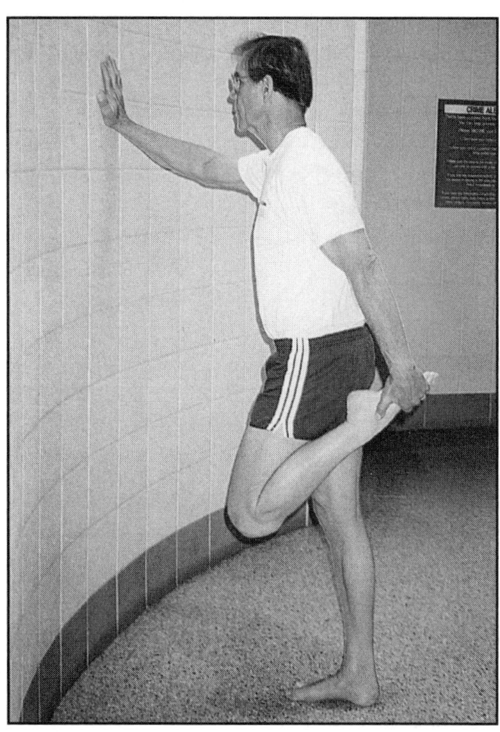

Hip Flexor Stretch (for Rectus Femoris, Iliopsoas Muscles)

Kneel down with one knee on the floor and the other knee bent with your foot flat on the floor. With a straight back, slowly lean your entire trunk forward until you feel a stretch in the thigh of the knee-down leg.

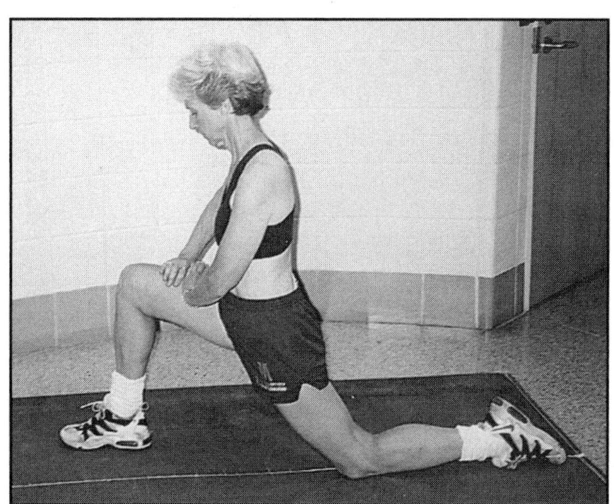

Alternative Hip Flexor Stretch

Kneel over therapy ball, with one foot placed beside ball and one foot extended behind until a stretch is felt in the front thigh of the extended leg.

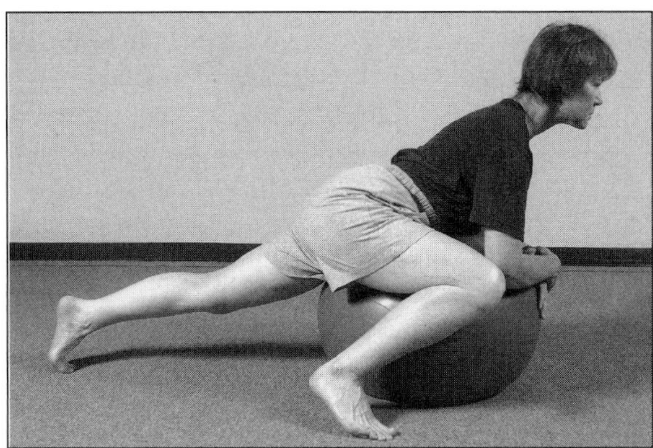

Sitting Calf Stretch

Sit with one leg extended, looping a towel or band around the ball of the foot. Gently pull on band, keeping knee straight and stretching your calf muscle.

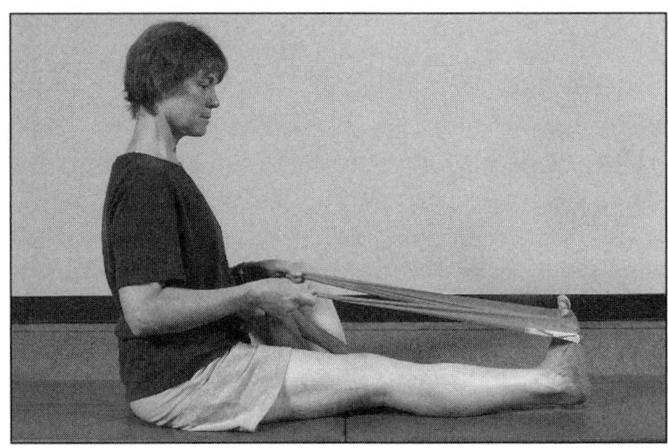

Hip Adductor (Groin) Stretch

Sit with knees bent and the soles of your feet together. Keeping your back straight and elbows on your legs, slowly lean forward and press knees down. You should feel a stretch along the insides of both thighs.

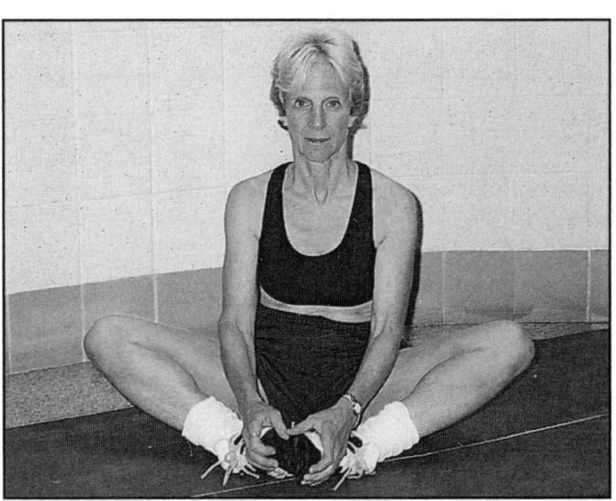

Calf Stretch (for Gastrocsoleus Muscles)

Stand facing a wall or holding on to a fixed surface. Place one foot in front and the other behind your hips, with toes of both feet pointing forward. Bending the front knee and keeping the back heel down, slowly lean forward until you feel a stretch along your calf (gastrocnemius muscle). Follow these same directions, but at the end also slightly bend your back knee, feeling an even deeper stretch (soleus muscle).

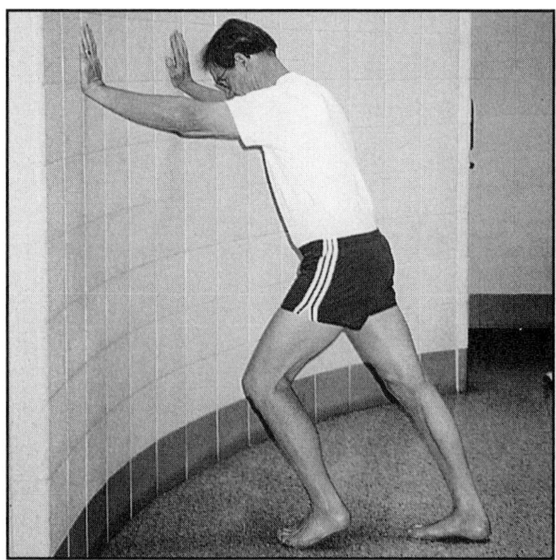

Tensor Fasciae Latae and Iliotibial Band Stretch

Stand sideways, holding on to a wall or stationary surface. Cross the leg next to the wall back behind the other leg. Turn the back foot onto its lateral surface and slowly lean your hip toward the wall, feeling a stretch along the side of your back thigh.

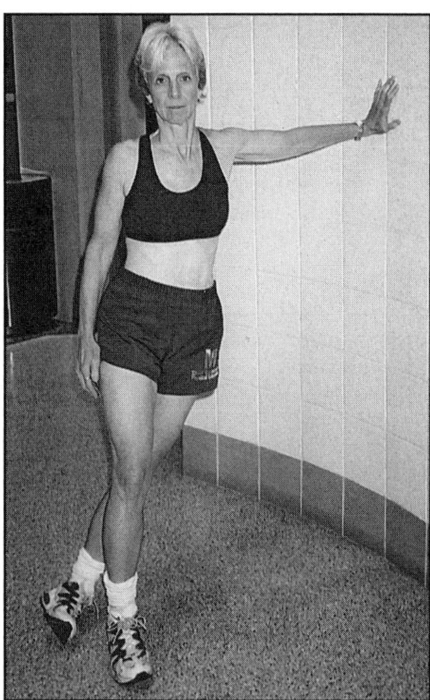

Piriformis Stretch

Lying on your back, flex one hip to 90° and cross that foot over the straight leg, with foot flat. Holding your pelvis down, slowly reach for the bent knee and pull it farther across your pelvis until you feel a stretch across your buttocks.

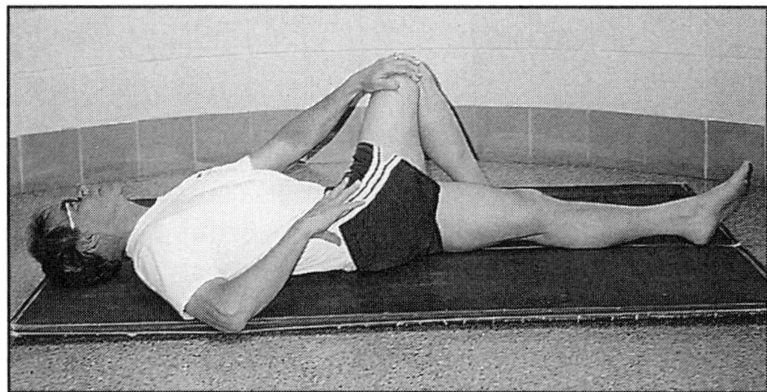

Trunk

Low Back Stretch

Lie on your back with one leg straight and slowly pull one knee toward your chest and hold, feeling a stretch along the back of that leg and buttocks. Repeat with the other leg and hold.

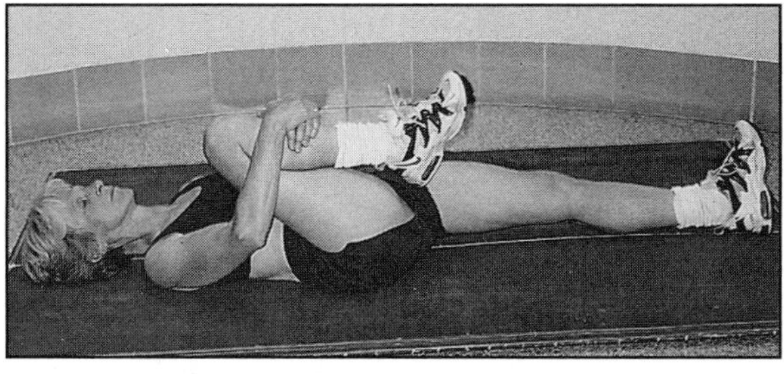

For a complete stretch of the low back, slowly pull both knees into your chest and hold.

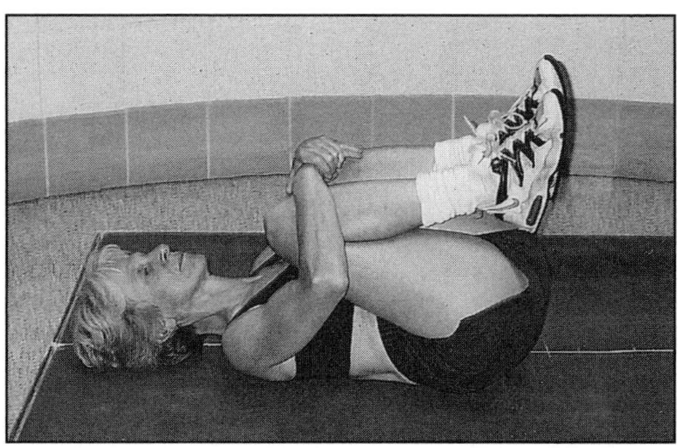

Pelvic Rotation (Cat/Camel)

Assume a hands-and-knees, or "all fours," position. Begin by arching your back up, tucking your tail bone under and looking at your thighs.

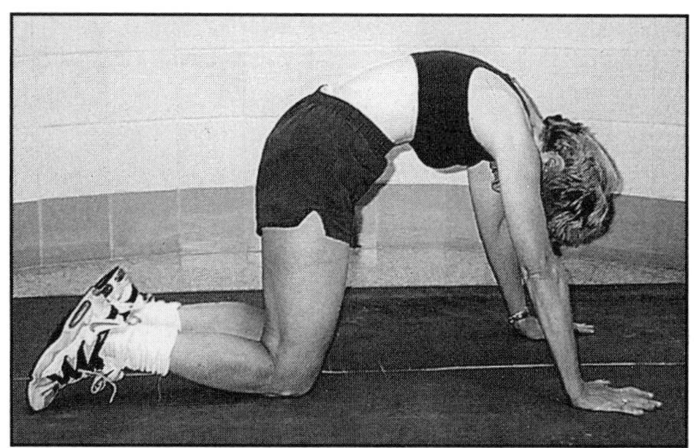

Then slowly let your back sink down toward the floor, with your buttocks and head held upward.

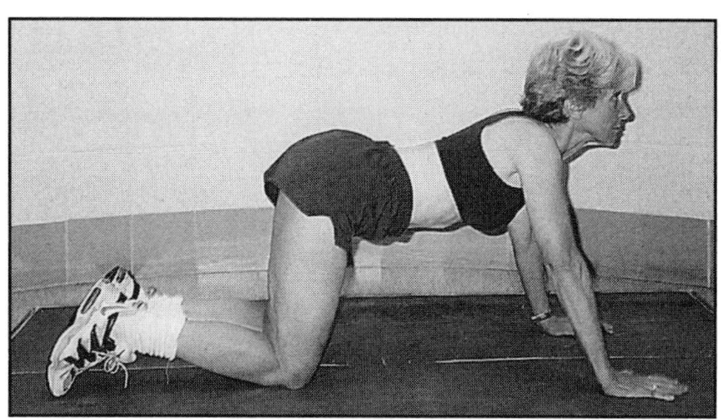

Case Study—Stretching

C.M. is a 56-year-old female who enjoys a variety of athletic activities. She has just begun to participate in local triathlons and so is including swimming, cycling, and running in her exercise regimen. C.M. has recently been experiencing right knee pain following her longer training runs and bike rides. Swimming has produced no pain in her knee (note: C.M. mainly swims the freestyle stroke). C.M. is a full-time manager in an information technology firm. Upon examination, C.M. was found to have decreased flexibility in her hamstring muscles bilaterally and in her right tensor fasciae latae (TFL) muscle group.

Before beginning her home exercise program, C.M. was provided educational materials emphasizing the concepts of

- elevated muscle temperature prior to stretching (general activity or warm shower/bath),
- low-force stretch, and
- long-duration stretch.

A self-stretching program was prescribed to include the following schedule:

- Hamstring stretch, holding for 30 s, four times on each leg (position in "Hamstring Stretch—Sitting") done in the evening at home daily
- Hamstring stretch, holding for 20 s, two times on each leg prior to training runs or bike rides and competitions (position in "Hamstring Stretch—Standing")
- TFL stretch, holding for 30 s, two times done in the evening at home daily
- TFL stretch, holding for 20 s, two times prior to training runs or bike rides and competitions

C.M. was also encouraged to avoid sitting for prolonged periods of time by taking short, regular walking breaks at work and thus decreasing periods of knee flexion.

At her three-week follow-up visit, C.M. reported decreased overall knee pain with her sport activities. She did feel mild discomfort upon returning from a three-day business trip (during which she was not compliant with stretching). Consistency with her stretching program was reinforced, and C.M. continues to successfully pursue triathlon events.

MASSAGE OR SOFT TISSUE MOBILIZATION

The use of massage in the treatment of musculoskeletal ailments, particularly related to sport and competition, can actually be documented back to the ancient Greeks and Romans. Massage was applied to render soft tissue more supple before and after gladiators underwent severe "tests of strength" (Kamenetz 1976; Tappan and Benjamin 1998). The Greek philosopher Aristotle, while serving as a tutor for Alexander the Great, is reported to have recommended rubbing with water and oil to resolve the famous ruler's fatigue (Kleen 1921). Massage can be defined as "the intentional and systematic manipulation of the soft tissues of the body to enhance health and healing" (Tappan and Benjamin 1998, p. 3).

Massage, or soft tissue mobilization, can encompass various types of techniques depending upon the desired therapeutic outcome. Sport massage reflects a combination of traditional forms of massage individually applied to the characteristics of an athlete's training and performance. The venue for providing an athlete with massage may vary from regular private sessions to a group event as part of a large competition. Just as sport massage is helpful for athletes in general, it is useful for mature patients who wish to remain active in sport or recreation. The soft tissues targeted for massage will be those directly used for the sport performance.

Western Massage Strokes

Classic western massage is the mainstay of today's therapeutic massage and was developed through the work of Europeans Ling and Metzger in the 19th century (Tappan and Benjamin 1998). Their system of active and passive movements was used initially to treat a variety of medical conditions. These techniques have since reached a wide range of populations to achieve goals of healing, injury prevention, and well-being. The most commonly used western massage techniques include the following strokes:

- Effleurage—a basic massage stroke also called "stroking." It is performed by passing the palmar surface of the hand (or a portion) over a body segment. Pressure may be deep or superficial (figure 4.2).
- Petrissage—also referred to as "kneading." This stroke consists of grasping the muscle bulk and applying intermittent pressure along the length of a muscle or muscle group (figure 4.3).
- Tapotement—consists of administering a series of claps or blows to the body part being treated. This stroke, also called percussion, can be utilized in chest physical therapy to decrease lung congestion.
- Friction—performed by rubbing one surface repeatedly over another. Friction can result in enhanced circulation and stimulation to a very

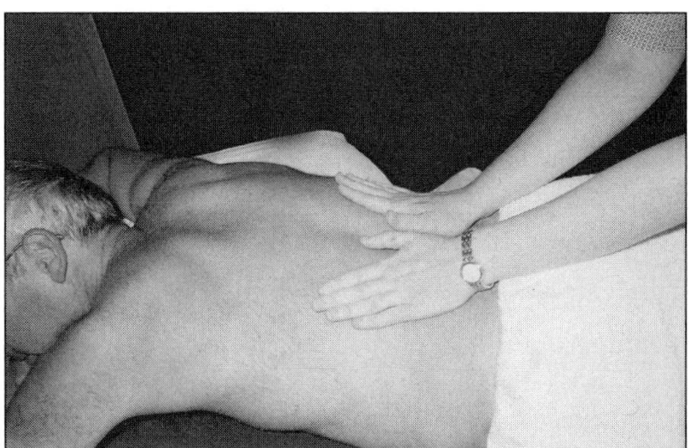

FIGURE 4.2 Effleurage.

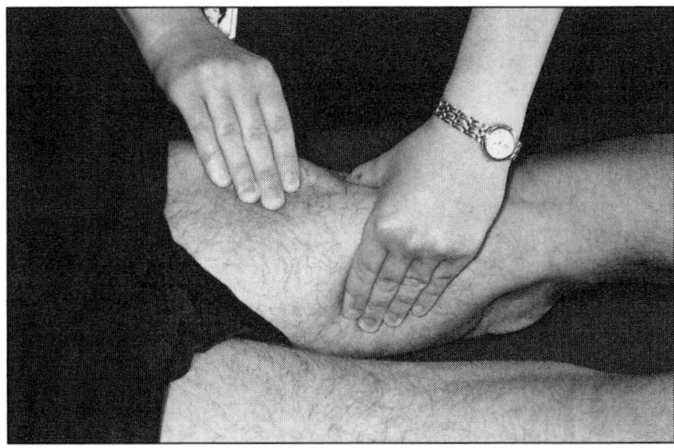

FIGURE 4.3 Petrissage.

specific area of soft tissue.

- Vibration—a trembling motion created when one or two hands are placed over soft tissue and stay on that one area. Depending on how fine or coarse the oscillations are, vibration can have either a stimulating or a relaxing effect.

Effects of Massage

Massage is recognized as a significant intervention to promote health and healing. Much of the literature describing the effects of massage reflects the specific technique being used; and in the majority of studies, western massage techniques provide the intervention. Specific physiological and psychological effects of massage accepted by most practitioners include enhanced blood flow and lymph circulation, muscle relaxation, increased joint mobility, increased psychological and emotional relaxation, reduced inflammation, and improved skin function. In addition, massage may be used to increase mental clarity, decrease anxiety levels, and help stimulate feelings of general well-being and aid in emotional release (Tappan and Benjamin 1998). Massage is believed to improve the performance of fatigued muscles by decreasing the amount of spasm in the muscle fibers, increasing the force of the muscle contraction, and enhancing endurance of the fibers (Goats 1994).

Thus massage would appear to have many potential benefits for the older active patient in terms of improving the state of soft tissue during exercise, training, and performance. Muscle tension in the athlete can be normalized by massage (Travell and Simons 1992); this produces a sedative effect following strenuous activity. Soft tissue massage can result in increases in muscle length and flexibility. Crosman and colleagues (1984) demonstrated significantly increased hamstring length or range of motion following western massage techniques. Investigations of the effects of therapeutic massage on specific patient populations demonstrate solid positive changes, including decreased blood pressure, decreased resting heart rate, decreased pain, decreased anxiety and stress hormones, and increased relaxation (Ferrell-Torry and Glick 1993; Field et al. 1996; Hernandez-Reif et al. 2001; Preyde 2000).

General health benefits from these responses that may be especially attractive to senior athletes include the following:

- Decreased oxygen consumption and metabolic rate, therefore reduced strain on the body's energy resources
- Increased frequency and intensity of alpha brain waves associated with deep relaxation
- Reduced blood lactates, substances associated with pain and anxiety
- Significantly reduced blood pressure in hypertensive individuals
- Reduced heart rate and rate of respiration
- Decreased muscle tension
- Increased blood flow to arms and legs
- Decreased anxiety, fears, and phobias and increased positive mental health
- Improved quality of sleep (Tappan and Benjamin 1998)

One of the major goals of massage in sport and exercise is to reduce muscle soreness. In 1974, Hovind and Nielsen investigated the effects of petrissage strokes on muscular blood flow and found mixed results of increased flow following 2 min of treatment. When the technique incorporated more vigorous tapotement technique, the blood flow of skeletal muscle significantly increased (35%) compared to the baseline. This increase in circulation can assist in removing metabolic waste products and restoring nutrients to the area receiving the massage. Massage has also been found to be more effective than rest during recovery from fatigue by reducing the pooling of waste products (Smith et al. 1994; Weber et al. 1994). Most of the studies involving the use of massage specifically with athletes focus on athletes under the age of 50 years. Some of the results are mixed, particularly with respect to comparisons of massage and active recovery in decreasing muscle soreness. Most investigators do, however, acknowledge that massage techniques particularly are difficult to control and replicate. They also concede that the many positive comments made by successful athletes who have received sport massage are strongly supported by coaches and national sport organizations. In addition, no harmful effects of massage were noted by any investigators (Bell 1999; Cafarelli and Flint 1992; Martin et al. 1998; Tappan and Benjamin 1998; Tiidus and Shoemaker 1995).

Keeping in mind the normal soft tissue changes occurring in the mature patient as well as the potential history of past injuries, the mechanical and physiological effects of massage may be a powerful therapeutic intervention. Not only can the patient's soft tissue be made more pliable and therefore more flexible with massage, but circulation—which may be impaired through the aging process—also can be improved. Many people over 50, whether physically active or not, are beginning to experience problems such as increased blood pressure or impaired sleeping. Massage may be one tool to improve these symptoms without side effects and may contribute to more effective exercise, training, and performance. Generalized anxiety, unrelated to the exercise or sport, may also be present in an active individual over 50. Life is often a complex mixture of work, family, and community obligations; and massage can certainly assist in diminishing stress and worry.

Friction Massage and Trigger Point Therapy

Additional massage techniques frequently used in sport massage are friction massage and acupressure or trigger point therapy. As described here, friction massage provides deep strokes *across* the muscle fibers in order to realign connective tissue and increase soft tissue healing (figure 4.4). In deep transverse friction massage, the fingers and skin move together directly over the lesion, focusing on friction rather than amount of pressure.

This is a common technique used in treating chronic tendinitis in which the fibers of the tendon have developed adhesions, limiting motion. As the soft tissue heals, deep friction helps the fibers realign in a more parallel fashion, allowing for enhanced freedom of movement (Cyriax and Cyriax 1983). This technique may be uncomfortable initially and should be used with care by a practitioner who has a thorough understanding of the connective tissue pathology and healing process.

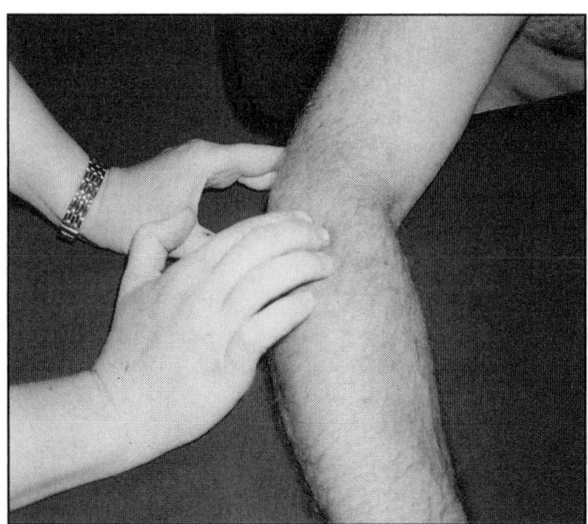

FIGURE 4.4 Friction massage.

Trigger points have been described as tender knots felt particularly in muscles that are being extensively used. Travell and Simons (1983, p. 4) define a trigger point as a "focus of hyperirritability in a tissue that, when compressed, is locally tender and, if sufficiently hypersensitive, gives rise to referred pain and tenderness, and sometimes to referred autonomic phenomena and distortion of proprioception." Trigger points can be perceived as local pain as well as referred pain or a "radiating" discomfort. For example, a person with a trigger point in the upper trapezius muscle may also describe pain going up into the neck and head, with a subsequent headache. Individuals such as athletes, musicians, or physical laborers who overexert, repeatedly use, or traumatize muscles may be prone to having trigger points.

Ideally, the treatment of trigger points would include solving the precipitating factors such as poor posture, muscular imbalance, or overtraining. In addition to other therapies, trigger points may respond to deep ischemic compression of the tissues at the trigger point site.

Sustained digital pressure to a trigger point should last for 20 s to 1 min. The pressure is slowly increased as the trigger point becomes less sensitive and less tense. When the practitioner feels the trigger point relax or the pain subsides, pressure is released. This type of manual therapy should be followed by appropriate stretching of the soft tissue in question unless hypermobility is a concern (Travell and Simons 1992).

Precautions With Massage

As with stretching, massage may help the active older individual maintain soft tissue health. It is essential that the person applying stretching or massage techniques be trained and competent in evaluating the soft tissue restrictions and in selecting and applying the appropriate type of intervention. In addition, the practitioner should recognize general contraindications to massage. These include, but are not limited to, compromised or insufficient peripheral circulation (thrombus, embolus), injured vessels (bleeding, acute phlebitis), acute infection or inflammation (rheumatoid arthritis), irritating skin conditions (impetigo, poison ivy), and metastatic cancers (melanoma, bony metastasis) (Bell 1999; Tappan and Benjamin 1998).

Applications of Massage With the Mature Active Patient

In order to effectively apply massage as both a prevention and treatment tool, the practitioner should understand the biomechanics of the exercise or sport as well as the patient's training and performance schedule. For example, in providing massage for a competitive cyclist, the practitioner should appreciate the training schedule of hard versus easy days, mileage and terrain (hills or flats), and the possible team strategy. The lower extremities in this case would be a target for pain reduction and lactic acid removal. In addition, following very long rides, the cyclist may benefit from upper body work, particularly for the trapezius muscles since they remain forward and tense for long periods. If a patient enjoys recreational tennis but is diagnosed with epicondylitis or "tennis elbow," the mechanics of the tennis swing should be analyzed and strength of the wrist extensor muscles should be assessed. One intervention for treating this problem may be to apply friction massage over the wrist extensor tendons to break up scar tissue and realign fibers.

Many active patients over the age of 50 are very competitive athletes. One goal of massage for the senior athlete may be to prepare the muscle groups for maximum efficiency through increasing circulation of oxygen supply to tissue. A different goal would be to reduce muscle tension, soreness, and swelling following an event or training period. Therefore both the timing of massage and the techniques used are variable. Although these concepts are described with the competitive athlete in mind, many of the applications relate to exercise bouts in general. Four different strategies in which massage may be incorporated into the senior athlete's soft tissue health include

- pre-event massage,
- intercompetition massage,
- post-event massage, and
- preventive or maintenance massage.

- **Pre-event massage.** A warm-up or pre-event massage may occur up to 2 h prior to an athletic event and should be invigorating and positive. The goal is to aid in the general warm-up or preparation for specific muscle activity. The intervention itself should last only 10 to 20 min, and the strokes should be light, general, and pain free. Techniques such as tapotement and effleurage may be used, avoiding friction or deep, heavy strokes.

- **Intercompetition massage.** When an athlete competes more than one time in a day or when some type of extended break occurs in the midst of a competition, light but invigorating massage may be applied. As in pre-event massage, the techniques should not cause pain and should focus on the particular muscle groups being used. The goal here is to assist in recovery and invigorate for further competition.

- **Post-event massage.** From minutes to several hours following an athletic activity, massage can reduce muscle tension and soreness by "flushing" sport-specific areas. General techniques such as effleurage and petrissage can be used to assist the muscles in recovery. Massage techniques can stimulate muscle fibers to minimize myofascial adhesions. This may also be a point at which injuries begin to be assessed and either treated or referred to the appropriate practitioner. Post-event massages are often available for groups of athletes (e.g., following a marathon, triathlon, soccer match) and should be pain free and promote general well-being.

- **Maintenance or preventive massage.** Maintenance or preventive massage can also be thought of as preconditioning for maximum activity. This type of intervention should occur on a regular basis, up to one day before or after a competition. In addition, this comprehensive massage approach may be a useful option for the active patient who does not compete as an athlete. A full-body massage, concentrating on specific areas as needed, may last from 30 to 60 min. Effleurage and petrissage techniques are used, and deep strokes can be directed toward those muscle groups used in the sport activity. The experienced practitioner may also use this setting to identify and treat "trigger points" or tender spots, using deep acupressure techniques, or additional soft tissue mobilization strategies.

Additional Considerations With Use of Massage

The massage medium refers to any topical substance, such as oil or lotion, that is used to facilitate the strokes applied during massage. Typically, the practitioner and the individual receiving the massage collaborate on what is best, depending on such factors as skin integrity, odor, or allergies. For areas of the body with more hair, increased lubricant is required to allow smooth gliding strokes. If little to no motion is desired, as in friction massage, no lubricant would be indicated. One basic guideline for using topical substances in massage is to use the least amount of lubricant possible to achieve the goals of the massage.

Ideally, all forms of massage are provided in an environment that contributes toward the goals of this soft tissue work. Warmth is important to help facilitate relaxation, circulation, and recovery. Either the ambient temperature should be warm and comfortable, or sheets, towels, or blankets may be provided to keep the patient's entire body warm during the massage. In some cases, the patient may wish to rest following massage, particularly if symptoms such as muscle soreness, anxiety, or tension have been reported.

Patients who exercise or train regularly understand the importance of fluids in their training and competition regimens. Certainly the mature individual should recognize that proper hydration is critically important for soft tissue health. In addition to drinking fluids prior to exercise and replenishing fluids following a workout or event, people need to remember that hydration is an important consideration during massage or soft tissue work. Since one effect of massage may be to increase circulation, the water surrounding cells is moving nutrients in and waste products out at an enhanced pace, requiring replenishment of fluids.

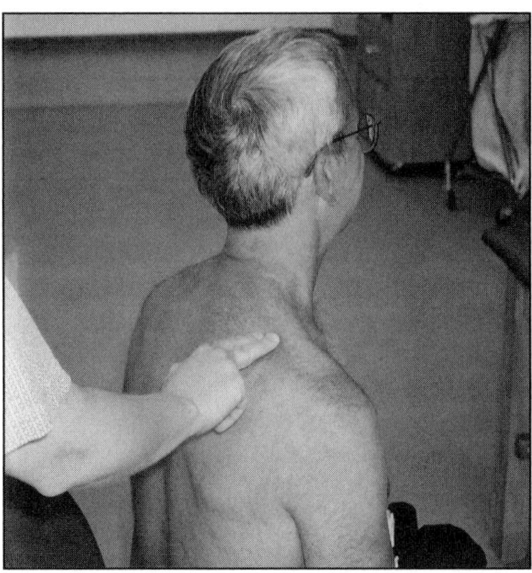

FIGURE 4.5 Trigger point therapy.

Case Study—Masters Swimmer

R.P. is a 60-year-old male who has competed for many years as a masters swimmer. He complains of chronic "achy" pain in his right upper trapezius muscle and general soreness in both of his shoulders, particularly during the heavy part of his training schedule. R.P. swims five days a week, alternating sets of endurance and sprinting workouts. He receives a preventive or preconditioning massage on one of his "off" days. The focus of this massage is his upper body and begins with R.P. positioned comfortably on a massage chair or table. A brief general effleurage covers the upper quadrant of primarily trapezius and deltoid muscles. Petrissage or a deep kneading stroke is applied to each section of these muscle groups.

A tender spot is palpated at the midpoint of his right upper trapezius muscle (figure 4.5). During the massage to this area, the practitioner uses deep circular strokes until sensing that this "trigger point" melts away. R.P. initially feels increased tenderness and then the sensitivity resolves. Finally, petrissage and effleurage are applied to R.P.'s paraspinal muscles, continuing up into their attachment to the occiput. Tension in the cervical paraspinals is noted and these muscles receive gentle petrissage. (Forward head posture and cervical tension may have been contributing to his "shoulder" soreness.) The massage ends with a repeat of the initiating general effleurage stroke, covering the entire upper quadrant.

Massage has become a standard component of R.P.'s training and well-being. He is able to schedule regular sessions of soft tissue work as well as educate teammates and family on using deep pressure over the trigger point in his upper trapezius muscle. Finally, R.P. also is becoming more conscious of factors that may be contributing to his shoulder and neck pain, such as poor posture, tight pectoral and cervical extensor muscles, and overstretched or weak upper back muscles.

SUMMARY

The active patient over 50 may have benefited from years of physical activity, all of which have contributed to improved overall health (Mazzeo et al. 1998). Utilizing conservative techniques such as stretching and massage makes it possible to treat soft tissue concerns as well as prevent future injuries. Motivation to exercise, train, or compete in sporting events is much more internal for the senior athlete as compared with a younger athlete, who may be driven by financial or institutional demands. This self-motivation can provide a perfect opportunity for taking charge of health promotion and injury prevention.

The senior athlete or mature active patient may bring experience and proven strategies to sport and exercise that a younger individual does not have. While the aging process may present new challenges through changes in soft tissue, regular attention to muscle flexibility and pliability through stretching and massage can help keep the older patient active and competitive. Through years of exercise as well as general life activities, the mature active patient has learned to "listen" to what the body is saying with regard to aches, pains, stiffness, and instability. Using this body knowledge, it is possible for active seniors to be proactive in selecting approaches that will add many more years of physical fitness, activity, and sport to their lives.

CHAPTER

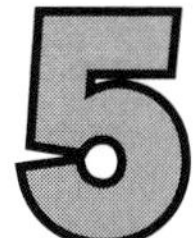

Nutrition and Pharmacology

Franca B. Alphin, MPH, RD, LDN
Daryl C. Osbahr, BS

Thanks to modern science and technology, we are living longer and healthier lives. There are approximately 34 million Americans over the age of 65, and it is estimated that by the year 2030 there will be 57 million, with the fastest growing segment constituting the 85 and older group (Food Insight 1998b). This implies, of course, that the healthy aging physically active population will be growing significantly.

There may be no set formula for maintaining optimum health and increasing longevity, but ample data support that after a good genetic pool for longevity, lifestyle modification—which includes regular physical activity and healthy eating habits—may be the next best thing. Areas of nutrient and dietary concerns for the graying athlete are calcium, vitamin D and bone health, fluids and dehydration, adequate B12 and B6 intake due to decreased absorption, protein intake and muscle integrity, and supplement and antioxidant use. Additional nutrition-related concerns are promoting weight control and decreasing risk of chronic disease.

One might think that younger and older active people would have vastly different dietary needs, but in actuality their needs are quite similar. The greatest differences are in the amount of food needed and the malabsorption of certain nutrients that may occur with aging. Sarcopenia (loss of muscle mass) associated with aging decreases caloric need and increases need for dietary protein. However, studies continue to show that aerobic activity along with a strength training program can slow the rate of lean muscle tissue loss, thereby slowing the decline in basal metabolism (Bonnefoy, Constans, and Ferry 2000; Evans and Cyr-Campbell 1997). Perhaps appetite, which often wanes with aging, may be stimulated through regular physical activity as well.

Because of the higher level of physical activity in the younger athletic population, neither appetite nor food volume is usually considered problematic. In the active aging, however, the focus with respect to nutritional needs should be on nutrient density.

DIETARY CONCERNS

Rather than focus on the basics, which are often perceived as boring, people frequently gravitate to "quick fixes," "magical cures," or other trends. It is human nature, and especially in view of the progressive nature of aging, for people to want quick results. However, quick results are often costly, both financially and physically, as well as unsustainable. They are also not necessary if one has a good understanding of the basics and how to apply them.

What You Should Know About Dietary Recommendations

Dietary recommendations for all Americans are based on the guidelines set forth jointly by the U.S. Department of Agriculture and U.S. Department of Health and Human Services. The foundation of the food pyramid is starches that are dense in nutrients, rich in antioxidants, and adequate in fiber, assuming that the complex carbohydrates chosen are predominately whole grains and less-processed foods. Fewer calories should come from the fattier protein foods and the fat group, which can be high in saturated fats (figure 5.1).

In the past few years the pyramid has come under much scrutiny, with many experts maintaining that it does not reflect an ideal diet. Criticism has intensified with the ever rising trend of obesity in this country.

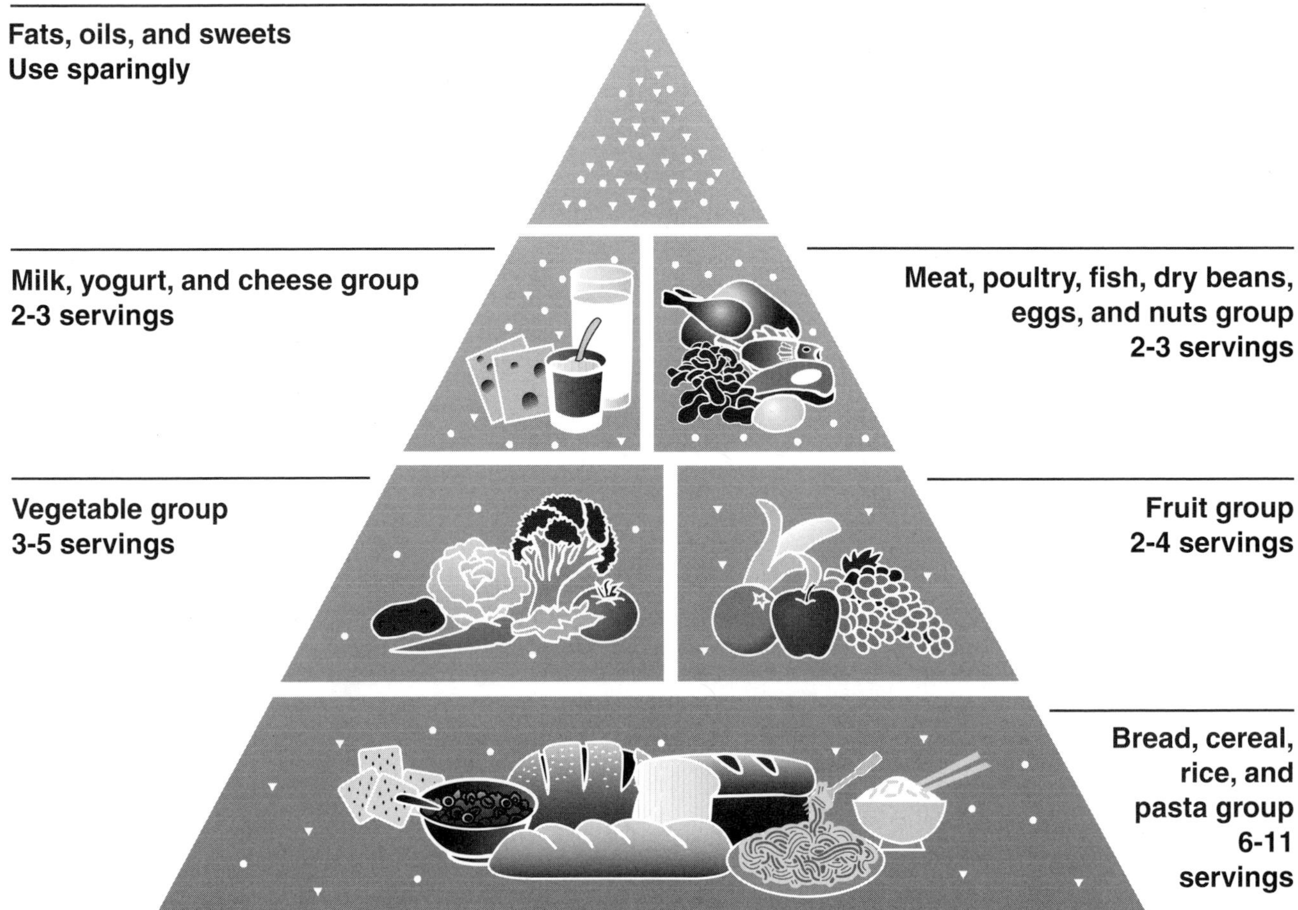

FIGURE 5.1 The food guide pyramid.

United States Departments of Agricultre and Health and Human Services.

According to critics, for example, the pyramid does not address fluid or exercise needs and gives an overly negative impression of fats, whereas in fact some fats are tremendously beneficial and fats are a necessary component of any diet.

Recently, the National Academy of Sciences (September 2002) issued new macronutrient guidelines as well as physical activity targets to reduce chronic disease risk. These recommendations are slightly different from those of the food pyramid. The two tools, however, address slightly different issues. The National Academy of Science guidelines are intended to help reduce risk of the most prevalent chronic diseases, address risk factors for those diseases, and suggest how they can be changed through diet and exercise. The food guide pyramid is intended more as an educational tool for the consumer. The greatest difference between the new and the earlier macronutrient guidelines is that the new guidelines recommend *ranges* of nutrient intake versus set percentages of nutrients in the diet. These ranges are more encompassing than the earlier recommendations: 45% to 65% of total calories of the diet should come from carbohydrates, 20% to 35% from fat, and 10% to 35% from protein. Obvious is the decrease in total carbohydrate (the range allows for a lower intake than the previous guidelines), although a recommended increase in fiber, as well as an increase in both protein and fat, is certainly appropriate for the aging active person. Unfortunately, though, one of the recommendations does allow for a higher percentage of added sugars, having gone from 10% to 25% of carbohydrate calories. From both the athletic and the aging standpoint, as discussed later, it would not be advantageous to increase added simple sugar intake.

Healthy elderly persons have macronutrient requirements very similar to those of the younger population. The greatest difference lies in the inability of older people to absorb all of the necessary nutrients due to age-associated physiological changes. According to the food guide pyramid, the bulk of calories should come from complex carbohydrates (50% for the general population and 55% or greater for athletes).

Simple sugars should not contribute more than 10% of total carbohydrate calories; approximately 15% to 18% of calories should come from protein (with both elderly persons and athletes requiring more); and no more than 30% of total calories should come from fat. Alcohol recommendations are one drink of an alcoholic beverage per day if one wishes to drink alcohol (a drink is defined as one 12-oz beer, 5-6 oz of wine, or 1.5 oz of hard liquor).

Carbohydrates

Carbohydrates are essential to healthy living, improved immune system functioning, and optimum sport performance (ACSM Joint Position Statement 2000; Nieman 2000). The majority of calories should come from the three food categories composing the carbohydrate group: fruits, vegetables, and starches. Carbohydrates are the preferred source of energy for the brain and the muscles and provide fiber, vitamins, minerals, and antioxidants, along with other nutrients. They are also associated with heightened hormonal and immune responses. Nieman (2000) found that only carbohydrates, versus vitamins, minerals, and glutamine, are effective countermeasures for exercise-induced inflammation and immunosuppression. For optimum health and sport performance, total carbohydrates should be predominately fruits, vegetables, and whole grains, with an emphasis on lower-fat starches.

Complex Carbohydrates

Starches, vegetables, and few fruits are complex carbohydrates. Because of their more complex or longer molecular structure (and thus the name), these foods are broken down more slowly than simple sugars. Because less refined complex carbohydrates are also rich in fiber, they can slow stomach emptying, which in turn helps moderate blood sugars and minimizes blood sugar spiking. Fiber, found only in carbohydrates, is essential for regularity, decreasing the recurrence of diverticulitis and possible risk of colon/rectal cancer.

Carbohydrates are good sources of many B vitamins, in particular B12 when fortified, a key vitamin often found to be malabsorbed with aging. Carbohydrate absorption, barring illness, remains almost unchanged with aging (Saltzman and Russell 1998).

Complex Carbohydrates and Weight Control

To control weight and decrease likelihood of weight gain, moderation in consumption of all nutrients is advised. Contrary to popular belief, carbohydrates are not fattening when eaten in appropriate quantities and should compose the bulk of the diet. In addition, when the emphasis is on whole grains and less refined starches, along with ample fruits and vegetables, weight gain can be less problematic. Only people with syndrome X (a group of heart-threatening abnormalities in individuals with hyperinsulinemia; term coined by Dr. Gerald Reaven, professor of medicine at Stanford University) are advised to reduce carbohydrate consumption, due to insulin resistance, to as low as 40% versus the recommended higher levels (Reaven 2000).

Antioxidants

Carbohydrates are also a rich source of antioxidants—a compound that can donate electrons to electron-seeking compounds (oxidizing), thereby minimizing the negative effects of oxidizing compounds (Wardlaw 2003). In relation to exercise, free radicals (oxidizing compounds) have been hypothesized to affect energy production, muscle contraction, and thus physical performance (Subudhi et al. 2001). Even though much more research is needed on the potential benefits of the specific dietary compounds, a body of sound scientific research already indicates that these compounds may be beneficial. Several types of antioxidants are found in carbohydrates:

- Carotenoids, contained in plant pigments, are found in fruits and vegetables including carrots, fresh tomatoes, tomato products, green vegetables, peppers, and squash.
- Vitamin C is found in citrus fruits, potatoes, strawberries, green bell peppers, broccoli, tomatoes, and other fruits and vegetables.
- Vitamin E is found predominately in nuts, seeds, fats, and plant oils (corn, soybean, safflower, wheat germ) and to some degree also in green leafy vegetables. With the emphasis on the need to decrease fat intake because of the high rate of obesity in this country, it is possible that some diets may be low in vitamin E. The Recommended Dietary Allowance (RDA) for vitamin E for adults is 15 mg alpha-tocopherol (αTE) per day. Alpha-tocopherol is the active form of vitamin E. Reference amounts, however, for vitamin E can be expressed as any of the following: International Units (IU), milligrams, and alpha-tocopherol (αTE). For comparison's sake, 1 αTE = 1 mg of active vitamin E; 1 IU is equal to 0.67 mg αTE if from natural sources and 0.45 mg αTE if from synthetic vitamin E. The synthetic form or dl version is usually found in supplements and is less active. Safe recommended supplemental amounts range from 100 to 400 mg of active vitamin E and up to 800 or 1000 IU of synthetic. Even though vitamin E is a fat-soluble vitamin, it has not been found to be toxic for healthy individuals (Fogelholm 2002).

Vitamin E supplements may be warranted due to limited dietary intake. But caution is advised with any supplement use. For example, vitamin E has a blood-thinning effect, so people on blood-thinning medication are not good candidates for these types of supplements. People should always check with their doctor before taking any of these products.

Many products geared to athletes, such as energy replacement bars and shakes, are fortified with higher levels of these antioxidants, which may make it unnecessary to supplement these vitamins separately. The fact that most antioxidants come primarily from the fruit and vegetable groups further supports the desirability of ample produce in the diet. Fruit and vegetable intake has also been found to have a positive relationship with bone density (Incledon 2001), partly because of the high mineral content of these foods, which play a key role in bone metabolism. Antioxidants also play a key role in minimizing the likelihood of cataract formation.

Simple Carbohydrates

Sugars and most fruit, made of one or two units in contrast to their more complex counterpart, make up the simple carbohydrate group. Simple sugars are either monosaccharides (only one sugar unit) or disaccharides (two units). Fructose, glucose, and galactose are the monosaccharides; sucrose, lactose, and maltose are the disaccharides. Some sugars can "spike" blood sugar levels, which in turn initiates insulin release. Insulin excites cells to promptly use or store the necessary sugars, which can then result in a sugar "slump." It is advised that people eat simple sugars in conjunction with other foods, such as protein, to help minimize this sugar high. Note that added simple sugars, mainly sucrose-based beverages or foods, often have little nutrient value and are a ready source of calories. They are not recommended in large quantities, and especially not before any recreational activity or event as they can induce symptoms of hypoglycemia. Postexercise, simple sugars may be ingested to help replenish carbohydrate stores.

The Controversial Glycemic Index

The theory of the glycemic index (GI) has been around for many years. It wanes in popularity and eventually surges back. The GI was originally used to help people with diabetes in maintaining even blood sugar values.

The index attributes numerical values to foods as indicators of how high blood sugar rises after ingestion of a high-carbohydrate load (using 50 g of carbohydrate as the standard). The key in this context is *food*, not *meal*, and herein lies a controversy. Foods with GI values equal to that of glucose or white bread (depending on which reference food is used) are considered high GI foods. They are assigned a value of 100. The higher the number, the quicker the response, and the more likely that blood sugar will spike and the energy will be used quickly. Thus the goal would be to consume foods with lower GI values such as lentils, popcorn, and oranges, to name a few. However, the index is controversial in that when more than one food is eaten at the same time, the GI values change. Whole grain bread, for example, which has a GI value of 51, would have a much lower value if eaten along with margarine, cream cheese, or peanut butter; these additional nutrients slow digestion. Regardless of this controversy, low GI foods still assist in decreasing blood sugar postprandially and are still advisable.

Part of the resurgence in popularity of the index has been in connection with sport performance. Lower GI foods provide sustained energy, which is highly beneficial to the endurance athlete. Thus it may be helpful to use the GI to evaluate a pregame or pretraining snack.

The currently popular GI is a slightly different version, taking the form of glycemic loading (Webb 2002). This refers to the blood sugar response after consumption of a normal-size serving of a food rather than the 50-g amount used in the previous index. Use of this version of the GI, or glycemic loading, could be beneficial for reducing obesity and onset of diabetes. Although much more research is needed in these areas, studies show that people eating high GI foods tend to be hungry more often and to have higher spikes in blood sugar, which in turn, because of the subsequent insulin release, could promote fat storage and also chronic overuse of the pancreas. For optimum health, the timing, portion, and type of carbohydrate can make a difference. It is advisable to eat small, combination meals (containing protein, carbohydrate, and small amounts of fat) often and to use less-processed, lower GI carbohydrates that are also higher in fiber, such as whole wheat, whole grains, brown and wild rice, and beans, along with vegetables and fruit.

Protein

Protein requirements may be calculated as a percentage of total caloric consumption (often 15-18% of total calories) or more accurately determined as grams of protein per kilogram body weight. The average recommended intake is 0.8 g of protein per kilogram body weight. However, athletes and elderly persons have higher requirements. Sarcopenia, primarily affecting the skeletal muscle, results in a reduction of the body's major protein pool. Protein is essential for maintaining muscle mass; therefore adequate protein must be ingested to replace obligatory nitrogen losses as well as support protein turnover (Bonnefoy, Constans, and Ferry 2000). Loss of muscle mass accounts for the decrease in metabolic rate, muscle strength, and activity levels often seen in aging.

A minimum of 1 to 1.25 g per kilogram body weight is suggested for older individuals, as well as a starting point often for athletes. Higher levels are dependent on body size, lean muscle mass, intensity, and amount of activity. Using the guideline of 1 g per kilogram body weight, people with weights from 120 to 250 lb would require 54 to 113 g of protein per day. Good protein sources are meat, fish, skinless poultry, shellfish, milk, yogurt, cottage cheese, cheese, soy products, nut butters, nut and seeds, and eggs. Beans (legumes) are also excellent sources of protein as well as of carbohydrates and fiber. One-half cup of cooked beans provides approximately 1 oz (7 g) of protein, 9 g of fiber (depending on bean), and 120 low-fat calories.

Fat

Because of the high rate of heart disease in this country, which is more prominent later in life, and the increase of obesity seen over the past 10 years, fat in the diet plays a key role both in healthy aging and in sport performance. Interestingly, Evans and Cyr-Campbell (1997) have found that the amount of fat that athletes of all ages store is directly related to the amount of time they spend exercising and not their age. Again, it is inactivity that promotes fat storage, not the mere fact of aging.

Fatty acids stored in adipose tissue and used within the muscle cells serve as an important energy source for exercise metabolism. Of the recommended 30% or less of total calories coming from fat, it is advised that no more than 10% come from each type of fat: saturated, monounsaturated, and polyunsaturated. Saturated fat intake has been linked to an increase in serum cholesterol, thereby increasing risk of heart disease. Foods high in saturated fats are primarily foods of animal origin or processed foods using tropical oils such as palm and coconut.

More active people, who require a higher caloric intake, will also have a higher fat intake. Shirley Gerrior's poster presentation (2001a) on dietary intakes of active men and women over 65 showed that men meeting American College of Sports Medicine (ACSM) guidelines for activity had lower intakes of total and saturated fat than their counterparts who were less physically active. However, total fat consumption was about 30% of total calories and saturated fat consumption was above 10%. The women Gerrior studied were divided into two groups, ages 51 to 64 and above 65. Overall, as with the men, the women's intakes of total and saturated fat were above 30% and 10%. However, the older group that engaged in light activity ate significantly less fat than the younger group that was moderately active (Gerrior 2001b).

To improve performance, endurance athletes may resort to severe fat restriction. This is not advised, as fat is a primary fuel source for endurance activities and also a source of fat-soluble vitamins and essential fatty acids. Athletes consuming very low-fat diets are in jeopardy of impeding performance and incurring health risks (Rosenbloom 2000). Performance can be impeded in two ways: (1) if meat protein is decreased to address the saturated fat concern, the athlete could also be low in protein; (2) by decreasing fat, calories are also decreased, which can impact energy level. Fats are essential to well-being, particularly healthy fats such as omega 3 fats and monounsaturated fats found in olive oil, canola oil, peanut oil, and avocados, for example.

Nutrition and Bone Health

According to the National Institutes of Health, 10 million people in the United States have osteoporosis and another 18 million have low bone mass, with the odds favoring that these individuals will also develop osteoporosis (Incledon 2001). Osteoporosis, most often seen in later life, is a disease characterized by a decrease in bone mass that results in an increased susceptibility to bone fracture.

The development of osteopenia in the elderly is dependent on lifetime calcium intake. Bone is metabolically active tissue that is continually undergoing change. The amount of bone mass attained at skeletal maturity is a major factor in determining risk of osteoporosis. The denser the bone prior to ages 40 to 45, when bone loss begins to occur, the less likely that bone mass will diminish to a level that would increase risk of fracture. Major factors affecting bone loss are aging, menopause, decreased intestinal calcium absorption, and medications. Whether or not high protein intakes promote calcium excretion continues to be controversial. Atrophic gastritis, type B, is due to environmental conditions and shows no clear inheritance patterns (Saltzman and Russell 1998). This condition produces a lack of stomach acid, which hinders calcium absorption from calcium carbonate. In addition, older persons tend to have a poor intake of dietary calcium, which can be explained, in part, by lactose intolerance. Although lactose intolerance can start at any age, it not uncommonly begins to develop in the 30s or 40s.

Some evidence suggests that phytoestrogens affect bone turnover. Phytoestrogens are plant-based substances such as isoflavones, found in soy, that appear to mimic some of the effects of synthetic estrogen, though at much milder levels. Soybeans and flaxseed (oil or meal) are excellent sources. Since it is the isoflavones in soy that are thought to generate the positive effects, it is important to take care that soy products contain adequate amounts of these. Studies often use up to 40 g/day of isoflavones; but according to Food and Drug Administration (FDA) recommendations, 25 g of soy protein per day, within a diet low in saturated fat, may reduce risk of heart disease. Isoflavone content is often noted on the label. Caution is advised for women having or having had breast cancer, as soy can mimic the effects of estrogen. One cup of soy milk contains approximately 20 g of isoflavones.

Saltzman and Russell (1998) found that a major contributor to decreased absorption of calcium is poor vitamin D intake and activity (i.e., how the body utilizes vitamin D once it's taken in). This recognition that vitamin D plays a key role in calcium absorption is reflected in the new recommended levels. Vitamin D is needed for absorption of calcium but enough calcium must be present. It is difficult to achieve these levels of calcium from the diet alone, especially given that many older people may be lactose intolerant (table 5.1). Therefore, a general recommendation is that people take a calcium supplement (citrate or carbonate) along with vitamin D or a calcium supplement with a multivitamin containing D. Calcium supplements taken in smaller amounts, two to three times per day, are more readily absorbed. As stomach acid enhances absorption, it is ideal to take these supplements around mealtimes; however, calcium supplements should not be taken at the same time as any iron supplements.

Vitamins

Even though vitamin requirements are influenced to some degree by subtle age-related physiological changes, the predominant reason for poor vitamin nutriture is inadequate dietary intake (Saltzman and Russell 1998). The RDAs, once the standard for preventing dietary deficiencies, are being replaced with the newer Dietary Reference Intakes (DRIs). The DRIs focus on dietary intakes necessary to reduce chronic disease as well as to prevent deficiencies. Dietary Reference Intakes are slowly beginning to address the fact that extrapolation of nutrient needs from the younger populations to the needs of the elderly is not sufficient.

As many as 30% of people aged 65 and older in the United States develop atrophic gastritis type B, the number ranging from 11% to 50% of the population (Saltzman and Russell 1998). Atrophic gastritis is a decrease in or lack of stomach acid production, associated with the development of atrophy of the stomach. Gastric acid is one of the major mechanisms for deterring bacterial overgrowth in the upper intestinal tract and is also vital for efficient absorption of folic acid, calcium, iron, and vitamin B12. Bacterial overgrowth of the small intestine can hinder the absorption of fat-soluble vitamins A, D, E, and K and lead also to generalized malabsorption of fat (although vitamin K levels are not often impacted, as more K is produced through the increase in bacterial numbers). Fat malabsorption may be due to the deconjugation of bile salts by the bacteria, which can result in passive absorption of free bile acids and in turn fat malabsorption (Saltzman and Russell 1998). Although up to 30% of people over 65 develop this problem, the percentage is lower among the physically active because regular exercise helps maintain the integrity of many systems.

Vitamin A

Vitamin A (retinol) plays a key role in maintaining vision (especially night vision), regulating cell growth and division, and maintaining immune system efficiency. Its malabsorption due to aging and increased intake through supplements can be problematic. As we age, vitamin A is cleared more slowly from the blood and tissues, leaving levels in the bloodstream that may result in toxicity. The RDA for vitamin A is 700 RAE for women, 900 μg for men (1 μg = 1 Retinol Activity Equivalent (RAE) = 3.3 IU = 12 μg beta-carotene = 24 μg of other provitamin A). Retinol Activity Equivalents (RAEs) are now the standard unit used for vitamin A, where International Units (IUs) were previously used. Because of their increased nutrient needs, elderly people are advised to use supplements. In the case of vitamin A (retinol), however, it is important to ensure that the supplement does not contain more than the recommended amounts of vitamin A in the form of retinol. The upper limit for vitamin A is 3,000 RAE. It is not unusual to find supplements containing 25,000 IU. Beta-carotene, which is nontoxic and is converted by the body to vitamin A, is the recommended source for a person who is taking higher levels.

Dietary sources of vitamin A in retinol form are liver, fish, fish liver oils, margarines, milk, milk products, butter, and eggs. Good dietary sources of vitamin A (carotenoids) are dark green leafy vegetables (broccoli, Swiss chard, kale, spinach, romaine lettuce, endive) and yellow/orange vegetables and fruits (carrots, sweet potatoes, pumpkin, winter squash, apricots, cantaloupe, papaya, and peaches).

Individuals on blood-thinning agents should avoid consuming large amounts of dark green vegetables, as high vitamin K content of these foods can influence the effect of the medication. People consuming diets

TABLE 5.1 Dietary Calcium

Source (dairy)	Amount	Milligrams
Yogurt, plain nonfat	1 cup	450
Yogurt, plain, low-fat	1 cup	415
Yogurt, fruit	1 cup	315
Milk, skim	1 cup	300
Milk, 2%	1 cup	295
Milk, whole	1 cup	290
Milk, chocolate, 1%	1 cup	285
Milk, chocolate, 2%	1 cup	285
Milk, soy, calcium-fortified	8 oz	250-300
Cheese, Swiss	1 oz	270
Ice cream	1/2 cup	85
Cheese, cheddar	1 oz	205
Cheese, mozzarella, part-skim	1 oz	185
Pudding	1/2 cup	150
Cottage cheese	1/2 cup	75
Pizza, cheese (average)	1/8 of a 15-inch pizza	220
Frozen yogurt	1/2 cup	105
Quark	1 oz	24
Source (non-dairy)		
Orange juice, calcium fortified	3/4 cup	225
Orange, navel, raw	1	52
Macaroni and cheese (average)	1/2 cup	180
Blackstrap molasses	1 tablespoon	170
Salmon, canned with edible bones	3 oz	205
Tofu (processed with calcium sulfate)	1/2 cup	260
Turnip greens	1/2 cup	100
Sardines with edible bones	1 oz	90
Dried figs	3	80
Broccoli	1/2 cup	45
Tempeh	1/2 cup	75
Mustard greens	1/2 cup	55
Collard greens	1/2 cup	115
Scallops	3 oz	21
Shrimp	3 oz	33
Okra	1/2 cup	50
Whole wheat bread	2 slices	40

already high in vitamin A need to be careful about supplementing this nutrient.

Vitamin D

The older person may have an increased vitamin D requirement. With aging comes a tendency toward decreased exposure to sunlight (i.e., sunscreen is essential to minimize the risk of sunburn and skin cancer but also reduces the number of sun rays available to convert inactive D to active D; SPF above 8 allows minimal to no conversion), which can help the body synthesize vitamin D. In addition, the skin becomes less efficient in vitamin D synthesis, and the kidneys become less responsive to converting the inactive form of vitamin D to the active hormonal form. Thus overall, less vitamin D is available. At the same time, food volume can be considerably less in elderly than in younger people. Although physically active older people tend to have more sun exposure and better dietary habits than their inactive peers and thus better vitamin D levels, a daily multivitamin with D is recommended for everyone regardless of diet or physical activity.

The DRI for vitamin D is Adequate Intakes or AI. The AI for vitamin D is 5 µg/day (= 200 IU/day) for people under age 51. Individuals over the age of 51 are encouraged to consume two to three times this amount, or possibly more depending on sun exposure—600 to 800 IUs or 15 to 20 µg from a combination of vitamin D fortified foods and a multivitamin and mineral supplement (Wardlaw 2003). The diet continues to provide the best sources, however; good sources of dietary vitamin D are fortified cow's milk, egg yolks, butter, liver, some fatty fish, and fortified margarine.

Vitamin B12 (Cobalamin) and Folacin

As already noted, vitamin B12 absorption is often less efficient in people who are elderly because of the prevalence of atrophic gastritis (Russell and Mason 2000). When B12 is bound to food it is not absorbed efficiently. B12, when not fortified, is exclusively found (bound form) in animal products. Therefore, it is advisable for aging persons to receive vitamin B12 either through supplements or in the form of a fortified cereal or soy-based meat substitutes, in which the B12 is not bound.

Folacin is a water-soluble B vitamin. Deficiencies of either B12 or folate (also called folic acid when added to foods or in supplemental form) can cause a form of anemia that can result in increasing paralysis of the muscles and nerves. Because folacin and B12 work synergistically, supplementing folacin can clear up the early anemia but mask the underlying B12 deficiency. Therefore, supplemental over-the-counter folic acid is limited to 400 µg, which is the RDA, (an amount that will not mask the underlying deficiency). On the other hand, it is recommended (Russell and Mason 2000) that total daily intake of folate be targeted at about but not exceed 1 mg/day.

Another reason for aging active people to be sure they are getting enough folate is that elevated levels of homocysteine are associated with mildly depleted levels of folate. Although still controversial, it appears that hyperhomocysteinemia (elevated blood levels of homocysteine) is an independent risk factor in myocardial infarctions, peripheral vascular disease, and cerebrovascular diseases.

Good dietary sources of folate are leafy vegetables, liver, yeast, legumes, and some fruits. It is crucial to be aware that regular food processing in meal preparation can reduce the amount of folacin by 50%. Ideally, vegetables should be well cleaned but eaten raw or minimally cooked to preserve folacin content.

Vitamin B6 (Pyridoxine)

Vitamin B6, essential for new cell growth and a primary player in protein metabolism, provides a boost for the immune system while keeping blood glucose levels in check. B6 along with B12 and folate also helps decrease homocysteine levels in the blood. According to extensive government studies (Webb and Ward 1999) there appears to be a greater risk of vitamin B6 deficiency with aging. This is attributable to a decrease in protein intake (B6 and protein occur together), and to an increase in B6 requirements with age because of an increased metabolism of the compound.

Current dietary recommendations, RDA, for vitamin B6 ranges from 1.3 mg to 1.7 mg/day. Athletes may need slightly more B6 because of increased use of glycogen (carbohydrates) as fuel. Good dietary sources of vitamin B6 are liver, oatmeal, banana, chicken, potatoes, avocado, halibut, wheat germ, pork chop, brown rice, canned corn, hamburger, prunes, peanut butter, and vegetables such as cauliflower and Brussels sprouts. Apples, breads, and cheese also provide some B6.

Other Special Needs of the Older Active Person

Among other functional foods (term implies that food provides health benefits beyond those normally found in its nutrients) are oats, which not only contribute insoluble fiber that may help reduce risk of colon/rectal cancer but also soluble fiber which helps in reducing serum cholesterol (Wardlaw 2003). Oats are an excellent addition to any older person's diet. Soy is also beneficial for lowering serum cholesterol levels (Greaves and Thomson 2001). The FDA has approved a Heart Health Claim regarding consumption of soy and lowering risk of heart disease. In addition, soy is a good source of calcium for people who are lactose intolerant or do not consume many dairy products. The recommendation is a minimum of 25 g of soy protein daily as part of a low-fat diet.

Selenium, a mineral, is found mostly in seafood and organ meats such as liver and kidney. Like vitamins A, C, and E, it is an antioxidant and is thus helpful in reducing the damage that free radicals may cause to cell membranes. These protective effects may help boost the immune system. Moreover, selenium may help reduce the risk of prostate, lung, and colon cancer. The RDA for selenium is 55 μg/day for adults. In general, adults meet the RDA but for some, selenium supplements may be warranted due to limited dietary intake.

Fluids

Water accounts for approximately 50% to 70% of total body mass. The largest single component of the human body, water is the nutrient that has the greatest single impact on sport performance and human functioning. A few days of fasting, assuming ingestion of liquids, has very little impact on functional capacity. However, cessation of water intake has debilitating consequences after times ranging from 1 to 2 h to a few days (Maughan and Nadel 2000). Both the aging and athletic populations are high-risk groups for dehydration. Athletes and physically active individuals who

Summary of Recommendations for the Graying Athlete

- Fluid intake should be adequate to meet daily needs and replenish losses due to sweat and daily functioning (rest: six to eight 8-oz glasses; activity: 10 to 12+ depending on intensity of exercise, environmental conditions, and sweat losses). Some replenishment fluids should come from energy drinks, which contain small amounts of carbohydrate and sodium to help with restoring glycogen and fluid retention. This is essential when exercising more than 30 to 45 min.
- Ensure adequate caloric intake to maintain healthy weight and sport performance.
- Obtain the majority of calories from unrefined, complex carbohydrates and from simple carbohydrates in the form of fruit and those added to fluid replenishment beverages. Small amounts of simple carbohydrates may come from occasional desserts, ideally postexercise to replenish glycogen stores.
- Protein requirement is at least 1 g protein per kilogram body weight.
- Total fat calories should not exceed 30% of total calories with no more than 10% coming from saturated fat. If weight is not a concern, fat intake may be increased to 35% if the fats are predominately monounsaturated or omega 3 fats; if maintaining optimum body weight is problematic, fat is more calorically dense.
- Ensure adequate B12 and B6 intake by incorporating foods that have been fortified with B12 and are rich in B6.
- Ensure adequate calcium intake by striving to include more dairy products in the diet and supplementing in the range of 1,000 to 1,200 mg/day.
- It is imperative for people to address any stress incontinence issues they have, as this condition can limit one's intake of fluids and increase the risk of dehydration. If fluid intake is already a concern, people should be sure not to consume caffeinated beverages, as these will increase the need to urinate more frequently.
- Environmental conditions also play a key role in hydration. Hot, humid conditions can deplete fluid reserves quickly and need to be considered prior to exercising. Following recommended guidelines for hydration can be difficult or even impossible for aging people because of medical concerns regarding stress incontinence. Therefore the recommendation is that each individual increase fluid intake to a personally tolerable level.

Recommended Fluid Intake for Optimum Hydration

Night before:*	500 ml or 16 fluid oz of fluid prior to bedtime (2 cups)
Morning:	500 ml or 16 fluid oz of fluid (2 cups)
One hour before activity:	500 to 1,000 ml or 16 to 32 fluid oz (2-4 cups)
Twenty minutes before:	500 ml to 1,250 or 8 to 16 fluid oz (1-2 cups)
During activity:**	Every 15 to 20 min another 250 ml or 8 oz of fluid (1 cup)
After activity:	Drink fluids until amount and color of urine have returned to normal (light color, large volume)

Fluid intake recommendations vary depending on weather conditions, level of perspiration, and intensity and length of exercise. Remember that humid weather requires a greater, more frequent intake of fluids, as it is more difficult for fluid to evaporate and therefore cool the body down.

* Only if inadequate fluid has been taken in during the day or in anticipation of strenuous physical activity the next day.

** Very important in strenuous events or events lasting more than 45 to 60 min.

begin to exercise with less than normal body water are more likely to experience adverse effects on cardiovascular function, temperature regulation, and exercise performance (Lamb and Helmy Shehata 1999).

Lean body mass contains about 75% water by mass, whereas adipose tissue, consisting mainly of fat, has very little water content. Leanness or muscle mass increases water storage capabilities, whereas the onset of sarcopenia as seen in the elderly and a possible increase of adipose tissue increase the risk for dehydration. In conjunction with this increased risk, it appears that elderly people may appreciate thirst less readily (Kendrick, Nelson-Steen, and Scafidi 1994; Stout, Kenny, and Baylis 1999). Ayus and colleagues, comparing healthy elderly men to younger controls, found differences in their response to water deprivation. The older men showed deficits in both the intensity and threshold of their thirst response (Ayus and Arieff 1996). Stout, however, has shown that healthy elderly people may be able to compensate for this with an enhanced vasopressin response to osmotic stimulation compared to younger counterparts (Stout, Kenny, and Baylis 1999). This is significant because vasopressin is an antidiuretic hormone.

With aging, therefore, it becomes extremely important for people to make greater efforts to drink adequate fluid throughout the day and before, during, and after exercise. Thirst in and of itself cannot be used as a guide for adequate fluid intake.

Caffeine, a diuretic, has been linked to poor hydration status prior to and during exercise. Caffeine has also been used as an ergogenic aid to enhance sport performance. Gordon et al. did not find any changes in core body temperature, sweat loss, and plasma volume during exercise following caffeine consumption (Maughan and Nadel 2000). However, these findings were from a younger, well-hydrated population group. It is advised that coffee or caffeinated products not compose the bulk of fluid intake for aging active people. Recommended fluids for optimum hydration are water, skim milk (if tolerated), diluted fruit juice, or energy drinks. Energy drinks are often recommended not only for their fluid replenishment properties, but also for their carbohydrate, sodium, and potassium contents. Carbohydrates help replenish glycogen losses, and sodium helps in retention of the ingested fluid (Lamb and Helmy Shehata 1999). Diluted fruit juices can also serve this function.

Hyponatremia, an electrolyte imbalance due to too much fluid consumption, has become more of a concern as athletes become more aware of hydration needs. Know your own needs, perspiration rates, urine color, and weather conditions prior to overindulging in fluids.

Some of the newest research on recovery nutrition for athletes shows that a beverage combining carbohydrate and protein is more advantageous than carbohydrate alone for replenishing glycogen stores and promoting muscle development (Zawadzki, Yaspelkis, and Ivy 1992). However, because many of these beverages do not promote adequate fluid replenishment, water or other fluids need to be taken also.

HERBAL SUPPLEMENTS

The herbal industry in the United States has boomed over the last 10 years. Even though the industry is still in its infancy in the United States, herbs have been used successfully for medicinal purposes in other countries for hundreds of years.

Effectiveness and Regulation of Herbal Supplements

Unfortunately, the effectiveness of many herbs has not been well documented in clinical research trials. At this time the Commission E documents from Germany provide the only significant clinical data on many herbal preparations. Until more recent research is available, these documents remain the most reliable source of data on herbs.

In addition, dietary supplements such as herbals and vitamins, unlike medicines and other drugs, are very loosely regulated in the United States. The FDA is actually prevented from closely monitoring these products by the Proxmire Amendment to the 1938 Food, Drug, and Cosmetic Act, along with the follow-up legislation, the Dietary Supplement Health and Education Act (DSHEA), which was passed in 1994. At the time, it was argued that herbs and vitamins are foods and not drugs and therefore that the FDA should not be allowed to regulate them closely. However, the FDA does require a standardized supplements fact label on herbs and other related products (Wardlaw 2003).

Should any significant side effects or harm be reported to the FDA in regard to a supplement, the government may intervene and have the product removed from the market. However, this still leaves the consumer without knowledge about the purity of the product and the amount, if any, of active ingredient, as virtually very little testing is done on these products. Some Web sites may be of help, but since the purpose of most of these sites is to "sell" products rather than provide consumer health-related information, their value is very limited. ConsumerLab.com, one of the first reputable sites—an independent laboratory that tests the purity of many of these products—recently indicated that of 25 brands of glucosamine, chondroitin, and combined products, nearly one-third did not pass testing for adequate levels of active compound (ConsumerLab.com 2000). So, in effect, even though herbals may be beneficial, any positive results from the product versus placebo are unknown at present.

Many herbals claim to invigorate and improve sport performance. Claims of invigoration usually refer to ingredients such as caffeine, guarana (a paste made from herbs that also has caffeine-like effects), or Ephedra, which has now been banned by the FDA. Caution is advised for people considering herbal supplements. Such supplements are not recommended for people allergic to flowers in the daisy family, individuals on blood-thinning medication, anyone with any type of immune disorder, or individuals already on prescription medications (which can be a large part of the active aging population). With these exceptions, herbal use appears to be relatively safe.

Some theories have suggested that ginseng may enhance muscle glycogen synthesis after exercise, help sustain muscle creatine phosphate levels during exercise, and decrease lactic acid (Williams 1998). However, all of these claims remain theories until reputable scientific evidence proves otherwise.

Because of the quantity of faulty information on these preparations worldwide, people should carefully research the product or check with credible sources before taking or recommending any herbals or other questionable supplements.

Supplement Shopper Know-How

Three population subgroups at high risk for health scams are athletes, the aging Baby Boomers, and the elderly: Athletes are always looking for an "edge" to improve performance, people who are aging wish to find a "magical" cure to slow the process, and elderly persons are often looking for ways to minimize their aches and pains. For all these reasons the active aging are particularly susceptible to misinformation. Thus practitioners cannot emphasize enough to patients in these categories that when they shop for supplements, whether herbal, ergogenic, or just vitamins and minerals, they should be well informed, both about the products themselves and about the credentials of the sellers.

People working in stores that sell supplements are rarely appropriately trained in the United States. Most often the health and nutrition information they pass on is not scientifically based but instead based on employer information, hearsay, or their own experience. In addition, it is important to know that anyone can use the title "nutritionist" and that use of this title is not regulated by any agency and does not imply that the person is a nutrition expert. In contrast, the title Registered Dietitian (RD) can be used only by people who have undergone extensive training, participated in an internship, and passed a state exam.

Herbals and sport supplements may have their place, but they are not cures. Multivitamin and mineral preparations that provide 100% of the RDA are rarely if ever problematic; but supplementation of individual nutrients often poses a greater threat, since the amounts people take are often significantly above the upper limits. We are repeatedly cautioned not to use supplements to cure a problem that could be prevented with better self-care. For example, people should warm up and cool down before and after exercise to encourage blood flow to the muscles, and thus minimize occurrence of injury, rather than relying on protein supplements to heal torn muscle tissue or taking glucosamine and chondroitin to prevent bone injury.

Prevention is the key, but education is also our ally. Refer to reputable Web sites and journals for scientific information about supplements. The National Institutes of Health (www.health.nih.gov) has an office on complementary medicine (nccam.nih.gov) that addresses herbs and other forms of complementary medicine, as well as a Web site on aging (www.nia.nih.gov). Gatorade Sports Science Institute (www.gssiweb.com) is a reputable site for sport information, along with the ACSM (www.acsm.org). Should you wish to consult a dietitian, the American Dietetic Association (eatright.org) provides information about dietitians in your area. And as a final word of caution, the more prescription medications one takes, the more likely are problems with supplement use resulting from medication–supplement interaction. Also, the larger the quantity taken, the more likely the side effects. People who choose to pursue the supplement route need to be well informed.

NSAIDs AND COX-2 INHIBITORS

Nonsteroidal anti-inflammatory drugs (NSAIDs) and COX-2 inhibitors are used in orthopedic patients to minimize pain and inflammation caused by musculoskeletal injury, especially in the older population. In 1992, the COX enzyme was discovered to have two different forms, COX-1 and COX-2, which has revolutionized the utility of NSAIDs in the treatment of musculoskeletal pathology (Holtzman, Turk, and Sharnick 1992). The COX-1 enzyme was determined to be constitutively active in many cell lines and associated with many essential body functions while the COX-2 enzyme is inducible in most cells during situations of pain and inflammation. Therefore, the selective inhibition of COX-2 was thought to provide analgesic and anti-inflammatory effects yet avoid many of the adverse side effects associated with traditional NSAIDs that also inhibit the COX-1 enzyme.

NSAIDs in the Older Population

Nonsteroidal anti-inflammatory drugs are used by both competitive and recreational older exercisers because of their ability to reduce muscle soreness as well as minimize inflammation associated with exercise. However, the older population is also more prone to complications associated with medication usage and medical comorbidities than the younger population. A few studies have linked NSAID use to acute renal failure during exercise, and therefore a conservative approach to use is advised (Farquhar and Kenney 1997). However, Farquhar and Kenney (1997) found that with appropriate doses of over-the-counter medication or prescription drugs there were no apparent adverse renal effects. Further support for conservative use, on the other hand, comes from research showing that NSAIDs inhibit platelet aggregation and cause gastropathy, which could lead to gastrointestinal bleeding and peptic ulcer (Reents 2000). Pahor and colleagues (Reents 2000) found that the risk of gastrointestinal bleeding was lower in older subjects who exercised than in those who did not. Even though the incidence of renal failure during exercise is low and the incidence of other complications, including gastropathy, also appears to be low, it is advisable for people to use NSAIDs prudently and for exercisers to be well hydrated, especially in warm climates, prior to exercising.

Use of COX-2 Inhibitors With the Older Population

COX-2 inhibitors, COXIBs, were introduced into widespread clinical use in 1999 with the approval of two drugs by the FDA: celecoxib (Celebrex, Searle, Chicago, IL, and Pfizer, New York, NY) and rofecoxib (Vioxx, Merck & Co., West Point, PA). COXIBs have been subjected to several clinical trials that have consistently demonstrated efficacy similar to that of traditional NSAIDs and superior to that of a placebo for the treatment of both pain and inflammation in older active and inactive patients with musculoskeletal injury, including arthritis. With its greater specificity for the COX-2 enzyme, rofecoxib has demonstrated higher efficacy in arthritis patients in particular when compared to celecoxib (Bingham 2002; McMurray and Hardy 2002). However, rofecoxib has been withdrawn from the market by Merck due to preliminary results from the Adenomatous Polyp Prevention on Vioxx (APPROVe) research study which showed a higher incidence of thromboembolic events in those patients taking rofecoxib (Fitzgerald 2004). COXIB alternatives, such as celecoxib and valdecoxib, must now be used with caution as well, especially in the older population who have potential comorbidities (e.g., cardiovascular risk factors), and celecoxib should not be prescreibed in those patients with a sulfonamide allergy.

Arthritis and COX-2 Inhibitors

It is estimated that by the year 2020, the prevalence of arthritis in the United States will extend to over 60 million people affected by a severity of disease that influences work performance, activities of daily living, or both (Lawrence et al. 1998). Considering the substantial number of arthritis patients, especially within the older population, control of associated symptoms with medication is becoming increasingly important in both conservative and surgical management settings.

Arthritis is most commonly described by two major categories of disease: osteoarthritis (OA) and rheumatoid arthritis (RA). The clinical hallmarks of OA and RA include pain and inflammation resulting from the conversion of arachidonic acid into prostaglandins by the cyclooxygenase (COX) enzyme. Nonsteroidal anti-inflammatory drugs, including ibuprofen, naproxen, and diclofenac, have traditionally been prescribed to inhibit the COX enzyme and provide analgesic and anti-inflammatory relief to older active and inactive patients with and without arthritis; however, they have also been associated with many significant adverse reactions, which COXIBs have been proposed to possibly minimize.

COXIBs and Drug Interactions

Although older active people are not as susceptible to age-related declines and are less likely than older inactive people to be affected by comorbidities or to be taking other medications, adverse reactions and drug interactions are a greater concern with older than with younger active people. Thus it is important to be aware of the possibility of negative drug interactions for older active clients, patients, or competitive athletes who are taking COXIBs. Such people should always be monitored for adverse reactions due to physiologic toxicities in all body systems, especially when risk factors are present. Some of the more common toxicities are gastrointestinal (GI), cardiovascular, and renal complications.

- **Gastrointestinal.** As GI risk factors are an important contraindication to traditional NSAID use, the decreased risk of GI toxicity associated with COXIBs as compared to that of traditional NSAIDs allows for more extensive use in the older population. However, concomitant aspirin use for cardiovascular prophylaxis reportedly results in a loss of the added benefit (Catella-Lawson et al. 2001; Silverstein et al. 2000).
- **Cardiovascular.** Evaluation of the overall effect of COXIBs on cardiovascular function still requires clinical studies; nevertheless, COXIBs, until recently, were thought to be an unlikely source of cardiovascular morbidity or mortality. In fact, naproxen had been shown to be associated with a lower incidence of thrombotic events than COXIBs, but this was attributed to the cardioprotective effect of naproxen. Thus, the concurrent use of low-dose aspirin was recommended in those patients on COXIBs with cardiovascular risk factors (Konstam and Weir 2002). From the preliminary results of the APPROVe study, our rationale concerning the effects of COXIBs on the cardiovascular system has been further elucidated as patients being administered 25 mg of rofecoxib per day had a significant increase in incidence by a factor of 3.9 of serious thromboembolic events, including myocardial infarction and thrombotic stroke (Fitzgerald 2004). COXIBs are being proposed to have this potential to cause thromboembolic events through a common mechanism beginning with a depression in prostaglandin formation which results in an elevated blood pressure and the potential for subsequent increase in atherogenesis. Therefore, all patients should judiciously utilize COXIBs, and patients with an increased risk for cardiovascular disease should avoid using COXIBs.
  - -When COXIBs are indicated in patients taking warfarin, especially older patients receiving treatment for atrial fibrillation, blood clotting defects, and thrombotic prophylaxis indicated by surgery, dosage adjustments are required because COXIBs increase the half-life of warfarin through several mechanisms (Stading, Skrabal, and Faulkner 2001).
  - -Given that over 20 million people in the United States are taking an antihypertensive along with an NSAID, the drug interactions between these medications are extremely important. In fact, an increase in blood pressure has been noted with use of a COXIB along with an antihypertensive, necessitating an adjustment in COXIB dosage, use of a non-NSAID like aspirin, or both.
- **Renal.** This hypertensive effect can also be influenced by renal function, as an age-related decrease in renal blood flow is accentuated in hypertensive patients (Crofford 2002). When one is evaluating overall renal toxicity, standard precautions associated with traditional NSAIDs apply to COXIBs as the two medications have similar effects. Although the prevalence of renal complications is low, people at high risk include the older population in general. Therefore, health care professionals should always be cautious in prescribing NSAIDs and COXIBs to either older active or inactive patients and should monitor renal function at yearly physical examinations through the assessment of the patient's past medical history, symptoms, signs, and appropriate laboratory tests (Schwartz et al. 2001; Swan et al. 2000).

In addition, older women, especially after menopause, are prone to bone loss (i.e., osteopenia and osteoporosis), and theory has suggested that this process may be prevented with COXIBs through the inhibition of prostaglandin formation that would otherwise promote bone resorption (Raisz 2001). An unrelated yet important side note concerning COXIB use involves their possible advantages in other disease processes that affect the older population, including colorectal cancer (Kawamori et al. 1998; Oshima et al. 2001), Alzheimer's disease (Eikelenboom et al. 2000; Frederickson and Brunden 1994), and breast cancer (Subbaramaiah et al. 2002). Future research is needed to delineate the exact mechanisms and the extent of benefit, however.

Overall, COXIBs remain an exciting alternative for analgesic and anti-inflammatory treatment in aging patients. However, their side effect profile must continue to be elucidated as they maintain decreased GI toxicity yet a potential source for thromboembolic events. The next generation of COXIBs, including valdecoxib (Searle, Skokie, IL), etoricoxib (Merck, West Point, PA), and parecoxib (Pharmacia, Peapack, NJ) is already in testing. With a proposed increased specificity of these drugs for the COX-2 enzyme, there is a strong possibility that they will provide even better alternatives for the treatment of pain and inflammation which must be balanced with future research on the worrisome relationship between COXIBs and thromboembolic events, expecially in the older active and inactive populations who are likely to have medical comorbidities.

OTHER POPULAR SUPPLEMENTS

Earlier sections of this chapter have covered the more common, less controversial types of supplements: vitamins and minerals as nutrients and herbals; herb derived. Glucosamine and creatine, two very popular and possibly effective supplements, fall into neither one of these categories.

Glucosamine Sulfate and Chondroitin Sulfate

Nonsteroidal anti-inflammatory drugs have been the standard in treating OA for the last 30 years. However, long-term use of these agents can cause gastrointestinal medical complications. Glucosamine sulfate, an aminomonosaccharide and a constituent of cartilage, and chondroitin sulfate nutritional supplements have recently emerged as an alternative in treatment of OA. However, considerable controversy surrounds questions of their effectiveness. A recent randomized, double-blind study using glucosamine sulfate as an analgesic in OA of the knee showed no significant difference between glucosamine sulfate and placebo as a symptom modifier (Carr 2002). Many of the studies have been criticized for methodological flaws as well as concerns regarding funding sources and positive outcomes.

Nevertheless, it is clear that many people experience pain relief when they take glucosamine and chondroitin sulfate. Also, supplementation of glucosamine, chondroitin sulfate, or both, along with NSAIDs, appears to provide the most optimal benefits initially, until the effects of the glucosamine and chondroitin are felt, after four to six weeks (Antonio and Stout 2001). Ideally one would then be able to stop taking the NSAIDs and rely only on the other supplements. In addition, these supplements appear to be safe alternatives (de los Reyes, Koda, and Lien 2000). Whether these results can be attributed to placebo effect or actual effectiveness of the drug is less important than the fact that these agents do appear to provide pain relief with no reported harmful side effects. It has been recommended that diabetics not use these supplements (McArdle, Katch, and Katch 2001). Chapter 11 provides an extensive discussion of the use of glucosamine and chondroitin sulfate in the treatment of arthritis (pp. 169-171).

Creatine

Creatine has received unprecedented attention in the field of sport ergogenics. It is classified as a physiological sport ergogenic or performance enhancer. The claims are that this natural dietary constituent provides physical power and strength. It has also been studied in relation to increasing body size. Creatine can be ingested through the diet, although not in nearly the amounts in the supplements. Meat, poultry, and fish are good sources of creatine, providing approximately 4 to 5 g of creatine per kilogram of food. In addition, the body synthesizes about 1 g daily. Creatine is a nitrogen-containing, organic compound made from nonessential amino acids. Because creatine is more readily found in animal products, vegetarians are at risk of not taking in adequate amounts from the diet. Thus, vegetarians tend to show greater improvements in strength when supplementing than does the carnivorous population.

Theoretically, supplementing creatine increases the body's creatine pool, thereby facilitating the generation of more creatine phosphate that in turn regenerates adenosine diphosphate (ADP) to adenosine triphosphate (ATP) to allow for more energy. This would allow for the rapid resynthesis of ATP (high energy bond), thereby providing more energy by delaying muscle fatigue (Williams 1998). Even though more and more researchers are examining the validity of these claims, controversy still surrounds this topic. Many believe that supplementing creatine is beneficial, and others believe it is not. Bermon and colleagues (1998) studied the effects of creatine ingestion in sedentary and weight-trained older adults. They concluded that

Meeting Nutrient Needs Through the Diet

Breakfast: High-fiber cereal fortified with B12
Skim milk or soy milk
Whole wheat toast with margarine and jam
Fruit and/or fruit juice
Coffee or tea if desired
1 glass of water

Lunch: Bowl of soup*
Sandwich on whole wheat or multigrain bread**
Small raw carrots
Small amount of chips if desired
Fruit and yogurt
Water to drink or milk or juice if no fruit is desired

Dinner: Broiled, grilled, or baked fish***
Steamed vegetables such as broccoli, cauliflower, Brussels sprouts, or medley of all three
Baked or mashed potatoes
Salad with lite dressing
Water, milk, or juice as beverage

Snack: **Pre- and/or postexercise:**
Peanut butter crackers with beverage
Low-sugar energy bar with beverage
Graham crackers with milk

* Soups such as bean or minestrone are excellent choices.
** Ensure that sandwich contributes protein in the form of a meat or meat substitute.
*** Fish makes for a very low-fat meal when grilled or baked. Substituting 3 to 4 oz of lean red meat or chicken, rather than fish, is fine two to three times a week.
Note: This "sample" diet is not based on any set caloric amount.

creatine supplementation did not provide additional benefits for body composition or maximal strength in healthy elderly subjects. However, according to a study in *Australian Family Physician* (2002), a review of the research suggested that creatine supplementation may not only provide symptomatic pain relief but also have a role in protecting chondroitin. At this time, it is still premature to recommend creatine supplementation for the general active population; however, some people may derive benefits with respect to increased muscle mass and improved energy in high-intensity, quick forms of exertion.

SUMMARY

Because of physiological changes associated with aging, it is apparent that the nutrient needs of the physically active aging are slightly different from those of their younger counterparts. However, this field of research is still very young, and there is much to learn about the specific nutrient needs of the active aging. It appears, though, that primary differences relate to decreased nutrient absorption of B12, possibly B6, and vitamin D; increased protein needs; increased calcium needs; and ample fluid intake. Emphasis should therefore be on consuming nutrient-dense foods with supplementation of calcium and B12 (if these are not taken with fortified foods) and adequate protein to promote retention or building of muscle tissue, or both, along with adequate fluid intake. Apart from these specific issues, nutrient recommendations remain the same for the healthy active aging person as for the younger athlete.

PART

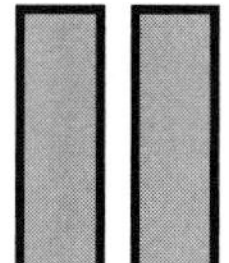

INJURIES AND CONDITIONS IN ACTIVE OLDER ADULTS

CHAPTER

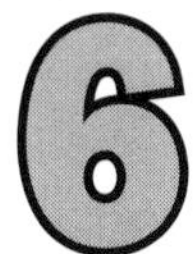

Shoulder Problems

Edward G. McFarland, MD
Hyung Bin Park, MD
Tae Kyun Kim, MD
Efsthathios Chronopoulos, MD
Atsushi Yokota, MD

Studies have shown an increasing incidence of shoulder problems as a person ages (Brewer 1979; Milgrom et al. 1995). This increasing predisposition to shoulder problems is magnified in the active and athletic older individual. Activities that might not have caused problems or symptoms in the past suddenly result in pain and loss of function. Some health care providers tend to dismiss these difficulties and urge the patient to avoid the activities that aggravate the condition, but this attitude ignores the desire and need of maturing individuals to be active. Older patients, whether they are training for the Senior Olympics or just playing recreational tennis, have the same desire to return to participation as active individuals of any age.

Any patient with shoulder problems should have a diagnosis of the condition and a determination of the severity of the limitations, expectations for function, and the rapidity with which the patient needs to recover. In this respect the active or athletic older individual does not differ from younger people who want to remain active in their sport and daily routines. However, there are some special considerations in the more mature athletic individual who presents with a shoulder problem or injury. Previous chapters have addressed some of the physiological, biomechanical, and biochemical changes that occur with aging. This chapter summarizes how age-related changes in the shoulder complex should influence evaluation and treatment of the older active person. We cover evaluation and management of acute and chronic disorders since the aging process affects the approach to these patients.

CHANGES IN THE SHOULDER COMPLEX WITH AGE

As people mature, the shoulder complex in most cases will continue to function without problems (figure 6.1). However, important changes occur in the shoulder with age that are helpful to understand when one is evaluating and treating this joint. First, the range of motion and laxity of the shoulder can decrease with increasing age (Barnes et al. 2001; Kibler et al. 1996). This loss can be subtle, but it should not be more than a few degrees in any direction. Increasing loss of motion indicates a more severe underlying process and should not be ignored because of aging.

Degeneration of the rotator cuff tendons increases with increasing age. Cadaver studies, magnetic resonance imaging (MRI) studies, and clinical studies have verified increasing rotator cuff pathology with increasing age (Brewer 1979; Sher et al. 1995). Almost everyone is affected to some degree, and the vast majority of persons over the age of 40 show some microscopic cuff degeneration grossly and microscopically (Sarkar and Uhthoff 1996). Histological studies reveal characteristic degenerative changes of the tendons. These include the presence of incomplete tendon tears (Nixon and DiStefano 1975; Uhthoff and Sano 1997), thinning of tendon fibers (Uhthoff and Sano 1997), presence of granulation tissue (Sano et al. 1999; Uhthoff and Sano 1997), disorganization of tendon collagen fibers (Brewer 1979; Nixon and DiStefano 1975), calcification (Uhthoff and Sarkar 1993), loss of staining properties (Brewer 1979), abnormalities of

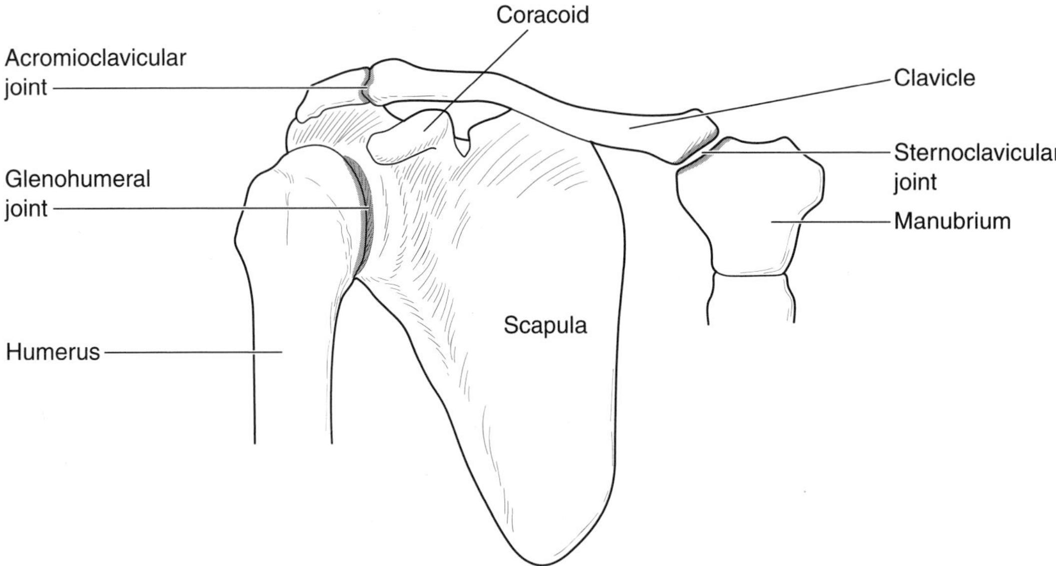

FIGURE 6.1 The shoulder joint, or glenohumeral joint, is composed of the humeral head and the glenoid, which is part of the scapula.

tidemark (Yamakata and Fukuda 1991), loss of cellularity (Brewer 1979), diminution of vascularity of tendon (Brewer 1979), and diminution of fibrocartilage at the tendon insertion site (Brewer 1979).

The exact etiology of gradual tearing of the rotator cuff tendons is not known, but the most prevalent ideas include normal senescence of the tendons; vascular insufficiency of the tendons near their attachment on the tuberosities; and wear of the rotator cuff tendons against the acromion (external or Neer impingement), against the coracoid (coracoid impingement), or against the glenoid (internal impingement) (Davidson et al. 1995; Dines et al. 1990; Gerber et al. 1985; Lindblom 1939; Liu and Boynton 1993; McFarland et al. 1999; Neer 1972; Paley et al. 2000; Rothman and Parke 1965; Walch et al. 1992). The histological studies support the hypothesis that the morphological changes weaken the tendon, so that the tear can occur insidiously and painlessly (Sano et al. 1997, 1999). The tears presumably go through phases and progress from tendinosis to partial tears and then on to full-thickness tears. With aging comes a slow loss of tendon substance with gradual retraction of the tendon away from the tuberosity. The supraspinatus tendon is the most commonly affected, followed by the infraspinatus and the subscapularis tendons. This wear occurs at different rates in different individuals. The prevalence of partial- or full-thickness tears was found by Milgrom et al. (Milgrom et al. 1995) to be 9% to 11% at 30 to 50 years, 50% at 60 to 70 years, and 80% at 80 to 99 years, which suggests that cuff pathology may be in part a natural consequence of aging.

Despite this high incidence of rotator cuff pathology with increasing age, the relationship to symptoms is inexact. The most common symptoms of rotator cuff dysfunction are pain and weakness. Symptoms of rotator cuff dysfunction include pain in the acromion region, biceps anteriorly, deltoid, or midhumerus. The pain may radiate from these areas down the arm. There is little correlation between tendon tear size and the presence of pain, but there is a relationship between strength and the size of the tendon tear. A small, full-thickness tear is defined as one that is 1 cm in size; a medium tear is 2 to 3 cm; a large tear is 3 to 4 cm; and a massive tear is one in which the whole tendon is missing, with dimensions of 3 to 4 cm in width and length. Some patients may have massive rotator cuff tears and have no symptoms at all. However, patients with massive tears commonly complain of weakness, particularly with overhead activities and lifting with their arm away from their body. The physical examination for rotator cuff pathology is inexact because of lack of sensitivity and specificity of commonly utilized tests (table 6.1).

Some physicians believe that loss of internal rotation of the shoulder contributes to symptoms of impingement and rotator cuff tendinitis by creating a "yo-yo" effect of the proximal humerus against the acromion and coracoacromial arch (Ticker et al. 2000). Using a database of patients who underwent shoulder surgery at our institution between 1994 and 2001, we examined the changes in internal rotation of the unaffected shoulder by decade (table 6.2). We found that both active and passive range of motion in internal rotation decreased with age. We also looked at the effects of age on shoulder laxity (table 6.3). Laxity was measured using a modified Hawkins scale (I: to the rim; II: over the rim but reduces; III: locks out) on the

TABLE 6.1 Diagnostic Values of Physical Tests According to the Arthroscopic Observation: Partial Tears and Full Tears

TEST	SENSITIVITY		SPECIFICITY	PPV*		NPV**		DIAGNOSTIC ACCURACY	
	Partial	Full		Partial	Full	Partial	Full	Partial	Full
Neer impingement sign	0.66	0.63	0.46	0.50	0.37	0.63	0.71	0.55	0.52
Hawkins impingement sign	0.72	0.77	0.45	0.51	0.41	0.66	0.79	0.57	0.56
Painful arc sign	0.48	0.71	0.66	0.53	0.66	0.61	0.70	0.58	0.68
Drop arm sign	0.26	0.32	0.81	0.51	0.49	0.58	0.67	0.57	0.62
Acromioclavicular adduction test	0.29	0.28	0.72	0.45	0.37	0.56	0.63	0.53	0.56
Acromioclavicular extension test	0.26	0.25	0.81	0.52	0.56	0.58	0.53	0.57	0.53
Speed's test	0.36	0.37	0.75	0.53	0.44	0.60	0.69	0.58	0.62
Apprehension test	0.16	0.05	0.67	0.27	0.07	0.50	0.58	0.44	0.46
Relocation test	0.23	0.18	0.70	0.41	0.36	0.50	0.47	0.48	0.45
Compression rotation test	0.30	0.21	0.76	0.51	0.45	0.57	0.50	0.55	0.49
Anterior slide test	0.15	0.12	0.82	0.42	0.33	0.52	0.56	0.51	0.52
Active compression test	0.49	0.61	0.64	0.54	0.55	0.59	0.69	0.57	0.63

* PPV = positive predictive value.

** NPV = negative predictive value.

TABLE 6.2 Changes in Internal Rotation of the Unaffected Shoulder by Decade

	RANGE OF MOTION (SD)	
Age in years (N)	Active internal rotation	Passive internal rotation
1-20 (68)	52 (27.4)	60 (23.4)
21-30 (76)	51 (27.2)	58 (23.1)
31-40 (84)	43 (26.5)	52 (25.7)
41-50 (111)	46 (27.7)	51 (24.3)
51-60 (119)	42 (26.6)	51 (23.3)
61-70 (90)	43 (30.6)	51 (26.7)
>70 (51)	34 (27.8)	41 (29.3)
Total (608)	45 (28.0)	52 (25.1)

TABLE 6.3 Changes in the Results of Laxity Testing by Decade

Age in years (N)	ANTERIOR TRANSLATION (%)			POSTERIOR TRANSLATION (%)			SULCUS SIGN (%)		
	Grade I	Grade II	Grade III	Grade I	Grade II	Grade III	Grade I	Grade II	Grade III
1-20 (75)	5 (7)	68 (91)	2 (3)	15 (20)	58 (77)	2 (3)	26 (35)	48 (64)	1 (1)
21-30 (93)	12 (13)	79 (85)	2(2)	18 (19)	72 (77)	3 (3)	59 (63)	27 (29)	7 (8)
31-40 (100)	22 (22)	76 (76)	2 (2)	34 (34)	66 (66)	0	68 (68)	31 (31)	1 (1)
41-50 (126)	38 (30)	87 (69)	1 (1)	57 (45)	68 (54)	1 (1)	98 (78)	25 (20)	3 (2)
51-60 (120)	23 (19)	97 (81)	0	57 (48)	63 (53)		89 (74)	29 (24)	2 (2)
61-70 (87)	28 (32)	59 (68)	0	41 (47)	46 (53)		71 (82)	14 (16)	2 (2)
>70 (38)	9 (24)	29 (76)	0	12 (32)	26 (68)		24 (63)	14 (37)	0
Total (639)	134 (21)	495 (77)	7 (1)	234 (37)	399 (62)	6 (1)	435 (68)	188 (29)	16 (3)

unaffected shoulder (Hawkins and Mohtadi 1991). We found that in all three planes (anterior, posterior, and inferior), the proportion of lower-grade translations increased over the 60s. Since there was no control group, the conclusions of our study are limited, but they do substantiate that decreasing internal rotation appears to be associated with rotator cuff pathology of aging.

Patients who tear their rotator cuff with trauma often have preexisting tendon tearing or degeneration that predisposes them to further injury. This explains the common history of a patient who has a trivial injury, such as one caused by putting on a coat or opening a door, that completes or extends the rotator cuff tear to the point that it becomes symptomatic. The shoulder may become inflamed if it is used too much or used for activities that the patient typically does not perform regularly. This explains why some patients who have rotator cuff tears present with insidious onset of pain with no trauma. In these instances the cuff tear was an attritional tear and not due to an acute traumatic event.

Degenerative changes in the acromioclavicular (AC) joint are also very common with increasing age (Bonsell et al. 2000; Keyes 1935). Recent MRI studies demonstrate that degenerative changes begin in the third decade and can affect up to 93% of shoulders over the fourth decade (Stein et al. 2001). Most of these degenerative AC joints are not symptomatic, and they do not warrant treatment. Also, degenerative arthritis of the glenohumeral joint occurs with increasing age, but it is not as predictable and inevitable as rotator cuff and AC joint degeneration.

Evaluation

Certain principles of orthopedic evaluation are constant regardless of age of the patient. However, as patients mature there is a greater possibility that chronic diseases or previous injuries will influence the shoulder joint.

History

The history of any patient should always include a history of other diseases, particularly a history of cancer. Neer in 1983 suggested that the main two differential diagnoses for rotator cuff tendinitis in the patient over 40 were cervical spine disease and cancer (Neer 1983).

A history of osteoarthritis in other joints or of rheumatological conditions such as rheumatoid disease, polymyalgia rheumatica, scleroderma, or ankylosing spondylitis should be obtained. A history of Crohn's disease, ulcerative colitis, psoriasis, and oral use of steroids should be ascertained since these can cause joint symptoms in the older individual. A history of osteoporosis, treatment for osteoporosis, or frequent fractures should be obtained. Since many conditions of the musculoskeletal system can be treated with anti-inflammatory agents, it is important to inquire about the use of anti-coagulants, a history of peptic ulcer disease or bleeding ulcers, and a history of renal disease or liver dysfunction. In patients who complain of weakness, we consider that symptom a neurological complaint and inquire about headaches, visual changes, dizziness, paresthesias, or weakness in other extremities. Parasthesias indicate nerve dysfunction, and careful questioning about the cervical spine is recommended. We utilize a general health questionnaire for all new patients in order to elucidate a more complete medical history.

Physical Examination

The examination of most musculoskeletal conditions should be guided by several basic principles, as shown in "Basic Shoulder Examinations." First, it is important to have the patient undressed in order to examine for atrophy or deformity. Subtle atrophy in the infraspinatus or supraspinatus fossa, which can be an important sign of long-standing rotator cuff disease or of occult nerve injury, cannot be seen in a clothed individual. Second, it is important to compare sides. This is not easy to do in female patients, since most offices do not have specialized gowns that allow visualization of both shoulders; and we recommend at a minimum placing the gown below the shoulder level (figure 6.2). Range of motion, strength, sensation, and reflex testing should be compared from side to side.

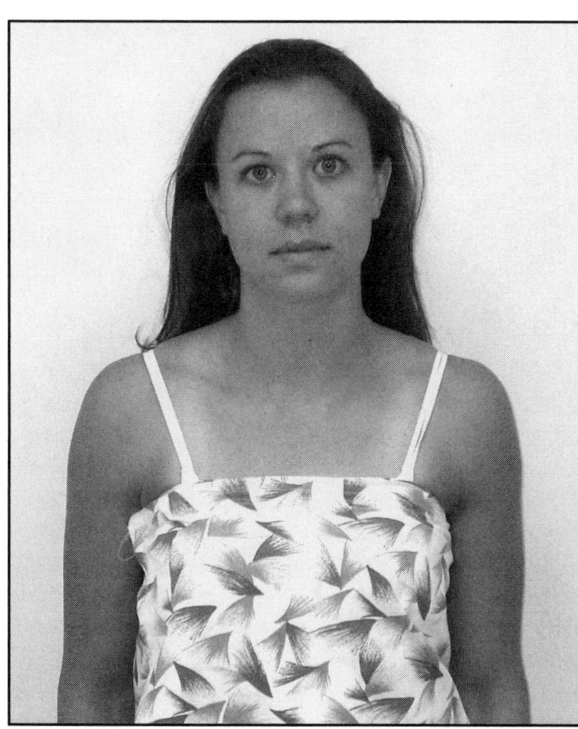

FIGURE 6.2 Specialized gown that allows visualization of both shoulders.

Basic Shoulder Examinations

- Observation
- Range of motion
  1. Elevation: normal range (170°-180°)
  2. External rotation at 90°: normal range (80°-90°)
  3. Internal rotation at 90°: normal range (50°-80°)
  4. External rotation arm at side: normal range (40°-70°)
  5. Internal rotation up back: normal range (T5-T10)
- Strength testing
- Tenderness
- Reflexes
- Provocative maneuvers
  1. AC joint
     - Crossed arm adduction
     - Active extension test
     - Active compression test
     - Local tenderness
  2. Impingement/Tendinitis
     - Neer impingement sign
     - Hawkins impingement sign
     - Speed's test
     - Coracoid impingement sign
  3. Instability signs
     - Anterior apprehension sign
     - Posterior apprehension sign
     - Increased external rotation sign
     - Sulcus sign
     - Relocation test
  4. Laxity signs
     - Anterior and posterior drawer
     - Load and shift test
     - Sulcus sign
  5. Superior labrum anterior and posterior lesion signs
     - Speed's test
     - Compression rotation
     - Active compression
     - Anterior slide test
     - Biceps load test II

The third principle is to examine the joint above and below the injured area. For the shoulder, the joint proximal is the cervical spine. The incidence of degenerative joint disease of the cervical spine increases linearly with age (ten Have and Eulderink 1981). As a result, pain that radiates from the neck down the arm or pain along the medial border of the scapula should be considered as possibly coming from the cervical spine. The next principle is to consider performing a neurological examination of the upper extremity when examining the shoulder. This helps to rule out more serious neurological causes of the pain or shoulder dysfunction and allows the proper diagnostic tests and treatments to be ordered.

Imaging

Lastly, radiographs of the shoulder should be ordered with regularity in the more mature patient to rule out conditions that might be contributing to the patient's complaints. In the more mature patient with chronic conditions, radiographs help to tell you not only what conditions are present but also what conditions are not present. Most orthopedists recommend radiographs in two views or directions, with the most common combination an anteroposterior radiograph and an axillary radiograph (Bateman 1978; Brewer 1979; DePalma 1983; McLaughlin 1952; Neer 1970; Neviaser 1987; Post 1978; Rowe 1988). A scapular "Y" view may be helpful in the acute traumatic cases seen in emergency rooms, but in the office setting an axillary view will give more information (figure 6.3*a*). In our office we use two techniques for obtaining this radiograph (figure 6.3, *b* and *c*). In patients with a history of cancer or with pain that is increasing, waking them up at night, or requiring increasing amounts of medication, we recommend repeat radiographs within 6 to 12 weeks.

Other special views may be obtained to evaluate the shoulder depending on the clinical situation. In patients with AC joint symptoms we recommend AC spot views that allow comparison of both AC joints (Demicis et al. 2000) (figure 6.4). This radiograph is performed by angling the radiographic beam down 20° as described by Zanca (1971). This radiograph is also beneficial when more detail is needed of the distal clavicle, such as in evaluation of distal clavicle fractures.

A modified scapular "Y" view is advocated by some physicians for evaluating the presence and size of the spurs on the anterior acromion. The exact role of acromial spurs in the generation of rotator cuff tendon pathologies is controversial. Neer believed that the spur was a cause of rotator cuff pathology and recommended partial acromioplasty to remove

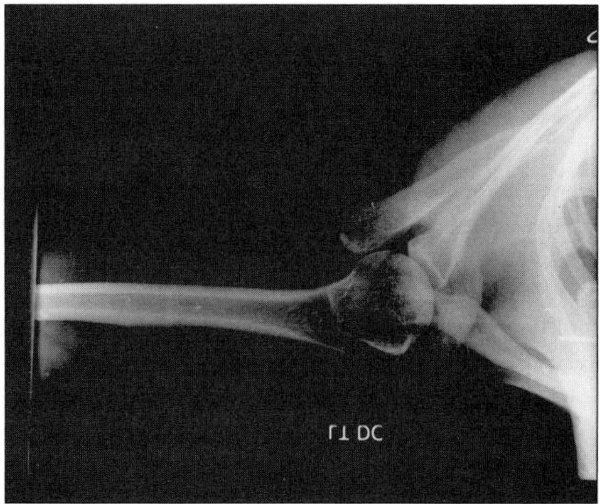

a

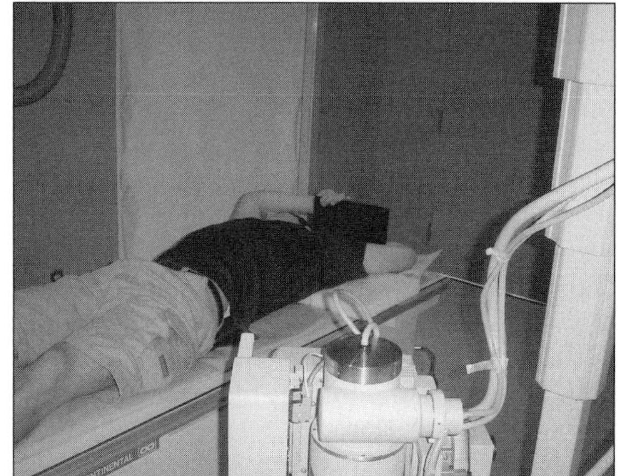

b

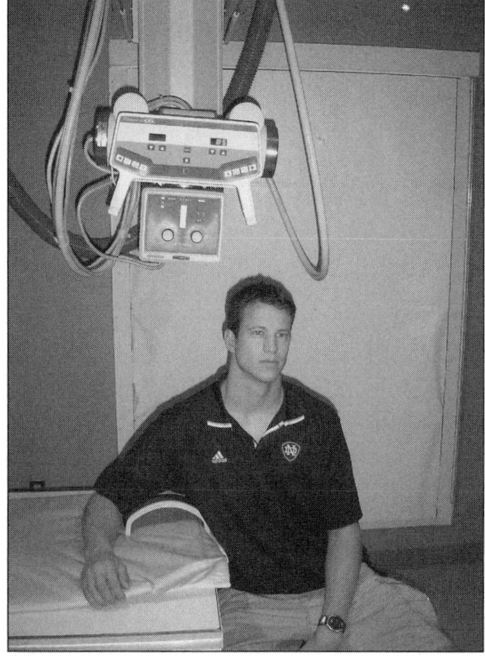

c

FIGURE 6.3 *(a)* An axillary lateral view, *(b)* the axillary lateral view obtained as the arm is abducted 70° to 90°, *(c)* modified technique for axillary lateral view.

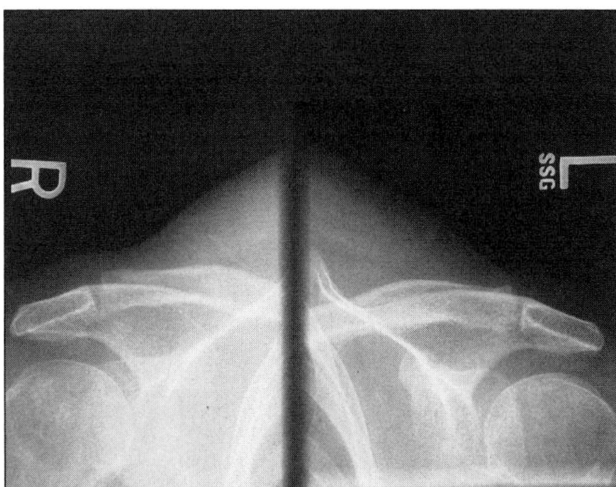

FIGURE 6.4 The acromioclavicular spot view.

the spur (Neer 1972). Bigliani and colleagues (Bigliani et al. 1986) used the modified scapular "Y" view to describe three acromial shapes (figure 6.5). They found an association of type III acromial shape with the presence of full-thickness rotator cuff disease. The association of increasing type III acromial morphology and rotator cuff tearing has been noted in many studies (Toivonen et al. 1995; Tuite et al. 1995). However, while there is an association between these entities with chronological age, a causal relationship between acromial spurs and rotator cuff tears has not been convincingly demonstrated. Also, there is increasing appreciation that the acromion and coracoacromial ligament serve to prevent superior migration and subluxation of the humeral head (Flatow et al. 1997; Lee et al. 2001). Consequently, the presence of spurs on the acromion is not necessarily an indication for an operation, and in some instances the acromial spurs should not be removed.

The decision to obtain further studies depends on the clinical situation. However, it is generally not the standard of care to order MRI or other studies prior to plain radiographs. For example, MRI should be performed judiciously only after careful consideration of the plain radiographs. A chest radiograph is indicated for scapular or thorax wall pain. In patients with a history of cancer, a bone scan may be indicated if the pain is atypical or if multiple sites of pain need to be evaluated.

In the acute situation in which a patient has sustained an injury, we typically order plain radiographs to rule out fractures. If the radiographs are negative, then the clinical examination and other factors determine the timing and choice of the next test. In patients who have severe pain and inability to use the arm after a period of symptomatic treatment, an MRI is the single best test to evaluate the rotator cuff and to detect occult fractures. However, the limits of MRI in the older patient must clearly be understood, as will be discussed further in the next section. In the mature patient, contusions of the greater tuberosity and occult fractures can be discovered when the plain radiographs are normal. In patients who have profound weakness after an injury, particularly with inability to lift the arm

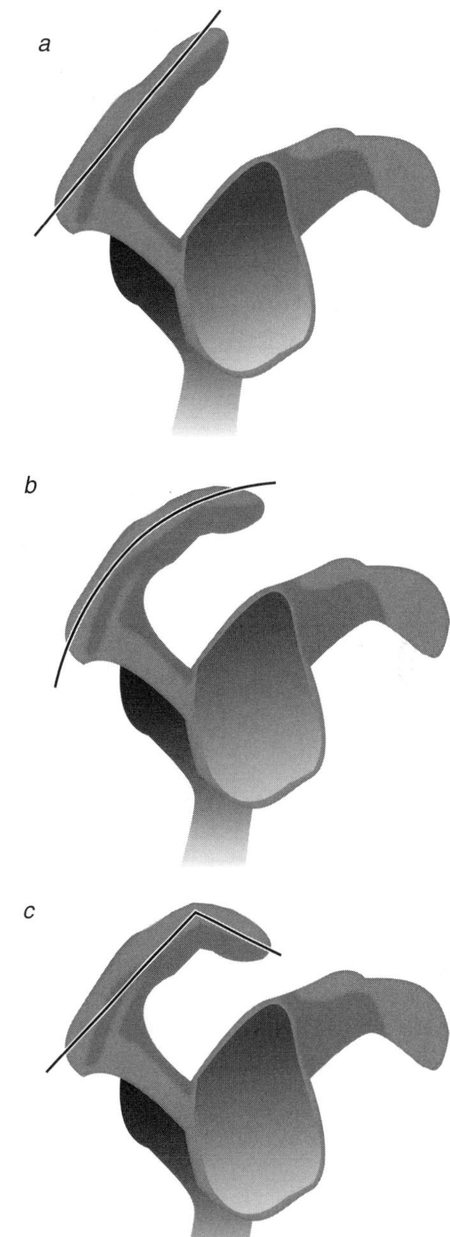

FIGURE 6.5 Bigliani et al. (1986) used the modified scapular "Y" view to describe three acromial shapes: *(a)* type I, flat; *(b)* type II, curved; *(c)* type III, hooked.

Reprinted, by permission, from L.U. Bigliani, D.S. Morrison, E.W. April, 1986, "The morphology of the acromion and rotator cuff impingement," *Orthopaedic Transactions* 10: 288.

or hold it elevated against gravity (called a "drop arm test"), an MRI is recommended within the first few weeks to evaluate whether more than one tendon has been torn (Yocum and Conway 1996). Arthrograms can be utilized in some instances in which the only concern is the status of the rotator cuff, but in general more information can be obtained from an MRI than with an arthrogram. Magnetic resonance images have the advantages of providing a more thorough evaluation of the size, extent, and number of tendon tears in the shoulder. They may detect either benign or malignant masses that would not be seen with arthrograms. Magnetic resonance images also allow the evaluation of intra-articular structures better than arthrograms. In instances in which the patient is having less pain and improving with treatment, further studies can be withheld until the clinical progress becomes clarified. The diagnostic values of MRI for full-thickness rotator cuff tear are summarized in table 6.4.

An imaging modality that has recently received more attention for the evaluation of rotator cuff disease is ultrasound (Teefey et al. 1999, 2000). The sensitivity and specificity have been reported to range between 57% and 100% and between 63.2% and 100%, respectively. The positive predictive value, the negative predictive value, and the accuracy have been reported to range between 82% and 100%, between 75% and 97%, and between 73% and 96%, respectively (Brandt et al. 1989; Brenneke and Morgan 1992; Drakeford et al. 1990; Mack et al. 1985; Martin-Hervas et al. 2001; Olive and Marsh 1992; Paavolainen and Ahovuo 1994; Pattee and Snyder 1998; Roberts et al. 2002; Swen et al. 1999; Teefey 2000; Vick and Bell 1990; Wallny et al. 1999) (table 6.5). The advantages of ultrasound are that it can be performed in the office and is not invasive. The disadvantages are that the reading of the scan depends on the experience of the examiner, that only the supraspinatus can be reliably imaged, and that other pathologies such as cysts or bone lesions cannot be assessed easily (Allen and Wilson 2001; Roberts et al. 2002).

ACUTE INJURIES

In the mature patient who has acute onset of shoulder problems with trauma, the most frequent diagnosis is a fracture of some portion of the shoulder girdle. The mechanism of injury is important since most fractures occur with a fall directly on the shoulder or an outstretched arm. An injury in abduction and external rotation can cause a fracture, a fracture-dislocation, or a rotator cuff injury.

Evaluation

In patients seen after an acute injury, a careful examination should be done to rule out any neurological injuries, since the incidence of nerve injury with fractures or dislocations of the shoulder increases

TABLE 6.4 Diagnostic Value of Magnetic Resonance Imaging Examination for Full-Thickness Rotator Cuff Tear

Study	Sensitivity	Specificity	NPV	PPV	Accuracy
Martin-Hervás et al. 2001	80.8%	97.1%	87.2%	95.5%	NS
Swen et al. 1999	81%	88%	74%	91%	83%
Sahin-Akyar et al. 1998	83-100%	NS	NS	NS	NS
Hirano et al. 1998	100%	76.9%	NS	NS	89.2%
Balich et al. 1997	84-96%	94-98%	NS	NS	92-97%
Bachmann et al. 1997	NS	100%	NS	NS	NS
Singson et al. 1996	100%	86%	NS	NS	NS
Quinn et al. 1995	84%	97%	NS	NS	93%
Iannoti et al. 1991	100%	95%	100%	92%	NS
Zlatkin et al. 1989	91%	88%	NS	NS	NS
Evancho et al. 1988	80%	94%	NS	NS	89%

NPV = negative predictive value.
PPV = positive predictive value.

TABLE 6.5 Diagnostic Value of Ultrasound Examination for Full-Size Rotator Cuff Tear

Study	Sensitivity	Specificity	NPV	PPV	Accuracy
Roberts et al. 2001	80%	100%	88%	100%	NS
Martin-Hervás et al. 2001	57.7%	100%	76.1%	100%	NS
Teefey et al. 2000	100%	85%	NS	NS	96%
Wallny et al. 1999	97.8%	63.2%	92.4%	86.3%	NS
Swen et al. 1999	81%	94%	77%	96%	86%
Read and Perko 1998	100%	97%	NS	NS	NS
Paavolainen and Ahovuo 1994	74%	95%	75%	95%	84%
Brenneke and Morgan 1992	95%	93%	NS	NS	NS
Olive and Marsh 1992	90%	91%	93%	87%	NS
Vick and Bell 1990	67%	93%	NS	NS	85%
Drakeford et al. 1990	92%	95%	97%	85%	NS
Brandt et al. 1989	57%	76%	NS	NS	NS
Pattee and Snyder 1988	77%	65%	NS	82%	73%
Mack et al. 1988	91%	98%	NS	NS	95%
Furtschegger and Resch 1988	91%	NS	NS	NS	NS

NPV = negative predictive value.
PPV = positive predictive value.

with increasing age (de Laat et al. 1994). Patients with fractures should be evaluated by an orthopedic surgeon or by health care professionals familiar with the care of these injuries. Patients with nerve injuries to the upper extremity after trauma should be carefully evaluated for cervical spine injuries as a cause of the symptoms. Further neurological evaluation should be sought as needed, depending on the clinical situation. Any suggestion of vascular injury or deep venous thrombosis should be immediately evaluated with consultation with experts in those fields.

Treatment and Pain Control

In patients with negative radiographs it is important to begin symptomatic treatment right away. This treatment includes application of ice to the shoulder for 20 to 30 min, which can occur as frequently as every 2 h. We usually recommend application of ice at least twice a day until the pain is gone or until the patient is reevaluated. Early range of motion of the elbow, wrist, and fingers should begin as soon as possible. In patients without fractures, pendulum exercises of the shoulder should begin as soon as the pain allows. A sling or support for a few days or a week may be indicated, but it should be removed once or twice a day so that the patient can perform pendulum exercises. One concern with long-term sling use is the development of a frozen shoulder.

Analgesics should be prescribed based on the degree of pain and discomfort. Acetaminophen with or without codeine, synthetic narcotics, or non-narcotic pain relievers (e.g., Ultram: tramadol hydrochloride, Ortho-McNeil, Raritan, NJ) can be prescribed for a short duration. However, increasing or prolonged use of narcotic pain medication is an indication for reevaluation of the patient. Nonsteroidal anti-inflammatory drugs (NSAIDs) can be used instead of or in conjunction with pain medication, but the patient must be carefully questioned about previous use of these NSAIDs and about risk factors for their use.

Physical therapy for a brief time should be considered to show the patient a range of motion program that he or she can perform at home. However, a physical therapy assessment should not be prescribed without a tentative or definitive diagnosis, which will allow the therapist and patient a clearer idea of the goals of the program.

Reevaluation

We typically reevaluate a patient with a shoulder injury and negative radiographs within 7 to 21 days. If the patient is not recovering at that time, then a decision should be made about further imaging studies or referral to other health care specialists. While there are no absolute rules about who should be referred, several general recommendations are appropriate. First, the patient should be having improvement in motion and strength with lessening of the pain. If the patient is progressing well and not showing signs of stiffness or weakness, then repeat follow-up takes place a few weeks later. If the patient has continued weakness, particularly in elevation of the arm or with resisted external rotation, then one should consider a nerve injury or a rotator cuff injury and either an MRI or referral.

The importance of frequent reevaluation of the patient cannot be overestimated. The patient should be making steady progress with resolution of symptoms over time. A gradual return of motion, strength, and function should occur over a six- to eight-week period. If the patient is not improving, then further studies or referral to other health care specialists should be considered.

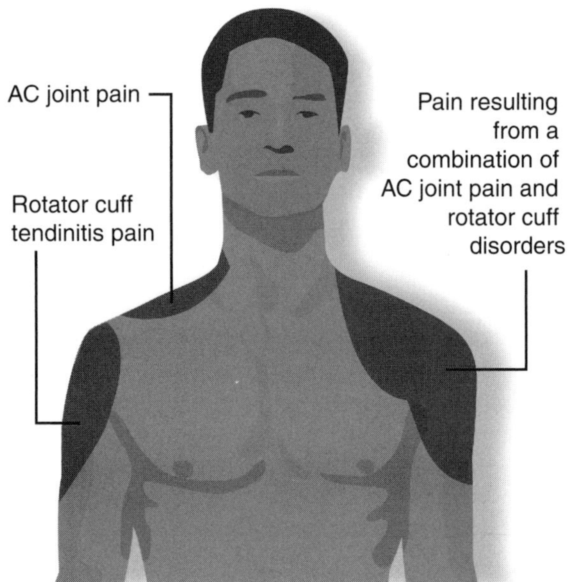

FIGURE 6.6 A patient experiencing acromioclavicular joint problems will most likely point directly to the joint when asked to identify the source of pain, whereas rotator cuff pain typically occurs in the deltoid lesion. These disorders can exist independently, as on the left side of the figure, or can coexist, resulting in a wider distribution of pain as shown on the right side of the figure.

ROTATOR CUFF INJURIES

The most common shoulder condition seen in active, older individuals is rotator cuff problems. The pain and loss of function can begin insidiously with no obvious inciting event, or it may be associated with an increase of activity or with beginning a new activity. Sometimes severe or even trivial trauma can initiate an inflammatory process in the rotator cuff. The first symptoms are typically pain into the deltoid region or into the mid-arm area. This distinguishes rotator cuff problems from AC joint pain, which usually is on the top of the shoulder (figure 6.6). The pain can radiate down the arm and can cause aching of the entire upper extremity. Often the pain waxes and wanes for no apparent good reason, or it may be increased by activities over shoulder level or with use of the extremity. Pain at rest and pain that awakens the patient from sleep are considered bad signs and warrant more aggressive evaluation and treatment.

Other factors can contribute to the development and propagation of rotator cuff dysfunction. These include chronic deconditioning due to favoring or disuse of the extremity. The patient may develop secondary scapular dysfunction and acquire motions that reinforce the pathological conditions (see chapter 3, "The Kinetic Chain"). It is not uncommon for patients who favor one extremity to develop symptoms in the other shoulder due to overuse and overcompensation for the involved extremity.

Evaluation and Treatment

Unfortunately there is no cookbook approach to the patient with shoulder pain. One must consider several variables when making a diagnosis, when deciding on imaging, and when deciding on treatment. These variables include the onset of the pain, the severity of the pain and loss of function, the dominance of the extremity, the health of the patient, and the need of the patient to recover quickly or less urgently. One must also add the findings upon physical examination to the equation when deciding on the next step of evaluation and treatment. Many of these factors are interrelated, and the treating health care provider must consider them carefully.

The most important historical factor is whether the pain began with trauma or not. Insidious onset of pain indicates a more chronic condition and suggests that the symptoms are due in part to age-related changes in the tendon. Patients with a traumatic cause of their symptoms typically warrant earlier studies than patients with insidious onset of pain.

The decision to obtain imaging studies early in the evaluation and treatment depends on multiple factors.

In patients who have weakness in abduction or external rotation, or who are not able to raise the arm after trauma, it is necessary to consider an MRI to evaluate the rotator cuff status. Occasionally we have Senior Olympic-level athletes who need an answer sooner than usual to help make decisions about participation in competitions and to plan their sport training.

Nonoperative Measures

If the patient is having only intermittent symptoms, then treatment should be symptomatic. Patients with rotator cuff tendinitis should moderate the activities that worsen the pain within the limits of their abilities and what they want to do. This is no different from the approach to younger active people. For pain, acetaminophen or NSAIDs are recommended for six to eight weeks. These should be taken daily. Application of ice packs directly to the shoulder daily, particularly after activity, should take place for six to eight weeks. For more severe symptoms we recommend ice pack three or four times a day and before bedtime to help the individual sleep. Immobilization is discouraged, and the patient is urged to maintain motion by stretching for 1 to 2 min daily to prevent a frozen shoulder.

Patients can receive a home program of rotator cuff exercises, but they should be counseled that these exercises should not be painful. If the exercises are painful, or if the patient is motivated to get back to a sport activity right away, formal physical therapy can be prescribed. However, for most cases of routine rotator cuff tendinitis, a prolonged course of physical therapy is not recommended unless the other measures fail.

Once these measures fail, the next step depends on the needs of the patient and the severity of the symptoms. In patients with insidious onset of symptoms that are interfering with activities of daily living or preventing activity, the next decision is between performing an MRI and giving the patient a cortisone shot into the subacromial space. In patients with insidious onset of pain who have severe symptoms that awaken them and generally are making them miserable, we may utilize a cortisone shot as the initial therapy. In this instance it is important that the diagnosis be accurate and that the patient be followed closely after the injection. We recommend after a cortisone shot that the patient go back on a routine of stretching, ice, and NSAIDs for another four to eight weeks. While cortisone shots for this condition were once commonly accepted, there is some controversy regarding their effectiveness. One study suggested that at three-month follow-up, patients who were injected with local anesthetic alone in the subacromial space had the same clinical success rate as patients who were injected with local anesthetic and cortisone (Vecchio et al. 1993). Most physicians recommend only two cortisone shots before surgical intervention is considered. Surgical intervention should be considered after nonoperative methods have failed and the symptoms are severe enough to warrant the risk of an operative procedure.

Surgery

The biggest dilemma for patients with rotator cuff tears is whether to have surgery or not. The exact natural history for rotator cuff tears that have occurred over time is not known. For example, it is not known if a 1-cm-diameter tear of the rotator cuff will progress into a larger tear; and if it does progress, there is no way to predict the rate at which it might progress. The one study that evaluated attritional rotator cuff tears showed that there was some progression over time (Yamaguchi et al. 2001). Another important variable is the number of tendons torn. If the tear is traumatic and more than one tendon is torn, then early surgery is recommended to repair the tendons. If multiple tendons are torn and the tears appear to be large and attritional, then surgery may not be as successful; and both patient and the surgeon must consider this. In active individuals who are young and want the best result possible, repair of the torn tendons might be indicated; but there is no way to predict the long-term result if no surgery is performed.

Fortunately, surgery for rotator cuff tendon pathology is successful in eliminating pain and returning function to the shoulder. Partial anterior acromioplasty for tendinosis or tendinitis gives good to excellent results in 85% to 90% of patients (Penny and Welsh 1981; Post and Cohen 1986; Tibone et al. 1985). Partial acromioplasty for partial tears of the rotator cuff gives positive results when the tear is less than halfway through the tendon, but when the tear is nearly full thickness partial acromioplasty is best performed with a formal repair of the tendon. Repair of torn rotator cuff tendons is generally a great operation for pain relief and in most cases will return mature patients to their activities. The most important factors in predicting the clinical result of surgery are the size of the tear, its chronicity, and whether more than one tendon is involved (Cofield et al. 2001). Larger tears tend to do less well with surgery than smaller tears. One study demonstrated that 80% of patients who underwent rotator cuff repairs were able to get back to tennis (Bigliani et al. 1992; Sonnery-Cottet et al. 2002). A vast majority of patients who undergo rotator cuff repair can return to their activities of daily living with few symptoms, and their ability to perform in sports generally is good (Bigliani et al. 1992; Sonnery-Cottet et al. 2002). We warn patients that rotator cuff repairs do not make their arms bionic, and that if they return to activity too fast or if they overexercise the shoulder they may still get tendinitis periodically. In instances in which symptoms of tendinitis occur after surgery, the patient is counseled to return to the program outlined earlier: relative rest, cryotherapy, and NSAIDs.

The prognosis for larger tears of the rotator cuff that have been surgically repaired is more guarded (Calvert et al. 2001; Yamaguchi et al. 2001). In their study of open repairs using ultrasound, Calvert et al. (2001) found that 50% of repairs of large to massive cuff tears had retorn. Galatz et al. (2004) found using ultrasound that 94% of massive tears repaired with arthroscopic techniques had failed at one year follow-up. In both of these studies, despite the high re-tear rate, the patient satisfaction rate was still high, which suggests that factors other than an intact rotator cuff tear are involved in the pathogenesis of rotator cuff symptoms.

ACROMIOCLAVICULAR JOINT DISORDERS

The most common condition affecting the AC joint in the maturing athlete is degenerative arthritis. While the incidence of degenerative arthritis increases linearly with age, the presence of symptoms is highly variable (Petersson 1983; Petersson and Redlund-Johnell 1983). As a result, the degenerative changes do not need to be treated unless the joint is symptomatic. The most common symptom of AC joint inflammation is pain, particularly when the arm is placed across the body as in a golf swing. Exercises known to provoke the AC joint include push-ups, dips, and bench press.

Upon examination the patient may or may not have increased swelling over the AC joint compared to the opposite side. Typically the pain radiates into the neck or trapezius region, but sometimes the pain may be difficult to localize (Gerber et al. 1998). Patients who have radiation into the deltoid or down the arm should be examined carefully for signs of rotator cuff problems. However, patients with isolated AC joint problems will point directly to the AC joint, a sign we call the "one-finger test" (figure 6.7). The physical findings for AC joint irritation upon examination are summarized in table 6.6 (Chronopoulos et al. 2004). If there is any doubt about the diagnosis, then an injection of local anesthetic into the joint should eliminate all or most of the pain.

The treatment of AC arthritis includes relative rest, avoidance of the activities that aggravate the shoulder, cryotherapy, and anti-inflammatory medications. Most patients have resolution of their symptoms, or the symptoms may be diminished enough that they can remain functional and active. In some patients cortisone shots into the joint and periarticularly can alleviate the symptoms. One study suggested that 93% of patients obtained relief with cortisone shots for AC joint problems (Jacob and Sallay 1997).

For a majority of patients with continued symptoms, distal clavicle excision produces good results (table 6.7). Indications for surgery include failed non-

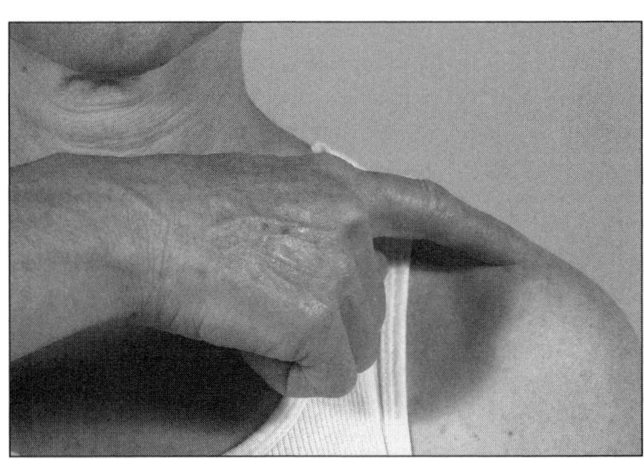

FIGURE 6.7 The one-finger test for AC joint problems.

TABLE 6.6 Physical Examination of Symptomatic AC Joint Patients Who Underwent Resection

Test	Sensitivity	Specificity	PPV	NPV	Diagnostic accuracy
Acromioclavicular (AC) joint tenderness	92% (35/38)	74% (412/557)	19% (35/180)	99% (412/415)	75% (447/595)
AC adduction test	76% (29/38)	79% (410/518)	21% (29/137)	98% (410/419)	79% (439/556)
AC extension test	80% (16/20)	85% (279/330)	24% (16/67)	99% (279/283)	84% (295/350)
Active compression test	47% (9/19)	95% (291/308)	35% (9/26)	97% (291/301)	92% (300/327)

PPV = positive predictive value.

NPV = negative predictive value.

Adapted, by permission, from Chronopoulos, E., T.K. Kim, H.B. Park, D. Ashenbrenner, E.G. McFarland, 2004, "Diagnostic value of physical tests for isolated chronic acromioclavicular lesions." *American Journal of Sports Medicine* 32(3): 655-661.

TABLE 6.7 Review of the Results of Isolated Distal Clavicle Excision

OPEN PROCEDURES			
Study	**Cases**	**Follow-up (years)**	**Results**
McFarland et al. 2002	41	1.9	83%
Blazar et al. 1998	8	2.7	NS*
Gurbuz 1998	11	1.1	100%
Jacob and Sallay 1997	27	NS*	NS*
Eskola et al. 1996	73	9	69%
Novac et al. 1995	21	2.7	78%
Petchel et al. 1995	18	3	72%
Bassett 1994	40	27	100%
Slawski et al. 1994	17	2.5	100%
Flatow et al. 1992	6	2.5	100%
Worland 1992	38	3.4	70%
Cook and Tibone 1988	23	3.7	96%
Scavenius et al. 1987	5	NS*	80%
Peterson et al. 1983	50	7	62%
Cahil 1982	21	>2	74%
Worchester 1968	56	4.5	100%
Sage and Salvatore 1963	13	26.3 weeks	84.6%
Wagner 1953	22	8	91%
ARTHROSCOPIC PROCEDURES			
Study	**Cases**	**Follow-up (yr)**	**Results**
Zawadsky et al. 2000	41	6.2	92.7%
Blazar et al. 1998	9	2.7	NS*
Auge et al. 1998	10	1.6	100%
Flatow et al. 1995	41	2.6	83%
Snyder et al. 1995	50	2	94%
Kay et al. 1994	10	1.6	100%
Tolin et al. 1994	23	1.5	87%
Jerosch et al. 1993	65	0.5	86%
Gartsman et al. 1993	20	2	85%
Flatow et al. 1992	4	1.5	100%

*NS = not stated.

operative treatment with continued pain that affects activities of daily living or prevents the patient from being active in sport or other avocations. Distal clavicle excision routinely in patients undergoing surgery for rotator cuff problems is generally not warranted. The role of the AC joint in the generation of rotator cuff pathology is controversial, but the added morbidity of distal clavicle excision is not necessary in rotator cuff repairs or acromioplasties unless the patient is symptomatic at the AC joint.

BICEPS TENDON RUPTURES AND TENDINITIS

The proximal end of the biceps muscle turns into a tendon about the size of a pencil that runs through a small area of the rotator cuff tendon into the glenohumeral joint (figure 6.8). Once inside the joint it attaches to the top of the glenoid. In more mature individuals, the biceps tendon can become frayed and painful.

The exact etiology of biceps tendonitis and tearing is not known, but it is known that it frequently accompanies rotator cuff problems (Neer 1983; Slatis and Aalto 1979; Walch et al. 1998). Some physicians suggest that biceps lesions are in part due to disruptions of the ligamentous "pulley" system that guides the biceps in the groove near its entrance into the joint (Bennett 2001; Gerber and Sebesta 2000; Walch et al. 1998). However, there are several difficulties with this concept. First, the pain distribution of isolated biceps pathology is not unique to the biceps tendon, and since biceps tendon pathology frequently coexists with rotator cuff disease, it is difficult to verify the role of the biceps pathology in producing pain. Secondly, while there have been tests upon physical examination that supposedly diagnose biceps tendinitis, these tests have not been validated as actually producing pain from the biceps. For example, Speed's test has been considered pathognomonic for biceps pathology, but it has never been validated (figure 6.9). However, in our study of these superior labrum lesions (also known as SLAP or superior labrum anterior and posterior lesions), we found that Speed's test had a 28% sensitivity and 72% specificity for biceps tendon lesions. Lastly, imaging studies of biceps pathology tend to have a low sensitivity. Even gadolinium arthrogram MRI of the shoulder may miss a large percentage of biceps pathologies, and arthroscopic evaluation of the shoulder remains the gold standard for detecting partial tears or detachments of the biceps.

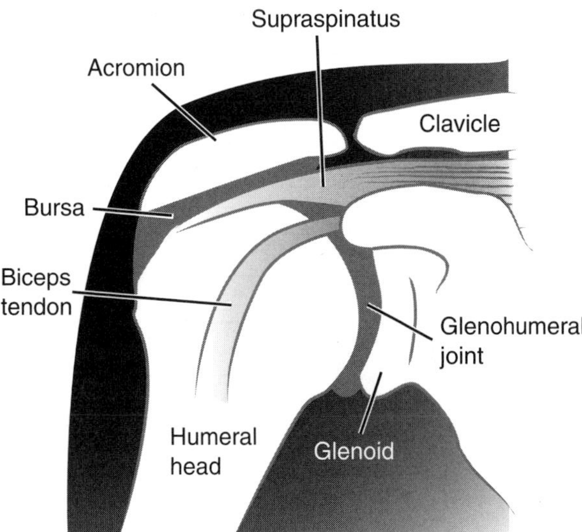

FIGURE 6.8 The proximal end of the biceps muscle turns into a tendon about the size of a pencil that runs through a small area of the rotator cuff tendon into the glenohumeral joint.

Conservative Treatment

Clinically biceps tendinitis is treated like rotator cuff tendinitis with rest, ice, and pain relievers. We do not recommend injections into the biceps tendon directly but rather injecting the subacromial space, since it is congruent with the biceps sheath.

Occasionally the biceps tendon will rupture, and often the patient will not have had any prodromal symptoms at all. When the tendon ruptures, there is a characteristic "Popeye arm" due to the tendon and muscle balling up in the anterior arm. The initial treatment of a biceps tendon rupture is symptomatic, with ice, range of motion, and acetaminophen or NSAIDs. Most people recover within three weeks and can resume their normal activities. There are almost no long-term sequelae of this injury, and rarely is there

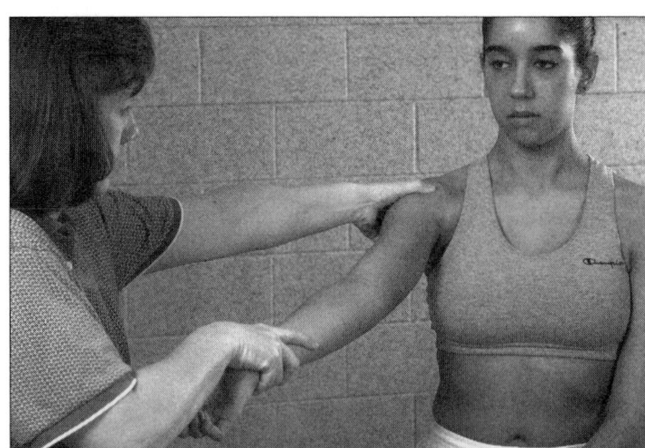

FIGURE 6.9 Speed's test.

any noticeable loss of strength at the shoulder. As a result, surgery is almost never indicated for biceps tendon ruptures. Rarely a patient considers surgery because of the cosmetic appearance, but this means trading a bump on the arm for a scar.

Surgical Treatment

Release of the biceps tendon at its attachment to the superior glenoid, also called biceps tenolysis, is a controversial treatment for biceps-related pathologies. The rationale for the release of the tendon is based on the observation that rupture of the biceps tendon often relieves shoulder pain in some patients. Walch et al. (1997) recommend biceps tenolysis in patients with anterior shoulder pain who have biceps tendon partial tearing and fraying observed at the time of arthroscopy. Biceps tenolysis was also recommended in patients with irreparable rotator cuff tears with pain. Gill et al. (2001) reported that pain relief could be accomplished in 96.7% of patients with biceps tenotomy. Another option for biceps tendon pathology is biceps tenodesis, which can be performed either open or arthroscopically. This should be considered in patients who would not favor the cosmetic deformity produced by biceps tenotomy.

STIFF AND FROZEN SHOULDERS

The concepts of the stiff and frozen shoulder are currently in transition. Some physicians suggest that idiopathic frozen shoulder is a distinct clinical entity that should be distinguished from other causes of a stiff shoulder, such as a fracture or after a surgical procedure (Beaufils et al. 1999; Nobuhara 1990; Warner 1997).

Etiology

It is important to recognize that in the mature active person, loss of motion can have many causes. The most common cause is post-injury immobilization, either due to the patient's reluctance to move the shoulder or due to health practitioners who instruct the patient to not move the joint. Consequently, except in those with fractures, most patients should be encouraged to begin immediate range of motion of their elbow, wrist, and fingers. They also should be encouraged to begin pendulum exercise (figure 6.10). Leaning over at the waist minimizes compressive forces, taking a substantial amount of stress off the shoulder so that the motion is much less painful. As the pain subsides, active motion in every direction and rotation can be performed as tolerated.

In patients who present with insidious onset of loss of range of motion without any trauma, the two most common causes are rotator cuff dysfunction and idiopathic frozen shoulder. The impulse of most patients when they have pain in the shoulder is to not move it, and the most common cause of pain in the shoulder of older patients is rotator cuff disease. It is important to do a good history and examination to rule out more serious causes of the pain. All patients with loss of motion should have plain radiographs as part of their initial evaluation. In these patients we typically do not order MRIs or other tests if the neurological examination is normal and if they have no history of trauma, cancer, or oral corticosteroid use. If the patient has signs of rotator cuff problems, we recommend treating the cuff problems as outlined previously.

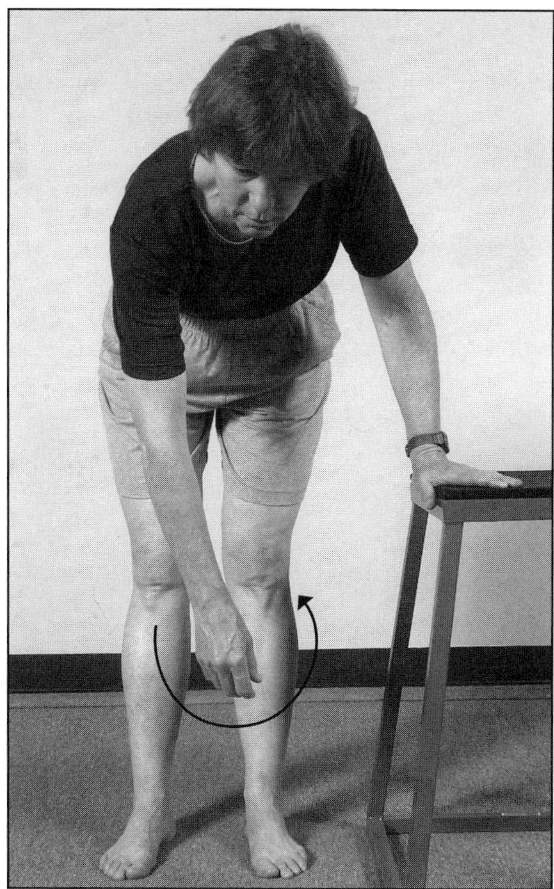

FIGURE 6.10 Pendulum exercise.

Idiopathic frozen shoulder tends to occur more frequently in females than males, and it is more common in people with diabetes than in the general population (Jando and Hawkins 1993; Ogilvie-Harris and Myerthall 1997; Warner 1997). While the exact etiology of this condition is unknown, at the time of arthroscopy these patients have a tremendous and florid synovitis. Synovial biopsies have shown intense vasculitis without any specific inflammatory changes and minimal papillary infolding without hyperplasia (Bunker and Anthony 1995; Wiley 1991).

Idiopathic frozen shoulder tends to be worse and more recalcitrant to treatment in people with diabetes, and some physicians consider it an organ manifestation of this disease like retinopathy or nephropathy.

Treatment Options

The recommended treatment of the stiff shoulder remains controversial because few controlled and randomized studies address this topic (Chambler and Carr 2003). Some have suggested that no treatment is necessary since the condition will spontaneously resolve in 12 to 18 months. However, most patients have symptoms requiring treatment, particularly pain and loss of motion that affects their daily living. Active patients often request treatment so that they can return to their sports and exercises.

Conservative Treatment

The protocol for the initial treatment of a stiff shoulder is similar to the techniques for treating rotator cuff tendinitis. It is difficult for an individual to move a painful shoulder, so the most important treatment goal is to decrease and hopefully eliminate the pain. The use of pain medication like acetaminophen or even a low-level narcotic, such as acetaminophen with codeine, is recommended for two reasons. First, it can help the patient sleep. Secondly, it can be used before or after stretching, and our philosophy is that patients should have some pain medication to take if the shoulder is sore so that they do not develop an aversion to stretching. Similarly, we recommend heat before stretching and ice afterward. Frequent application of ice helps to decrease pain and inflammation, and we recommend that it can occur several times a day and before bedtime. Nonsteroidal anti-inflammatory drugs are helpful in decreasing pain and do not tend to make patients drowsy, and we recommend them daily for three to six months or until the patient has full range of motion.

Physical therapy can be helpful in the management of the patient with a stiff shoulder. In some selected cases we show a patient a simple stretching program in the office, but in most instances we send the patient to a physical therapist for at least two visits to be taught a motion program. This should consist of primarily a stretching program with minimal strengthening. We feel that the patients benefit from spending more time stretching than from trying to get strong. With patients who are not making progress, who are not self-motivated, or who have severe loss of motion (namely elevation below 90°), we typically send them to therapy twice a week for several months. It is important that the therapists spend time stretching the patient manually and not spend inordinate time or money on modalities or machinery. This condition is improved by old-fashioned manual therapy, and the patients should be treated accordingly.

Second Level of Treatment

In patients who are not responding to this protocol after six to eight weeks, we carefully reconsider the diagnosis and do a careful examination. If there are any concerns, further imaging may be necessary. In patients with symptoms of rotator cuff pathology, a subacromial cortisone shot might be indicated. One of the diagnostic signs of a frozen or stiff shoulder is the lack of response to a cortisone shot in the subacromial space. The reason is that the inflamed synovium is inside the joint and the shot in the subacromial space will not communicate with the joint. Intra-articular injections of corticosteroids can provide relief, but they should be given under sterile technique and only by individuals who are familiar with the technique. Injection through a posterior approach with a spinal needle is recommended. Lastly, we have found oral steroids very effective for people who are not responding to the program just outlined. We typically recommend a cortisone taper, available commercially, that takes five to seven days. If it is helpful, we recommend a second pack within one to two weeks. Oral cortisone should be used with caution in patients with type 1 diabetes mellitus or ongoing sepsis or in those who are immunosuppressed.

Patients need to realize that nonoperative therapy should continue sometimes for six to nine months, and a vast majority of patients will not need surgery.

Surgical Treatment

In patients who have failed the program outlined and are not making progress, the next step is to consider manipulation of the shoulder. Prior to surgery an MRI is helpful to rule out underlying causes of the pain that might not have been manifest in the initial evaluations. The surgical options are a closed manipulation alone, a closed manipulation with diagnostic arthroscopy, and arthroscopy with arthroscopic release of adhesions. Which treatment is performed depends on the patient and the findings at the time of surgery. Arthroscopic evaluation may not be indicated in patients who do not have apparent intra-articular pathology, but in other cases it may be helpful if other conditions are suspected to be contributing to the patient's pain and loss of motion.

DEGENERATIVE ARTHRITIS

Arthritis of the shoulder joint is one of the less common causes of stiffness in the older active patient. It typically is insidious in onset and gradually worsens over years. However, if patients overexert themselves, they may get pain that causes them to lose motion relatively rapidly. The most common causes of arthritis of the shoulder in active older adults are primary degenerative arthritis and arthritis due to long-standing, large rotator cuff tears. Less commonly the arthritis may be due to previous injuries, such as multiple instability episodes of the shoulder when the patient was younger, or after a fracture.

Medical Treatment

The treatment of arthritis of the shoulder is either medical or surgical. The goals of medical treatment are to decrease the pain and maintain motion and function. To decrease the pain, activity modification is recommended. Although playing tennis or golf, running, cycling, and some other sports may not aggravate arthritis, patients should engage in these with caution. Those with arthritis in the upper extremity should lift weights with caution since the compressive force on the joint is so high that it may cause progressive wear of the joint. Generally upper extremity exercises are permissible as long as they do not increase pain or loss of motion. Soreness after activity can be treated either with modification of the amount of the sport or with the techniques used in the sport.

Arthritis of the shoulder can also be treated with acetaminophen or NSAIDs, but this too warrants caution, since hiding the pain may allow continued destruction of the joint. However, long-term use of NSAIDs is recommended for patients with symptomatic arthritis. Patients should use good judgment with their sports and other activities when taking these medications.

Patients should do range of motion exercises for a few minutes daily to prevent the insidious and gradual loss of motion that is typical of arthritis. In patients with long-standing arthritis and loss of motion, it is important that they and their therapists realize that increases in motion with stretching are uncommon. There are few patients more unhappy than those with arthritis who have been treated with aggressive stretching in physical therapy to increase their motion. The use of supplements such as glucosamine and chondroitin sulfate is acceptable, but we neither endorse nor counsel against these. Injections of corticosteroids into the joint are also not recommended except in unusual cases, since they do not provide long-term relief. Injections of hyaluronic acids into the shoulder have not been studied, but it is unlikely that they will provide long-term relief.

Surgical Treatment

Surgical procedures for patients with arthritis should be performed only after medical treatment has failed. The options include arthroscopic debridement, insertion of inert tissues into the joint (e.g., fascia lata or allograft tissue), and shoulder replacement (i.e., hemiarthroplasty or total shoulder arthroplasty). Arthroscopic debridement is recommended only for younger patients in cases in which there is some chance that it may delay further surgery (Weinstein et al. 2000). Arthroscopic debridement of the degenerative shoulder, as is done typically in the knee, does not seem to produce the same results in the shoulder. In very young patients with no bone destruction, some authors have reported good results for pain relief through implantation of tissues between the humeral head and the glenoid (Burkhead and Hutton 1995; Jones 1942; Spencer and Skirving 1986). The interposed tissue acts as a buffer, and the hope is that it may transform into a form of scar that will allow more activity. The tissues interposed are typically autograft tissues, although allograft tissues have been reported (Fink et al. 2001; Tillmann and Braatz 1989). The long-term results of this procedure are unknown.

Shoulder replacement surgery has been shown to be effective in relieving pain in over 90% of patients with degenerative arthritis and rheumatoid arthritis when the rotator cuff is intact. Patients typically see improved range of motion as well with a shoulder replacement. As a result, these operations are effective for improving activities of daily living by allowing patients more elevation and rotation of the shoulder. Heavy lifting and stressful repetitive motions, such as lifting weights or digging post holes, are not recommended since there is the possibility that loosening of the components may be hastened. Sport activities recommended after a shoulder replacement include swimming, walking, and golf (Healy et al. 2001; Mallon et al. 1996). Tennis is not recommended in most instances. The specific activities allowed after shoulder arthroplasty depend on many factors, and each case is considered individually.

SUMMARY

Shoulder conditions in the active older adult that interfere with activity and exercise are quite common. An accurate diagnosis and treatment plan can be made by following basic principles of examination and by synthesizing important information from the history, examination, and imaging studies. In the older adult it is important to distinguish normal loss of motion from pathological conditions. The treatment of atraumatic conditions requires a thorough knowledge of the variables that predict successful recovery. Traumatic injuries may require a more rapid assessment and treatment in the active adult, especially the older adult who needs and wishes to continue sports and exercises. Fortunately many shoulder conditions can be successfully treated to allow the more mature patient to stay active.

CHAPTER

7

Elbow Problems

Todd S. Ellenbecker, MS, PT, SCS, OCS, CSCS

Treating elbow injuries in active individuals requires an understanding of the mechanism of injury, the anatomy and biomechanics of the human elbow and upper extremity kinetic chain, and a structured and detailed clinical examination to identify the structure or structures involved. Treating the injured elbow of an older active patient requires this same approach, with the additional understanding of the effects of years of repetitive stress and the clinical ramifications of these stresses in the aging elbow joint. An overview of the most common elbow injuries and of the musculoskeletal adaptations of the elbow in the older athlete will provide a platform for a discussion of examining and treating patients in this age group. Additionally, the important interplay between the elbow and shoulder joints in the upper extremity kinetic chain is reviewed throughout this chapter to support the comprehensive examination and treatment strategies.

COMMON ELBOW INJURIES

Overuse injuries constitute most of the elbow injuries in the older active patient, and clearly one of the most common injuries in the athletic elbow is humeral epicondylitis (Ellenbecker and Mattalino 1997; Nirschl and Sobel 1981). The repetitive overuse reported as one of the primary etiological factors is particularly evident in the history of most older active patients with elbow dysfunction. Epidemiological research on tennis-playing adults demonstrates incidences of humeral epicondylitis ranging from 35% to 50% (Carroll 1981; Hang and Peng 1984; Kamien 1990; Kitai et al. 1986; Priest et al. 1977). This incidence is far greater than that reported in elite junior players (11-12%) (Roetert and Ellenbecker 1998; Winge et al. 1989).

Etiology of Humeral Epicondylitis

Reported in the literature as early as 1873 by Runge, humeral epicondylitis or "tennis elbow," as it is more popularly known, has been extensively studied by many. Cyriax, in 1936, listed 26 causes of tennis elbow (Cyriax and Cyriax 1983), while an extensive study of this overuse disorder by Goldie in 1964 reported hypervascularization of the extensor aponeurosis and an increased quantity of free nerve endings in the subtendinous space (Goldie 1964). More recently, Leadbetter (1992) described humeral epicondylitis as a degenerative condition consisting of a time-dependent process including vascular, chemical, and cellular events that lead to a failure of the cell matrix healing response in human tendon. This description of tendon injury differs from earlier theories that considered an inflammatory response a primary factor, thus using the term "tendinitis" as opposed to the term recommended by Leadbetter (1992) and Nirschl (1992).

Nirschl (1992, 1993) has defined humeral epicondylitis as an extra-articular tendinous injury characterized by excessive vascular granulation and an impaired healing response in the tendon, which he has termed "angiofibroblastic hyperplasia." In the most recent and thorough histopathological analysis, Nirschl and colleagues (Kraushaar and Nirschl 1999) studied specimens of injured tendon obtained from areas of chronic overuse and reported that these do not contain large numbers of lymphocytes, macrophages, and neutrophils. Instead, tendinosis appears to be a degenerative process characterized by large populations of fibroblasts, disorganized collagen, and vascular hyperplasia (Kraushaar and Nirschl 1999). It is not clear why tendinosis is painful, given the lack of inflammatory cells, and it is also unknown why the collagen does not mature.

Structures Involved in Humeral Epicondylitis

Nirschl (1992) has identified the primary structure involved in lateral humeral epicondylitis as the tendon of the extensor carpi radialis brevis. Approximately one-third of cases involve the tendon of the extensor communis (Kraushaar and Nirschl 1999). The extensor carpi radialis longus and extensor carpi ulnaris can be involved as well. The primary site of medial humeral epicondylitis is the flexor carpi radialis (figure 7.1), pronator teres, and flexor carpi ulnaris tendons (Nirschl 1992, 1993).

Recent researchers have described in detail the anatomy of the lateral epicondylar region (Boyer and Hastings 1999; Greenbaum et al. 1999). The specific location of the extensor carpi radialis brevis tendon is inferior to the tendinous origin of the extensor carpi radialis longus, which can be palpated along the anterior surface of the supracondylar ridge just proximal or cephalid to the extensor carpi radialis brevis tendon on the lateral epicondyle (Boyer and Hastings 1999). Greenbaum et al. (1999) describe the pyramidal slope or shape of the lateral epicondyle and show how both the extensor carpi radialis brevis and the extensor communis originate from the entire anterior surface of the lateral epicondyle.

These specific relationships are important for the clinician to bear in mind when palpating for the region of maximal tenderness during the clinical examination. While there are no detailed recent reports in the literature regarding the medial epicondyle, careful palpation can be used to discriminate between the muscle–tendon junctions of the pronator teres and flexor carpi radialis. Additionally, the clinician should perform palpation of the medial ulnar collateral ligament, which originates from nearly the entire inferior surface of the medial epicondyle and inserts into the anterior medial aspect of the coronoid process of the ulna (figure 7.2). Understanding of the involved structures, as well as a detailed knowledge of the exact locations where these structures can be palpated, can assist the clinician in locating the painful tendon or tendons involved.

Dijs et al. (1990) reported on 70 patients with lateral epicondylitis. They reported the area of maximal involvement in these cases, which identified the extensor carpi radialis longus in only 1% and the extensor carpi radialis brevis in 90%. The body of the extensor carpi radialis tendon was cited in 1% of cases, and 8% were over the muscle–tendon junction over the most proximal part of the muscle of the extensor carpi radialis brevis.

Epidemiology of Humeral Epicondylitis

According to Nirschl (1992, 1993), the incidence of lateral humeral epicondylitis is far greater than that of medial epicondylitis in recreational tennis players and in the leading arm of a golfer (left arm in a right-handed player); medial humeral epicondylitis is far more common in elite tennis players and throwing athletes due to the powerful loading of the flexor and pronator muscle–tendon units during the valgus extension overload inherent in the acceleration phase of those overhead movement patterns. Additionally, the trailing arm of the golfer (right arm in a right-handed player) is reportedly more likely to have medial symptoms than lateral.

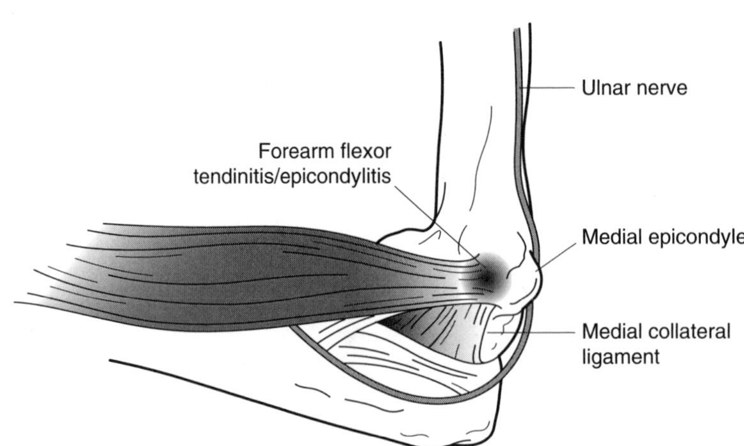

FIGURE 7.1 Anatomical site of medial humeral epicondylitis. The conjoin tendon of the wrist and finger flexors and forearm pronators at the medial epicondyle of the elbow.

Reprinted, by permission, from S.J. Shultz, P.A. Houglum, and D.H. Perrin, 2000, *Assessment of athletic injuries* (Champaign, IL: Human Kinetics), 132.

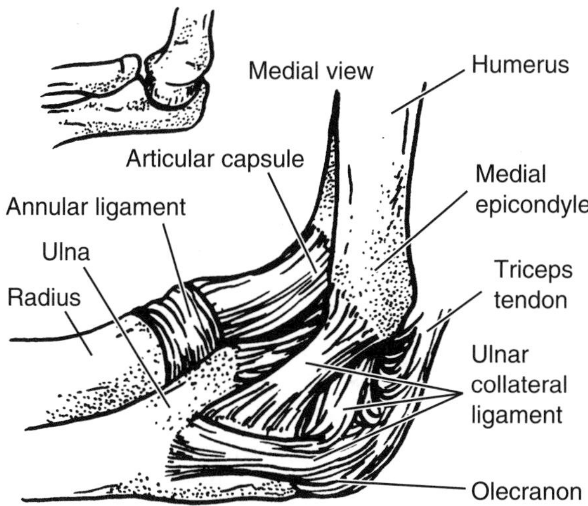

FIGURE 7.2 Medial view of the ligaments of the elbow. Note the extensive attachments of the ulnar collateral ligament to the inferior surface of the medial epicondyle.

Reprinted, by permission, from W.C. Whiting and R.F. Zernicke, 1998, *Biomechanics of musculoskeletal injury* (Champaign, IL: Human Kinetics), 190.

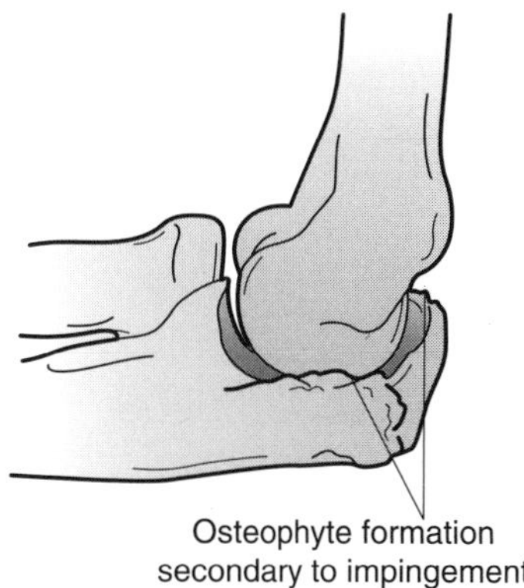

FIGURE 7.3 Anatomical diagram of the effects of valgus stress on the human elbow.

Reprinted, by permission, from S.J. Shultz, P.A. Houglum, and D.H. Perrin, 2000, *Assessment of athletic injuries* (Champaign, IL: Human Kinetics), 137.

ADDITIONAL OVERUSE ELBOW INJURY

Repeated overhead throwing or serving activity can lead to characteristic patterns of osseous and osteochondral injury in the older active patient. These injuries are commonly referred to as valgus extension overload injuries (Wilson et al. 1983). As a result of the valgus stress incurred during throwing or the serving motion, traction placed via the medial aspect of the elbow can create bony spurs or osteophytes at the medial epicondyle or coronoid process of the elbow (Bennett 1959; Indelicato et al. 1979; Slocum 1978). Additionally, the valgus stress during elbow extension creates impingement, which leads to the development of osteophyte formation at the posterior and posteromedial aspects of the olecranon tip, causing chondromalacia and loose-body formation (Wilson et al. 1983). The motion of valgus pressure combined with the powerful extension of the elbow leads to posterior osteophyte formation, due to impingement of the posterior medial aspect of the ulna against the trochlea and olecranon fossa. Joyce (Joyce et al. 1995) has reported the presence of chondromalacia in the medial groove of the trochlea, which often precedes osteophyte formation. Erosion to subchondral bone is often seen when olecranon osteophytes are initially developing.

Figure 7.3 shows the valgus loading of the athletic elbow and site of medial tension injury or valgus tensile overload response. Injury to the ulnar collateral ligament and medial muscle–tendon units of the flexor-pronator group can also occur with this type of repetitive loading (Indelicato et al. 1979; Wolf and Altchek 2003).

During the valgus stress to the human elbow during the acceleration phase of both the throwing and serving motions, lateral compressive forces occur in the lateral aspect of the elbow, specifically at the radiocapitellar joint. In the older adult elbow, the radiocapitellar joint can be the site of joint degeneration and osteochondral injury from the compressive loading (Indelicato et al. 1979). This lateral compressive loading is increased in the elbow with medial ulnar collateral ligament laxity or ligament injury (Ellenbecker and Mattalino 1997).

While many other injuries can occur in the older active elbow, the overuse stresses that result in humeral epicondylitis, as well as the characteristic injuries from valgus extension overload such as medial ulnar collateral ligament injury and osseous and osteochondral injury, form the bulk of the discussion in this chapter. As mentioned earlier, the older active elbow patient often presents with characteristic musculoskeletal adaptations that need to be addressed during examination and ultimately receive treatment. The following section on clinical examination includes discussion of these adaptations.

CLINICAL EXAMINATION

Structural inspection of the older active elbow patient must include a complete and thorough inspection of the entire upper extremity and trunk because of the reliance on the entire upper extremity kinetic chain for power generation and force attenuation during functional activities (Ellenbecker and Mattalino 1997). Adaptive changes are commonly encountered during clinical examination of the athletic elbow, particularly in the unilaterally dominant upper extremity athlete. In these athletes, use of the contralateral extremity as a baseline is particularly important to determine the degree of actual adaptation that may be a contributing factor in the patient's injury presentation.

Adaptive Changes in the Older Athlete's Elbow

Anatomical adaptation of the older athlete's elbow can be divided into four main categories: range of motion, osseous, ligamentous, and muscular. This section presents each within the context of the clinical examination of the patient with elbow dysfunction.

Range of Motion Adaptations

King et al. (1969) initially reported on elbow range of motion in professional baseball pitchers. Fifty percent of the pitchers they examined showed a flexion contracture of the dominant elbow, with 30% of subjects demonstrating a cubitus valgus deformity. Chinn et al. (1974) measured world class professional adult tennis players and reported significant elbow flexion contractures on the dominant arm, but no presence of a cubitus valgus deformity.

More recently Ellenbecker et al. (1998) measured elbow flexion contractures averaging 5° in a population of 40 professional baseball pitchers. Directly related to elbow function was wrist flexibility, which Ellenbecker et al. (1998) reported as significantly less in extension on the dominant arm due to tightness of the wrist flexor musculature, with no difference in wrist flexion range of motion between extremities. Ellenbecker and Roetert (1994) measured senior tennis players 55 years of age and older and found flexion contractures averaging 10° in the dominant elbow, as well as significantly less wrist flexion range of motion. The higher utilization of the wrist extensor musculature was likely the cause of limited wrist flexor range of motion among the senior tennis players, as opposed to the reduced wrist extension range of motion from excessive overuse of the wrist flexor muscles inherent in baseball pitching (Glousman et al. 1992; Ryu et al. 1988).

More proximally, measurement of range of motion of humeral rotation in the older overhead athlete is also recommended. Several studies have shown consistent alterations of shoulder rotational range of motion in the overhead athlete (Ellenbecker et al. 2002; Kibler et al. 1996; Roetert et al. 2000). Ellenbecker et al. (2002) showed statistically greater dominant shoulder external rotation and less internal rotation in a sample of professional baseball pitchers. Despite these differences in internal and external rotation range of motion, the total rotation (IR + ER) between extremities remained equal, such that any increases in external rotation range of motion were matched by decreases in internal rotation range of motion in this uninjured population. Elite-level tennis players had significantly less internal rotation and no significant difference in external rotation on the dominant arm, and an overall decrease in total rotation range of motion on the dominant arm of approximately 10°. Careful monitoring of proximal glenohumeral joint range of motion is recommended for the athlete with an elbow injury.

On the basis of the findings of these descriptive profiles, one can expect the finding of an elbow flexion contracture and limited wrist flexion or extension range of motion, as well as reduced glenohumeral joint internal rotation, during the examination of an older athlete from a unilaterally dominant upper extremity sport. Careful measurement during the clinical exam is recommended to determine baseline levels of range of motion loss and to ascertain whether rehabilitative interventions are needed or to assess progress of rehabilitation.

Osseous Adaptation

Priest et al. (1974) studied 84 world-ranked tennis players through use of radiography, finding an average of 6.5 bony changes on the dominant elbow of each player. Additionally, the authors reported two times as many bony adaptations, such as spurs, on the medial aspect of the elbow as compared to the lateral aspect. The coronoid process of the ulna was the number-one site of osseous adaptation or spurring. An average 44% increase in thickness of the anterior humeral cortex was found on the dominant arm of these players, with an 11% increase in cortical thickness reported in the radius of the dominant tennis-playing extremity.

Additionally, in a magnetic resonance imaging study, Waslewski et al. (2002) found osteophytes at the proximal or distal insertion of the ulnar collateral ligament in 5 of 20 asymptomatic professional baseball pitchers, as well as posterior osteophytes in 2 of 20 pitchers.

Ligamentous Laxity

Manual clinical examination of the human elbow to assess medial and lateral laxity can be challenging, given the presence of humeral rotation and small increases in joint opening that often present with ulnar collateral ligament injury. Ellenbecker et al. (1998) measured medial elbow joint laxity in 40 asymptomatic professional baseball pitchers to determine if bilateral differences in medial elbow laxity exist in healthy pitchers with a long history of repetitive overuse to the medial aspect of the elbow. A Telos stress radiography device was used to assess medial elbow joint opening, using a standardized valgus stress of 15 daN with the elbow placed in 25° of elbow flexion and the forearm in a supinated position. Results showed significant differences between extremities with stress application, with the dominant elbow opening 1.20 mm and the nondominant elbow opening 0.88 mm. This difference, while statistically significant, averaged 0.32 mm between the dominant and nondominant elbow and would be virtually unidentifiable with manual assessment. Previous research by Rijke et al. (1994) using stress radiography had identified a critical level of 0.5-mm increase in medial elbow joint opening in elbows with ulnar collateral ligament injury. Thus, the results of the study by Ellenbecker et al. (1998) support this 0.5-mm critical level and did identify small increases in medial elbow joint laxity on the dominant elbow in asymptomatic baseball pitchers.

Muscular Adaptations

Several methods can be used to measure upper extremity strength in athletic populations. These can range from measurement of anthropometric girths of an extremity to the use of a handgrip dynamometer and isokinetic dynamometers to measure specific muscular parameters. Increased forearm circumference was measured on the dominant forearm in world class tennis players (Chinn et al. 1974), as well as in the dominant forearm of senior tennis players (Kulund et al. 1979).

Isometric grip strength measured using a handgrip dynamometer has revealed unilateral increases in strength in elite adult and senior tennis players as well. Increases ranging from 10% to 30% have been reported using standardized measurement methods (Chinn et al. 1974; Ellenbecker 1991; Ellenbecker and Mattalino 1997; Kulund et al. 1979).

Finally, studies have used isokinetic dynamometers to measure specific muscular performance parameters in elite-level tennis players and baseball pitchers (Ellenbecker 1991; Ellenbecker and Mattalino 1997; Ellenbecker and Roetert 2003a, 2003b). Specific patterns of unilateral muscular development have been identified through review of the isokinetic literature from different populations of overhead athletes. Ellenbecker (1991) measured isokinetic wrist and forearm strength in mature adult tennis players who were highly skilled and found 10% to 25% greater wrist flexion and extension as well as forearm pronation strength on the dominant extremity, with no difference between extremities in forearm supination strength. No significant difference between extremities was found in elbow flexion strength in elite tennis players, but dominant arm elbow extension strength was significantly greater than in the non-tennis-playing extremity (Ellenbecker and Roetert 2003a).

Research on professional throwing athletes has identified significantly greater wrist flexion and forearm pronation strength on the dominant arm, by as much as 15% to 35% (Ellenbecker and Mattalino 1997), with no difference in wrist extension strength or forearm supination strength between extremities. Wilk, Arrigo, and Andrews (1993) reported 10% to 20% greater elbow flexion strength in professional baseball pitchers on the dominant arm, as well as 5% to 15% greater elbow extension strength.

These data illustrate the chronic muscular adaptations that may occur in the senior athlete who may present with elbow injury, and can also help the clinician determine realistic and accurate discharge strength levels following rehabilitation. Failure to return the stabilizing musculature to its often dominant status (10% to as much as 35%) on the dominant extremity in these athletes may represent an incomplete rehabilitation and prohibit the return to full activity.

Additional Clinical Examination Methods

In addition to the examination methods outlined in the previous section, several other tests should be included in the comprehensive examination of the elbow of the older active patient. A number of these are highlighted here based on their overall importance. See Morrey (1993) and Ellenbecker and Mattalino (1997) for more complete discussions solely on examination of the elbow.

Related Referral Testing

Clinical testing of the joints proximal and distal to the elbow allows the examiner to rule out referral symptoms and ensure that elbow pain is from a local musculoskeletal origin. Overpressure of the cervical spine in the motions of flexion/extension and lateral flexion/rotation, as well as quadrant or Spurling's test combining extension with ipsilateral lateral flexion and rotation, is commonly used to clear the cervical spine and rule out radicular symptoms (Gould and Davies 1985).

Additionally, clearing the glenohumeral joint, as well as determining the presence of concomitant impingement or instability, is highly recommended (Ellenbecker and Mattalino 1997). Use of the sulcus sign (McFarland et al. 1996) to determine the presence of multidirectional instability of the glenohumeral joint, along with the subluxation/relocation sign (Jobe and Kvitne 1989) and load and shift test, can provide valuable insight into the status of the glenohumeral joint. The impingement signs of Neer (1973) and Hawkins and Kennedy (1980) are also helpful for ruling out proximal tendon pathology.

Another recommendation, in addition to the clearing tests for the glenohumeral joint, is full inspection of the scapulothoracic joint. Removal of the patient's shirt or examination of the patient in a gown with full exposure of the upper back is strongly recommended. Kibler et al. (2002) have recently presented a classification system for scapular pathology. Careful observation of the patient at rest and with the hands placed on the hips, and also during active overhead movements, is recommended to identify prominence of particular borders of the scapula, as well as a lack of close association with the thoracic wall during movement (Kibler 1991, 1998). Bilateral comparison forms the primary basis for identifying scapular pathology; in many athletes, however, one can observe bilateral scapular pathology.

The presence of overuse injuries in the elbow occurring with proximal injury to the shoulder complex, or with scapulothoracic dysfunction, is widely reported (Ellenbecker 1995; Ellenbecker and Mattalino 1997; Morrey 1993; Nirschl 1992, 1993). Thus a thorough inspection of the proximal joint is extremely important in the comprehensive management of elbow pathology.

Overpressure and intercarpal mobilization are also recommended distally at the wrist joint to clear that segment of the upper extremity kinetic chain (Gould and Davies 1985).

Special Tests of the Elbow Joint

Several tests specific for the elbow are warranted to assist in the diagnosis of elbow dysfunction. These include Tinel's test, valgus and varus stress tests, milking test, valgus extension overpressure test, bounce home test, and provocation tests.

- **Tinel's test** involves tapping of the ulnar nerve in the medial region of the elbow, over the cubital tunnel retinaculum. Reproduction of paresthesias or tingling along the distal course of the ulnar nerve indicates irritability of the ulnar nerve (Morrey 1993).
- The **valgus stress test** is used to evaluate the integrity of the ulnar collateral ligament. The position used for testing the anterior band of the ulnar collateral ligament is characterized by 15° to 25° of elbow flexion and forearm supination. The elbow flexion position is used to unlock the olecranon from the olecranon fossa and decreases the stability provided by the osseous congruity of the joint. This places a greater relative stress on the medial ulnar collateral ligament (Morrey and An 1983). Reproduction of medial elbow pain, in addition to unilateral increases in ulnohumeral joint laxity, indicates a positive test. Typically the test is graded using the American Academy of Orthopaedic Surgeons guidelines of 0 to 5 mm, grade I; 5 to 10 mm, grade II; and greater than 10 mm, grade III (Ellenbecker et al. 1998). Use of greater than 25° of elbow flexion will increase the amount of humeral rotation during performance of the valgus stress test and provide misleading information to the clinician's hands. The test is typically performed with the shoulder in the scapular plane, but can be performed with the shoulder in the coronal plane to minimize compensatory movements at the shoulder during testing.
- The **varus stress test** uses similar degrees of elbow flexion and shoulder and forearm positioning. This test assesses the integrity of the lateral ulnar collateral ligament and should be performed along with the valgus stress test for a complete evaluation of the medial/lateral stability of the ulnohumeral joint.
- The **milking sign** is a test patients perform on themselves, with the elbow in approximately 90° of elbow flexion. By reaching under the involved elbow with the contralateral extremity, the patient grasps the thumb of the injured extremity and pulls in a lateral direction, thus imposing a valgus stress to the flexed elbow. Some patients may not have enough flexibility to perform this maneuver, and the examiner can impart a valgus stress to mimic this movement, which stresses the posterior band of the ulnar collateral ligament (Morrey and An 1983).
- The **valgus extension overpressure test,** as reported by Andrews et al. (1993), determines whether posterior elbow pain is caused by a posteromedial osteophyte abutting the medial margin of the trochlea and the olecranon fossa. This test is performed by passively extending the elbow while maintaining a valgus stress to the elbow. The test is meant to simulate the stresses imparted to the posterior medial part of the elbow during the acceleration phase of the throwing or serving motion. Reproduction of pain in the posteromedial aspect of the elbow indicates a positive test.
- **Provocation tests** can be applied during screening of the muscle–tendon units of the elbow. Provocation tests consist of manual muscle tests to reproduce pain. The specific tests used to screen the elbow joint of a patient with suspected elbow pathology include wrist and finger flexion and extension and forearm pronation and supination (Ellenbecker 1995). These tests can be employed to provoke the muscle–tendon unit at the lateral or medial epicondyle. Testing of the elbow at or near full extension can often recreate localized lateral or medial elbow pain secondary to tendon degeneration (Kraushaar and Nirschl 1999). Reproduction of lateral or medial elbow pain with resistive muscle testing (provocation testing) may indicate concomitant tendon injury at the elbow and would direct the clinician to perform a more complete elbow exam.

NONOPERATIVE REHABILITATION OF HUMERAL EPICONDYLITIS

Following the detailed examination of the older athlete with elbow pain, a detailed rehabilitation program can commence. Three main stages of rehabilitation should occur: the protected function, total arm strength, and return-to-activity phases.

Protected Function Phase

During the first phase in the rehabilitation process, care is taken to protect the injured muscle–tendon unit from stress, but not function. Nirschl (1992, 1993) cautions against the use of an immobilizer or sling, as either may lead to further atrophy of the musculature and have negative effects on the upper extremity kinetic chain. Protection of the patient from offending activities is recommended, however, with cessation of throwing and serving for medial-based humeral symptoms. Allowing the patient to bat or hit backhands provides continued activity while minimizing stress to the injured area. Very often, however, all sport activity must cease in order to allow the muscle–tendon unit time to heal and most importantly to allow formal rehabilitation to progress. Continued work or sport performance can severely slow the progression of resistive exercise and other long-term treatments in physical therapy.

Use of modalities is very helpful during this time period; however, agreement on a clearly superior modality or sequence of modalities has not been substantiated in the literature (Boyer and Hastings 1999; Labelle et al. 1992). A meta-analysis of 185 studies on treatment of humeral epicondylitis showed glaring deficits in the scientific quality of the investigations, with no significantly superior treatment approach identified. Although many modalities or sequences of modalities have anecdotally produced superior results, there is a tremendous need for prospective, randomized controlled clinical trials to identify optimal methods for initial treatment. Modalities such as ultrasound (Bernhang et al. 1974; Nirschl and Sobel 1981), electrical stimulation and ice, cortisone injection (Kamien 1990; Nirschl and Sobel 1981), NSAIDs (Rosenthal 1984), acupuncture (Brattberg 1983), transverse friction massage (Ingham 1981), and DMSO application (Percy and Carson 1981) have all been reported to provide varying levels of effectiveness. Boyer and Hastings (1999), in a comprehensive review of the treatment of humeral epicondylitis, reported no significant difference with the use of low-energy laser, acupuncture, extracorporeal shock wave therapy, or steroid injection.

The use of cortisone injection has been widely reported in the literature during the pain reduction phase of treatment of this often recalcitrant condition. Dijs et al. (1990) compared the effects of traditional physical therapy and cortisone injection in 70 patients diagnosed with humeral epicondylitis. In this research, 91% of patients who received the cortisone injection experienced initial relief, as compared with 47% who reported relief from undergoing physical therapy. The recurrence rate in the study, however, after only three months, showed that 51% in the cortisone injection group and only 5% in the physical therapy group had a return of primary symptoms. Similar findings were reported in a study by Verhaar et al. (1995) that compared physical therapy consisting of Mills manipulation and cross-friction massage with corticosteroid injection in a prospective randomized controlled clinical trial in 106 patients with humeral epicondylitis. At six weeks, 22 of 53 subjects reported complete relief with the cortisone injection, while only 3 subjects had complete relief from this type of physical therapy treatment. At one year, there were no differences between treatment groups regarding the course of treatment. This study shows the short-term benefit from the corticosteroid injection, as well as the ineffectiveness of physical therapy using manipulation and cross-friction massage.

Several additional recent studies can also direct clinicians in the development of appropriate interventions:

- Nirschl et al. (2003) examined the effects of **iontophoresis with dexamethasone** in 199 patients with humeral epicondylitis. Results showed that 52% of the subjects in the treatment group reported overall improvement on the investigators' improvement index, with only 33% of the placebo group reporting improvement two days after the series of treatments with iontophoresis. One month following the treatment, there was no statistical difference in the overall improvement between the patients in the treatment and control groups. One additional finding from this study that has clinical relevance was greater pain relief in the group that underwent six treatments in a 10-day period, as compared to subjects in the treatment group who underwent treatment over a longer period of time. While this study does support the use of iontophoresis with dexamethasone, it does not indicate substantial benefits during follow-up.
- Haake et al. (2002) studied the effects of **extracorporeal shock wave therapy** in 272 patients with humeral epicondylitis in a multicenter prospective randomized control study. They reported that extracorporeal shock wave therapy was ineffective in the treatment of humeral epicondylitis.

• Basford et al. (2000) used **low-intensity Nd: YAG laser irradiation** at seven points along the forearm three times a week for four weeks and reported this to be ineffective in the treatment of lateral humeral epicondylitis.

It appears, then, that no standardized modality or modality sequence has been identified that is clearly statistically more effective than any other at the present time. Clinical reviews by Nirschl (1992, 1993) and Ellenbecker and Mattalino (1997) advocate the use of multiple modalities, such as electrical stimulation and ultrasound, as well as iontophoresis with dexamethasone, to assist in pain reduction and encourage increases in local blood flow. Another recommendation is the copious use of ice or cryotherapy following increases in daily activity. The use of therapeutic modalities and also cortisone injection, if needed, can be seen only as one part of the treatment sequence, with increasing evidence favoring progressive resistive exercise.

Exercise is one of the most powerful modalities used in rehabilitative medicine. Research has shown increases in local blood flow following isometric contraction of the musculature at levels as submaximal as 5% to 50% of maximal voluntary contraction, both during the contraction and for periods of up to 1 min postcontraction (Jensen et al. 1995). One study has shown superior results in the treatment of humeral epicondylitis using progressive resistive exercise compared with ultrasound (Gam et al. 1998). In a recent study by Svernlov and Adolfsson (2001), 38 patients with lateral humeral epicondylitis were randomly assigned to a contract–relax stretching or eccentric exercise treatment group. Results showed a 71% report of full recovery in the eccentric exercise group as compared to the group that performed contract–relax stretching, only 39% of whom rated themselves as fully recovered. These studies support heavy reliance on the successful application of progressive resistive exercise in the treatment of humeral epicondylitis.

Total Arm Strength Rehabilitation Phase

Early application of resistive exercise for the treatment of humeral epicondylitis mainly focuses on the important principle stating that "proximal stability is needed to promote distal mobility" (Sullivan et al. 1982, 145-156). Thus the initial application of resistive exercise actually consists of specific exercises to strengthen the upper extremity proximal force couples (Inman et al. 1944). The rotator cuff and deltoid as well as the serratus anterior and lower trapezius force couples are targeted to enhance proximal stabilization using a low-resistance high-repetition exercise format (i.e., three sets of 15RM loading; RM = repetition maximum). Specific exercises such as side-lying external rotation, prone horizontal abduction, and prone extension, both with externally rotated humeral positions and prone external rotation, all have been shown to elicit high levels of posterior rotator cuff activation during electromyographic research (Ballantyne et al. 1993; Blackburn et al. 1990; Townsend et al. 1991). Additionally, exercises such as the serratus press and manual scapular protraction and retraction resistance can be safely applied without stress to the distal aspect of the upper extremity during this important phase of rehabilitation. The use of cuff weights allows performance of some of the rotator cuff and scapular exercises with the weight attached proximal to the elbow, to further minimize overload to the elbow and forearm during the earliest phases of rehabilitation if needed for some patients.

The initial application of exercise to the distal aspect of the extremity follows a pattern that stresses the injured muscle–tendon unit last. For example, the initial distal exercise sequence for the patient with lateral humeral epicondylitis would include wrist flexion and forearm pronation, which provides most of the tensile stress to the medially inserting tendons that are not directly involved in lateral humeral epicondylitis. Gradual addition of wrist extension and forearm supination, as well as radial and ulnar deviation exercises, occurs as signs and symptoms allow. Additional progression is based on the elbow position utilized during distal exercises. Initially, most patients tolerate the exercises in a more pain-free fashion with the elbow placed in slight flexion, with a progression as signs and symptoms allow to more extended and functional elbow positions. These exercises are performed with light weights, often as little as 1 lb or kg, as well as tan or yellow Theraband emphasizing both the concentric and eccentric portions of the exercise movement. According to the research by Svernlov and Adolfsson (2001), the eccentric portion of the exercise may actually have a greater benefit than the concentric portion. More research is needed, however, to establish a clearer understanding of the role isolated eccentric exercise plays in the rehabilitation of degenerative tendon conditions. Multiple sets of 15 to 20 repetitions are recommended to promote muscular endurance.

Once the patient can tolerate the most basic series of distal exercises (wrist flexion/extension, forearm pronation/supination, and wrist radial/ulnar deviation), exercises progress to include activities that involve simultaneous contraction of the wrist and forearm musculature with elbow flexion/extension range of motion. These include exercises such as exercise ball dribbling (figure 7.4), Body Blade (Hymanson, Inc., Playa del Rey, CA), Boing (OPTP, Minneapolis, MN), Theraband (Hygenic Corp., Akron, OH), resistance bar oscillations, and rowing. Additionally, closed kinetic chain exercise for the upper extremity is added to promote co-contraction and mimic functional positions with joint approximation (Ellenbecker and Davies 2001). Examples of closed kinetic chain exercises include quadruped rhythmic stabilization, step-ups, and push-up with a "plus" (Ellenbecker and Davies 2001).

In addition to resistive exercise, gentle passive stretching to optimize the muscle–tendon unit length is indicated. Combined stretches with the patient in the supine position are indicated to elongate the biarticular muscle–tendon units of the elbow, forearm, and wrist using a combination of elbow, wrist, and forearm positions. Additionally, stretching the distal aspect of the extremity in varying positions of glenohumeral joint elevation is recommended (Ellenbecker and Mattalino 1997). Mobilization of the ulnohumeral joint can also be effective in cases in which there are significant flexion contractures. Ulnohumeral distraction with the elbow near full extension will place tension selectively on the anterior joint capsule (Bowling and Rockar 1985).

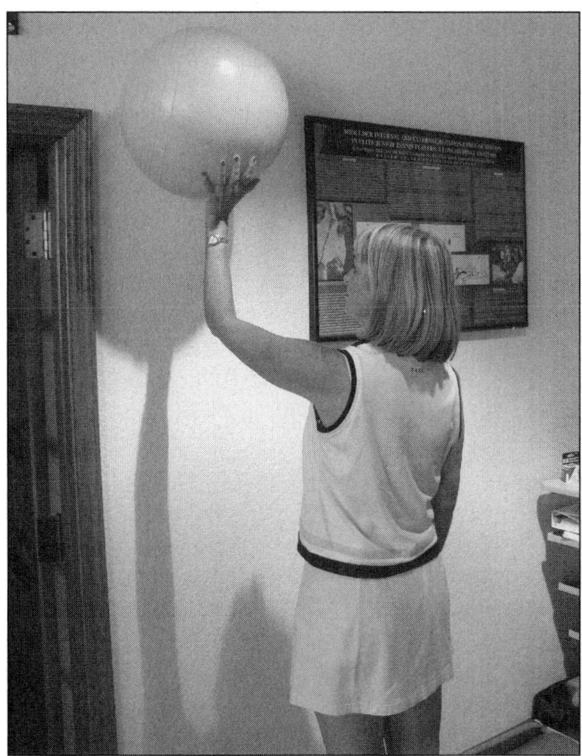

FIGURE 7.4 Ball dribbling exercise used during elbow rehabilitation as an example of low-resistance, high-repetition exercise programming.

As the patient tolerates the distal isotonic exercise progression pain free at a level of 3 to 5 lb or with medium-level elastic tubing or bands, and also tolerates the oscillatory-type exercises in this phase of rehabilitation, progression to the isokinetic form of exercise can take place. Advantages of isokinetic exercise are the inherent accommodative resistance and utilization of faster, more functional contractile velocities and the provision of isolated patterns to elicit high levels of muscular activation. The initial pattern of exercise used anecdotally has been wrist flexion/extension, with forearm pronation/supination added after successful tolerance of a trial treatment of wrist flexion/extension. Contractile velocities ranging between 180° and 300° per second, with six to eight sets of 15 to 20 repetitions, are used to foster local muscular endurance (Fleck and Kraemer 1987). In addition to the isokinetic exercise, plyometric wrist snaps (figure 7.5, *a* and *b*) and wrist flips (figure 7.6, *a* and *b*) are utilized to begin to train the active elbow for functional and sport-specific demands.

Return-to-Activity Phase

Of the three phases in the rehabilitation process for humeral epicondylitis, return to activity is the one that is most frequently ignored or cut short, resulting in serious consequences for reinjury and the development of a "chronic" status for this injury. Objective criteria for entry into this stage are

- tolerance of the previously outlined resistive exercise series,
- objectively documented strength equal to that of the contralateral extremity with either manual assessment (MMT) or preferably isokinetic testing and isometric strength, and
- a functional range of motion.

It is important to note that, especially in the older active elbow patient, full elbow range of motion is not always attainable, secondary to the osseous and capsular adaptations discussed earlier in this chapter. That being said, meeting those objective criteria leads the clinician to advance the patient to functional activity simulation and interval sport return programs (Ellenbecker 1995).

Characteristics of interval sport return programs include alternate-day performance and gradual progressions of intensity and repetitions of sport activities. For example, utilizing low-compression tennis balls such as the Pro-Penn Star Ball (Penn Racquet Sports, Phoenix, AZ) or Wilson Gator Ball (Wilson

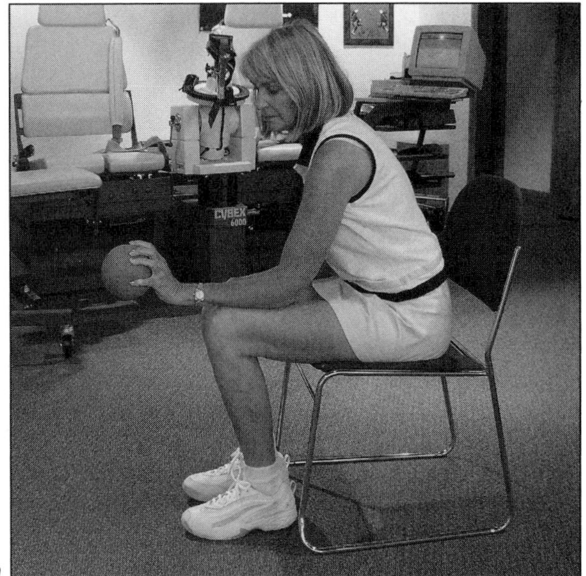

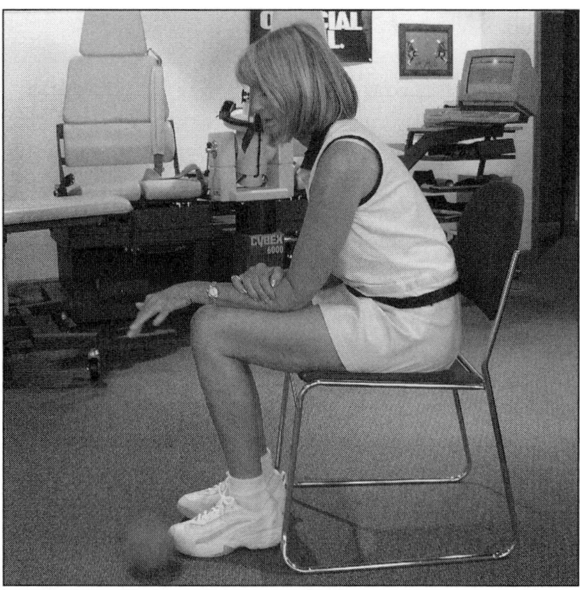

a b

FIGURE 7.5 Wrist snaps used during the total arm strength rehabilitation program: *(a)* beginning position and *(b)* ending position.

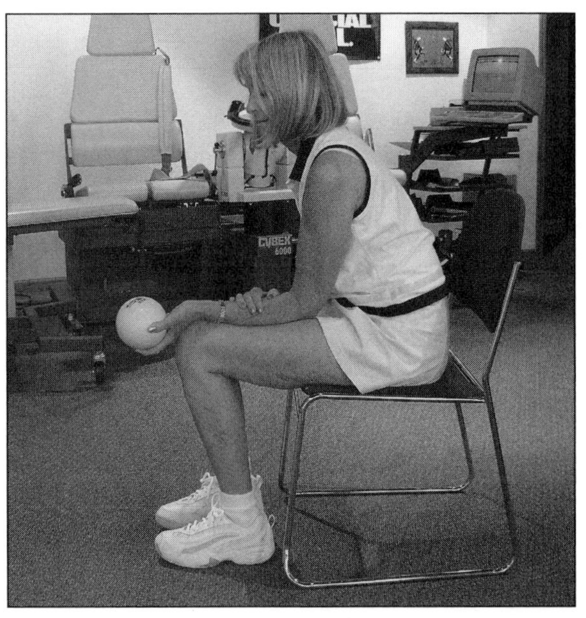

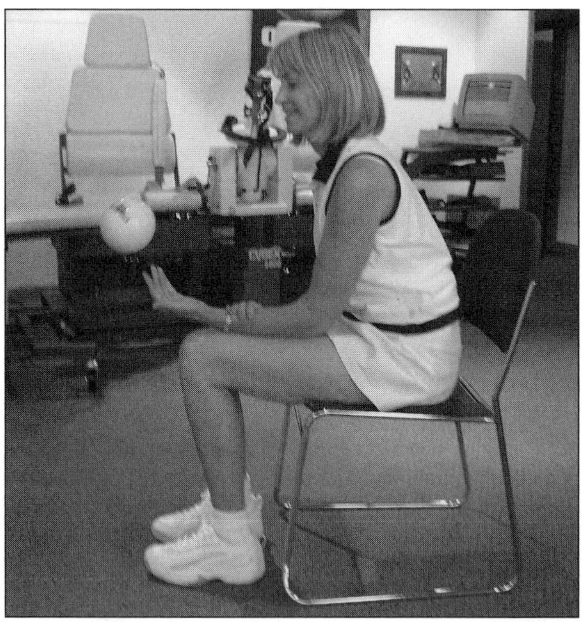

a b

FIGURE 7.6 Wrist flips used during the total arm strength rehabilitation program: *(a)* beginning position and *(b)* ending position.

Sporting Goods, Elk Grove Village, IL) during the initial contact phase of the return to tennis decreases impact stress and increases tolerance to the activity. Additionally, performing the interval program under supervision, either during therapy or with a knowledgeable teaching professional or coach, allows for biomechanical evaluation of technique and guards against overzealous intensity levels, which can be a common mistake in well-intentioned, motivated patients. Using the return program on alternate days, with rest between sessions, allows for recovery and decreases reinjury.

Two other important aspects of the return to sport activity are the continued application of resistive exercise and the modification or evaluation of the patient's equipment. Continuation of the total arm strength rehabilitation exercises using elastic resistance, medicine balls, and isotonic or isokinetic resistance is important to continue to enhance not only strength, but also muscular endurance. Inspection and modification of the patient's tennis racket or golf clubs are also important. For example, lowering the string tension several pounds and ensuring that the player uses a more resilient or softer string, such as a coreless multifilament synthetic string or gut, are widely recommended for tennis players with upper extremity injury histories (Nirschl 1992, 1993; Nirschl and Sobel 1981). Grip size is also very important, as research shows changes in muscular activity with alteration of handle or grip size (Adelsberg et al. 1986). Nirschl (1993) has characterized proper grip size as corresponding to the distance from the distal tip of the ring finger along the radial border of the finger to the proximal palmar crease. Nirschl has also recommended the use of a counterforce brace to decrease stress on the insertion of the flexor and extensor tendons during work or sport activity (Groppel and Nirschl 1986). Although there is a standard general placement for the counterforce brace, only the person wearing it can decide what precise location helps in his or her own case.

You will have noticed that although the advice given here is abundant, it is not step-by-step. The reason is that the course of recovery and the response to interventions vary so much among people experiencing this injury; it is impossible to provide a "cookbook" approach to rehabilitation. The therapist must listen carefully to the patient throughout the course of treatment and must base changes in activity levels and treatment strategies on frequent reevaluation. In short, the therapist must be extremely familiar with all the treatment options discussed in this chapter in order to respond appropriately to whatever variations different individuals may present during the course of rehabilitation.

SURGICAL TREATMENT

In a study of over 3,000 cases of humeral epicondylitis, Nirschl (1992) reported that 92% responded to nonoperative treatment. Characteristics of patients who often require surgical correction for this condition are failure of nonoperative rehabilitation programs, minimal relief with corticosteroid injection, and intense pain in the injured elbow even at rest. Surgical treatment for lateral humeral epicondylitis, as reported by Nirschl (1992), involves a small incision from the radial head to 1 in. proximal to the lateral epicondyle. Through this incision, Nirschl removes the pathologic tissue he terms angiofibroblastic hyperplasia, without disturbing the attachment of the extensor aponeurosis, to preserve stability of the elbow (Nirschl 1992). Vascular enhancement is afforded by drilling holes into the cortical bone in the anterior lateral epicondyle to cancellous bone level. Postoperative immobilization is brief (48 h), with early motion of the wrist and fingers on post-op day 1, progressing to elbow active assistive range of motion during the first two to three weeks. Resistive exercise is gradually applied after the third postoperative week, with a return to normal daily activities expected at eight weeks post-op and a return to sport activity several months thereafter (Nirschl 1992, 1993).

REHABILITATION FOLLOWING ELBOW ARTHROSCOPY

Repetitive stresses to the older active patient often result in loose-body formation and osteochondral injury, in addition to the more commonly reported tendon injury resulting in humeral epicondylitis. Andrews and Soffer (1994) report that the most common indications for elbow arthroscopy are loose-body removal and removal of osteophytes. Posteromedial decompression includes the excision of osteophytes, with or without resection of additional posteromedial bone from the proximal olecranon (Andrews et al. 2001). Early emphasis on regaining full extension range of motion is possible because of the minimally invasive arthroscopic procedure. The author's postoperative protocol following arthroscopic procedures of the elbow is presented in Postoperative Protocol for Elbow Arthroscopy and Removal of Loose Bodies (p. 118).

Outcomes following elbow arthroscopy for posteromedial osteophyte and loose-body removal were reported in a study by Ogilvie-Harris et al. (1995) in which 21 patients were followed an average of 35 months postoperatively. Good and excellent results were obtained in 7 and 14 patients, respectively. O'Driscoll and Morrey (1992) reported that arthroscopic removal of loose bodies was beneficial in 75% of all patients (71 arthroscopies performed in 70 patients); however, when loose bodies were not secondary to some other intra-articular condition, 100% of patients rated the procedure as beneficial. Andrews and Timmerman (1995) reviewed the results of 73 cases of arthroscopic elbow surgery in professional baseball pitchers. Eighty percent of the players were able to return to full activity, pitching at their preinjury level for at least one season. Further review of these patients showed that 25% returned for additional surgery, often requiring stabilization and reconstruction of the ulnar collateral ligament due to valgus instability. This important study shows the close association between medial elbow laxity and posterior medial osteochondral injury and also

Postoperative Protocol for Elbow Arthroscopy and Removal of Loose Bodies

Post-Op Days 1 & 2

A. Removal of bulky post-op dressing and replacement with Ace wrap

B. Electric stimulation and ice to decrease pain/inflammation

C. Initiation of range of motion exercise for the glenohumeral joint, elbow, forearm, and wrist

D. Initiation of submaximal strengthening exercises including:

1. putty
2. isometric elbow and wrist flexion/extension
3. isometric forearm pronation/supination

Post-Op Days 2 - 7

A. Range of motion and joint mobilization to terminal ranges for the elbow, forearm, and wrist. (Avoid over-aggressive elbow extension passive range of motion.)

B. Begin progressive resistance exercise program with 0 to 1 pound weight and three sets of 15 repetitions

1. wrist flexion curls
2. wrist extension curls
3. radial deviation
4. ulnar deviation
5. forearm pronation
6. forearm supination

C. Upper body ergometer

Post-Op Days 7 - 3 Weeks

Continue progressive resistance exercise program adding:

1. elbow extension
2. elbow flexion
3. isolated rotator cuff program (Jobe exercises)
4. seated row
5. manual and isotonic scapular program
6. closed chain upper extremity program

Post-Op 4 - 8 Weeks

A. Isokinetic exercise introduction using wrist flexion/extension and forearm pronation/supination movement patterns

B. Upper extremity plyometrics with medicine balls

C. Isokinetic test to formally assess distal strength

D. Interval Sport Return Program

Criteria for advancement

1. full, pain-free range of motion
2. 85-100% return of muscle strength
3. no provocation of pain on clinical exam

E. Upper extremity strength and flexibility maintenance program highlights the importance of identifying subtle instability in the athletic elbow.

Reddy et al. (2000) retrospectively reviewed a sample of 172 patients who underwent elbow arthroscopy and had a mean follow-up of 42 months. Fifty-six percent had an excellent result, which allowed them a full return to activity, with 36% having a good result. A 1.6% complication rate was reported, with an overall conclusion that this procedure is both safe and efficacious for the treatment of osteochondral injury of the elbow.

Ellenbecker and Mattalino (1997) measured muscular strength at a mean of 8 weeks post-op in eight professional baseball pitchers following arthroscopic removal of loose bodies and posteromedial olecranon spur resection. Results showed a complete return of wrist flexion/extension strength and forearm pronation/supination strength at 8 weeks following arthroscopy. This allows for a gradual progression to interval sport return programs between 8 and 12 weeks postoperatively.

SUMMARY

A comprehensive examination of the older active patient with elbow dysfunction is necessary to obtain baseline information for development of a rehabilitation program. Knowledge of the specific anatomic adaptations in the dominant upper extremity is needed for a better understanding of the level of range of motion and strength required for full recovery. A rehabilitation program that emphasizes the entire upper extremity kinetic chain is imperative for a return to full function.

CHAPTER

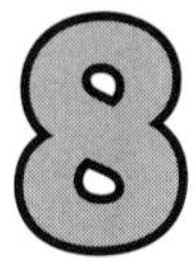

Hand and Wrist Problems

Jonathan Isaacs, MD
L. Scott Levin, MD, FACS

The incidence of degenerative and posttraumatic hand and wrist problems is related to age and not necessarily affected by activity (Caspi et al. 2001). However, the impact of these disorders may be more substantial in people trying to maintain an active lifestyle than in those who are not. In the past, treatment modalities for older patients were geared toward a more sedentary lifestyle, emphasizing activity modification and pain relief with little emphasis on returning to high-level function. A growing number of "aging athletes" find these limited goals unacceptable. Consider the 50-year-old avid female golfer. Although she has advanced first carpometacarpal (CMC) arthritis, she would rather play golf in pain than risk the potential adverse affects of surgery on her game! For these types of patients we must shift our paradigm. Although treating diseases indicative of advanced physiologic age, we must modify our tools to fulfill this group of patients' "youthful" needs.

Joints commonly affected by osteoarthritis in the hand include the distal interphalangeal (DIP), proximal interphalangeal (PIP), and thumb metacarpal-trapezial joints. In fact, up to 80% of elderly individuals have at least radiographic changes indicative of degenerative joint disease in their hands (Caspi et al. 2001). Involvement can range from asymptomatic radiographic changes to cosmetic deformity to disabling pain and instability.

Wrist disease may also be degenerative in nature but frequently is related to posttraumatic change following distal radius fractures, undetected scaphoid fractures, or previous disruptions of the scapholunate ligament. Characteristic degenerative changes that develop following these injuries may occur even despite "appropriate" treatment attempts. The symptomatology associated with these changes is quite variable and frequently minimal in the elderly low-demand patient. However, in the unique population of "high-demand" active seniors, further treatment options may need to be considered as these "old injuries" start to cause new problems.

Median nerve neuropathy at the wrist, or carpal tunnel syndrome (CTS), also shows an increased incidence with age (Phalen 1966; Yamaguchi, Lipscomb, and Soule 1965). While often seen in association with some of the degenerative and posttraumatic wrist and hand conditions already mentioned, idiopathic CTS is ubiquitous. Although advanced stages of CTS require aggressive treatment in most cases to avoid permanent nerve injury, the morbidity associated with even early CTS, while tolerable in the sedentary individual, may be bothersome enough to the active population to warrant a shift in our treatment algorithm.

HAND

The hand provides a crucial tool for interacting with the environment. In high-level activities, the demand placed on one's hands becomes even greater. The active adult will have trouble compensating for even minor hand disabilities. Arthritic changes in the interphalangeal (IP) joints are quite common, but symptoms and alterations in function can be quite variable. Treatments should focus on the relief of these symptoms.

Diagnosis

Diagnosis of osteoarthritis of the IP joints is based on clinical and radiographic findings. Pain may be chronic, or a previously asymptomatic joint may suddenly become quite painful. Loading activities, such as pinch and grip, or repetitive activities may exacerbate the condition. Physical findings include IP joint enlargement, loss of motion (both active and passive), and pain to palpation, motion, or stress. Lateral-directed stress may reveal instability or incompetence of the collateral ligaments in advanced stages of the disease. Small firm masses on the dorsum of the joint may represent mucoid cysts, which are often associated with arthritic changes. As with ganglion cysts at the wrist, verification of their cystlike nature can be demonstrated by transillumination (in a dark room, a small light source is placed flush against the mass and the entire cyst structure glows as this light radiates through the cyst).

Radiographic findings depend on the stage of disease. In early stages, loss of joint space may be the only positive finding. Later, bony changes include thickening of the subchondral bone (seen as sclerosis) and osteophyte formation (bony ridges at the periphery of both the proximal and distal sides of the joint). Instability or lateral deviation may also be confirmed by X-ray and contrasts with the hyperflexion or hyperextension deformities seen in some inflammatory conditions (figure 8.1). To confirm clinical suspicion of mucoid cyst formation, a dorsal osteophyte should be identified on the lateral X-ray (Eaton, Dobranski, and Littler 1973) (figure 8.2).

The clinical and radiographic findings reflect the ongoing pathologic process. In early arthritic disease, presumably related to both genetic and environmental factors, there is a loss of structural integrity to the cartilage. On a biologic level, this change involves alterations in proteoglycan, water, and collagen content and structure (Howell 1985; Mankin 1976; Mankin, Johnson, and Lippiello 1981). Continued wear on the softened cartilage results in fibrillation and gradual cartilage loss. Free cartilage particles probably account for some of the pain and synovitis seen even in this early stage. With the loss of cartilage, stress transmission to the bone increases and leads to characteristic subchondral thickening (sclerosis) and new bone formation at the joint periphery (osteophytes) (Howell 1985; Swanson and de Groot 1985). Interestingly, disease stage does not correlate well with symptom severity, and treatment must be tailored to the patient's complaints and demands.

Treatment objectives should address function-limiting pain, loss of motion, instability, or soft tissue compromise secondary to progressive mucoid cyst formation. As with most areas of the body affected by arthritis, conservative therapy is the appropriate initial approach.

Treatment of Distal Interphalangeal Joint Arthritis

In the case of the DIP joint, nonsteroidal anti-inflammatory drugs (NSAIDs) (especially now with improved gastrointestinal tolerability seen with COX-2 inhibitors), splinting, and even intra-articular steroid injections are all appropriate. Splints should immobilize only the affected joints and should be as low profile as possible to maximize patient acceptance. Modalities such as moist heat are occasionally helpful. Cortisone injections are particularly useful in acute flare-up situations. After prepping of the skin with betadine or alcohol, ethyl chloride ("cold spray") is

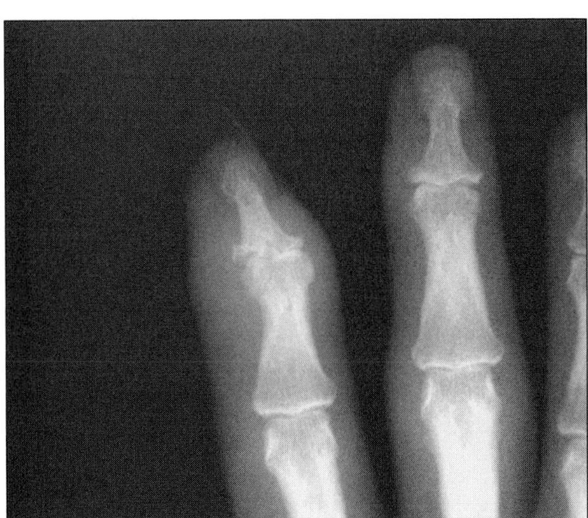

FIGURE 8.1 Arthritic distal interphalangeal joint (anteroposterior view). Note the loss of joint space associated with painful loss of motion.

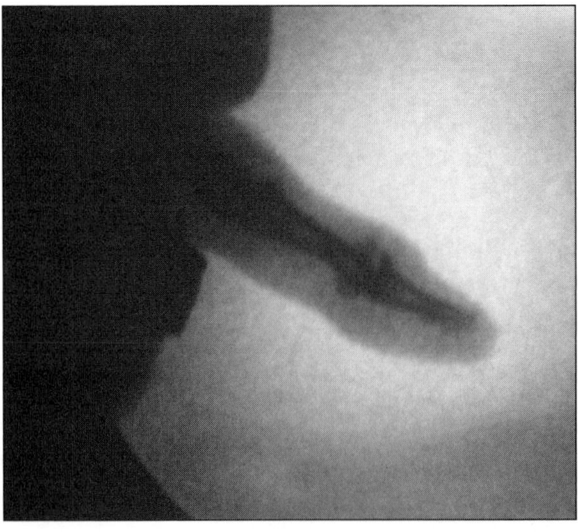

FIGURE 8.2 Arthritic distal interphalangeal joint (lateral view). Note dorsal osteophytes.

used to anesthetize the dorsal skin over the joint. A 25- or 27-gauge needle is introduced parallel to and under the extensor tendon into the joint. A 1-cc lidocaine-cortisone mixture can usually be infiltrated into the joint without difficulty.

Mucoid Cysts

Even asymptomatic mucoid cysts around the IP joints require at least close observation to avoid loss of skin integrity. Histological examination suggests that these cysts are the result of out-pouching of the synovial lining (Kleinert et al. 1972; Sonnex 1986) and, in the IP joints, are related to an osteoarthritic process. These cysts may be found distal or proximal to the joint but always have a stalk tracing back to an associated osteophyte (Eaton, Dobranski, and Littler 1973).

When found distal to the DIP joint, the mucoid cyst can cause pressure injury to the germinal and sterile matrix of the nail. Consequent nail plate deformity may range from a subtle groove to gross deformity (Brown et al. 1991) (figure 8.3). Often, again from pressure changes, the overlying skin may be quite thin and fragile (figure 8.4). Although some authors recommend injection and aspiration of these cysts (Brown et al. 1993), we feel that the risk of iatrogenic septic arthritis is too high. We discourage this approach and prefer to proceed directly to surgical excision if further treatment is necessary. Debridement of associated osteophytes is critical to excellent results, with minimal recurrence reported by multiple authors for this approach (Eaton, Dobranski, Littler 1973; Kasdan et al. 1994; Kleinert et al. 1972). Be aware that if the skin over the mucoid cyst is severely involved, skin graft or rotation flap may be necessary to obtain coverage.

Surgical Interventions for DIP

Pain and stiffness that continue to limit desired function despite conservative therapy require surgical treatment. Options include arthroplasty and arthrodesis. If motion is of paramount importance, a recent study by Wilgis (1997) suggests that DIP arthroplasty could maintain motion and stability. Wilgis reported on 38 digits following this surgery. Motion was maintained at an average of 33° and stability, a theoretical concern, was not an issue even in the index finger. Complications necessitating the removal of three implants included fracture, infection, or bony erosion (1997).

Distal IP motion is clearly less essential than PIP or MCP (metacarpophalangeal) motion to maintain high-level use of the hand. Occasionally, a patient such as a musician has unique needs requiring maintenance of maximum motion of the DIP joint. However, with this noted exception, our surgical treatment of choice is always arthrodesis. Usually by the time a joint has progressed to the point that this surgery is even being considered, stiffness is already present and further loss of motion in exchange for predictable pain relief and stability may be negligible. We have found that most patients, especially active ones, are quite satisfied. High union rates are likely regardless of technique, though a recent biomechanical study suggests that intramedullary screw fixation is more rigid than tension band or k-wire fixation (figure 8.5). This may translate to quicker return to activity. One warning with this technique is worth mentioning. The distal phalanx needs to be larger than the screw diameter (3.2 mm for the Herbert mini-screw) (Zimmer, Warsaw, IN) (Wyrsch et al. 1996).

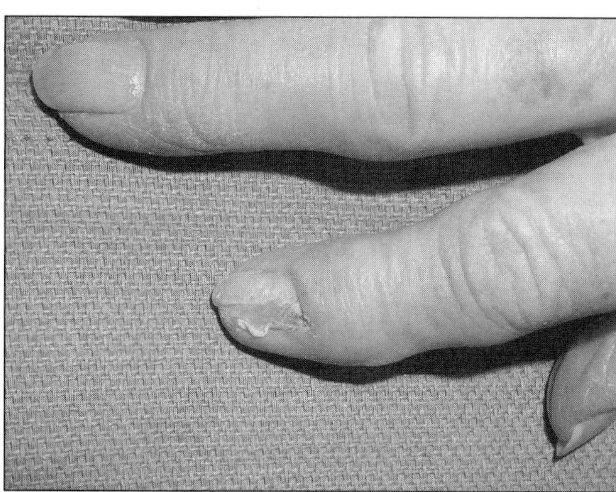

FIGURE 8.3 Nail groove secondary to mucoid cyst asserting pressure on germinal nail matrix.

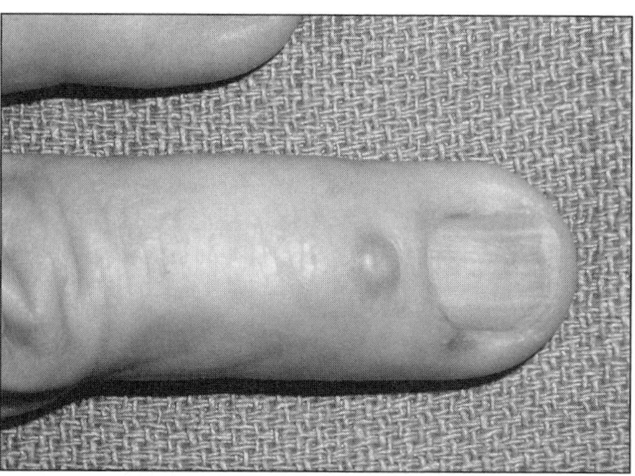

FIGURE 8.4 Mucoid cyst coming off arthritic distal interphalangeal joint. Note the thin, fragile appearance of the overlying skin.

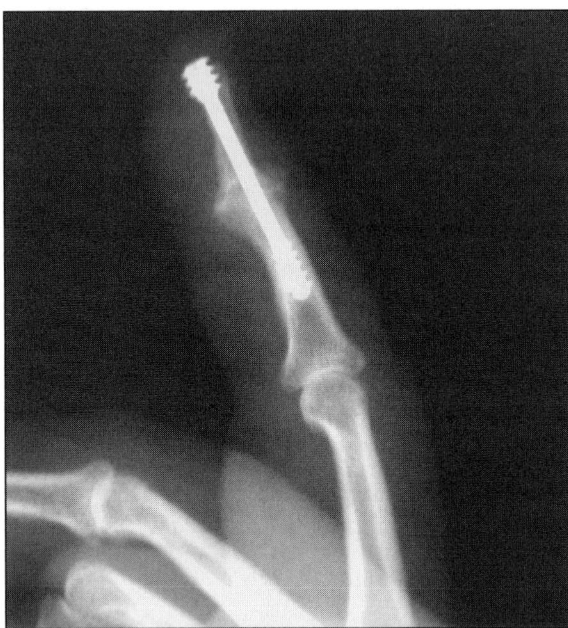

FIGURE 8.5 Distal interphalangeal joint following fusion with intramedullary screw. Because of the strength of this fixation, this patient required only brief immobilization.

Treatment of Proximal Interphalangeal Joint Arthritis

Proximal IP joint arthritis treatment may present a more difficult situation. Pain, stiffness, and sometimes deformity are again the activity-limiting symptoms.

Conservative Treatment

Conservative therapy consists of temporary splinting and rest, NSAIDs, and steroid injections. In some cases, debridement of osteophytes, synovium, and associated ganglions may offer relief while maintaining range of motion (Stern and Ho 1987). If more definitive treatment is necessary, arthroplasty and arthrodesis are the two standard options. Unlike what happens with the DIP joint, complete loss of motion at the PIP level can have significant impact on hand function, especially grip. This may be compounded by the fact that PIP and DIP arthritis are often seen together and DIP fusion may also be necessary.

Surgical Interventions

Arthroplasty, on the other hand, can maintain some motion and preserve grip but cannot provide the lateral stability to resist forces associated with pinch. The obvious (at least theoretical) solution is to develop a hinged or constrained implant to provide this additional stability. Unfortunately, designs incorporating this goal have resulted in implant fracture, bone loss, and high failure rates (Linscheid 2000; Pellegrini and Burton 1990).

Grip is important in the great majority of athletic activities and must be preserved to maintain desired function. Pelligrini and Burton (1990), I believe, offer a reasonable compromise. They divide the hand into two functional units. The radial side (specifically the index) is responsible for lateral pinch, and stability is more important here. For this digit, PIP arthrodesis is more appropriate. The ulnar-sided digits (the ring and little) are most essential for power grip, and lateral stability is less important. In addition, the fused radial digits would theoretically offer some protection from lateral forces. Arthroplasty in these affected joints would be appropriate. The long finger's role is more variable, and the patient and the desired activities need to be looked at critically to determine which approach would be better.

Of course, the elusive reconstructive goal of providing laterally stable PIP motion continues to be pursued, and innovative designs are continually introduced. Linscheid and colleagues, for example, have developed an articulating CrCo/ultra-high molecular weight polyethylene design (Linscheid et al. 1997). At this time, however, single-unit polymeric (silicone polymer either with or without a Dacron core) prostheses remain the most popular and well-studied design. Swanson's design was based on the idea that a silicon spacer would allow formation of a supportive fibrous capsule. Multiple clinical studies support its use, and it remains the joint replacement of choice. Predictable pain relief and moderate maintenance of strength (75% of contralateral side in one study) can be achieved. Although a slight extension lag should be expected, flexion should be around 40° and may be up to 70° (Hage et al. 1999; Swanson et al. 1985). Lateral instability has been reported as a complication occurring anywhere from 4% to almost 20% of the time (Pelligrini and Burton 1990; Swanson et al. 1985). Published incidence of other complications including bone resorption and implant fracture is quite variable (Mathoulin and Gilbert 1999; Pelligrini and Burton 1990; Swanson et al. 1985) but is not necessarily related to patient satisfaction. It is not clear how activity levels affect the incidence of these complications. Variations of the surgical approach have also been attempted to improve range of motion and stability, but there seems to be minimal difference with use of an anterior approach. We prefer a dorsal approach.

When joint destruction involves only the distal joint surface (as seen in early posttraumatic changes), volar plate arthroplasty offers a reasonable alternative to prosthetic implants. Eaton and Malerich (1980) found that this procedure was still applicable even two years out and reported good results, with predictable pain relief and almost 80° range of motion on average. Flexion contracture was not a problem, with an average of only 12° extension lag reported.

When arthrodesis of the index or middle PIP joints is necessary, multiple techniques offer predictable and reliable options. Chevron osteotomies with k-wire fixation, tension band technique, and Herbert screw fixation have all been associated with low failure and complication rates and high fusion rates (Ayres et al. 1988; Leibovic and Strickland 1994; Pribyl, Omer, and McGinty 1996; Stern, Gates, and Jones 1993). Usually the joint is fused at 30° to 40° of flexion, with slightly increased angles in more ulnar joints, but adjustments toward individual needs are appropriate. Reliable fusion rates have been reported for failed-arthroplasty salvage as well, though autologous bone graft, prolonged immobilization, and digital shortening were necessary (Pellegrini and Burton 1990).

Treatment of Thumb Carpometacarpal Joint Arthritis

After the DIP joint, the thumb-CMC joint is the second most commonly involved hand joint (Pellegrini and Burton 1990). This is especially common in middle-aged women, and as with other areas of the hand, degenerative X-ray changes may not correlate with the degree of disability.

Diagnosis

Symptoms usually include achiness around the thenar eminence and pain at the base of the thumb, most notably with gripping or pinching activities. Patients often note difficulty turning keys, opening jars, or turning doorknobs. Sports requiring grip strength such as golf or tennis are often affected. While the intensity of the symptoms tends to wax and wane, over time they progressively worsen.

Physical findings such as swelling around the thumb CMC joint, loss of pinch strength, and painful palpation of the CMC joint support the diagnosis. Axial load applied in a circumferential manner to the thumb (the "grind test") (figure 8.6) and forced adduction of the thumb metacarpal both usually reproduce pain (figure 8.7) as well. In advanced conditions, the base of the thumb metacarpal may be noticeably radially subluxed and the shaft fixed in an adducted position. Compensatory thumb IP joint hyperextension may also be noted.

Standard radiographs to confirm the suspected diagnosis must include standard anteroposterior (AP), lateral, and oblique views of the wrist, as well as a special AP view of the thumb CMC joint (figures 8.8 and 8.9). Radiographic changes have been well described by Eaton and Littler (1969). In stage I, the joint is still preserved and may actually be widened if an effusion is present. In stage II, narrowing and

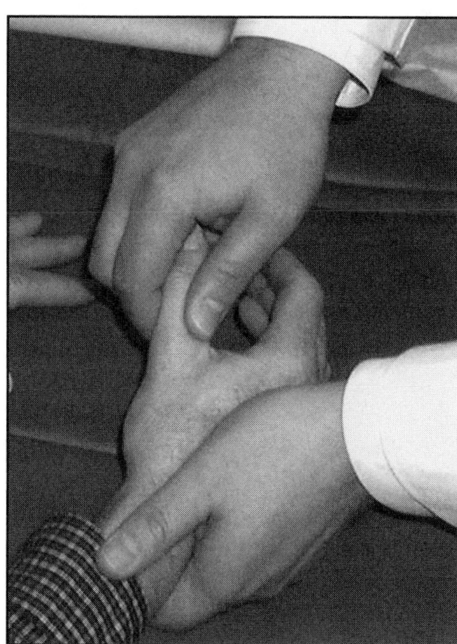

FIGURE 8.6 "Grind test" is performed by application of axial load to thumb metacarpal and moving the thumb in circumferential manner.

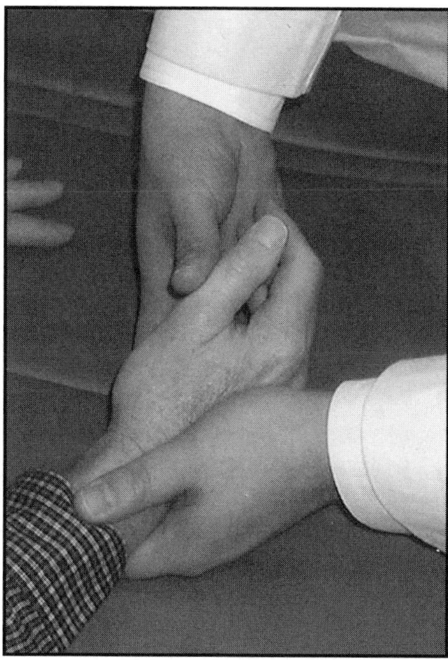

FIGURE 8.7 Thumb adduction test is considered positive if forced adduction of thumb metacarpal reproduces pain.

osteophytes less than 2 mm are present. By stage III, sclerosis, cystic changes, and osteophytes greater than 2 mm can be seen. Finally, in stage IV, pantrapezial changes have occurred as even the scaphotrapezial joints are affected.

Conservative Treatment

Conservative therapy includes NSAIDs, temporary splinting, and cortisone injections. These modalities may offer transient relief, delaying and occasionally preventing surgical treatment. Many over-the-counter and custom-made splints are available. To be useful, they must immobilize the thumb CMC joint, which necessitates marked limitation in thumb and wrist mobility (figure 8.10). For this reason, they are often poorly tolerated for long-term or repeat usage. Softer, more mobile straps are available. They may be more tolerable but are unable to immobilize or "rest" the painful joint.

Cortisone injections are useful on their own or in conjunction with other treatment modalities and help confirm the diagnosis. Significant relief can be achieved and may occasionally be surprisingly long lasting. Unfortunately, in advanced disease, joint narrowing and osteophyte formation make the injection particularly difficult and sometimes painful. After prepping the skin over the dorsum of the CMC joint, we anesthetize the skin with ethyl chloride ("cold spray") and introduce a 25-gauge needle directly into the joint. Less than 1 cc of lidocaine and cortisone mixture is slowly infiltrated into the small joint (figure 8.11). Patients should also be warned of

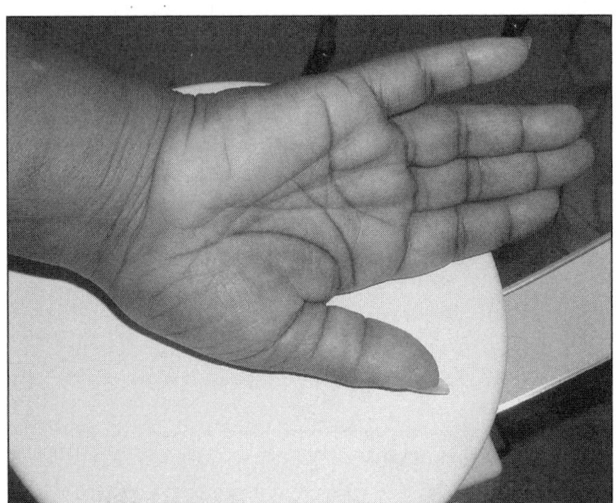

FIGURE 8.8 Positioning to obtain consistent good anteroposterior view of thumb carpometacarpal joint.

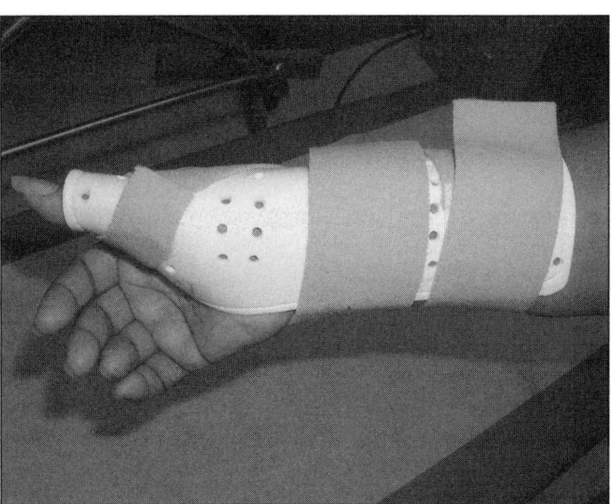

FIGURE 8.10 Splint to immobilize and "rest" arthritic thumb carpometacarpal joint.

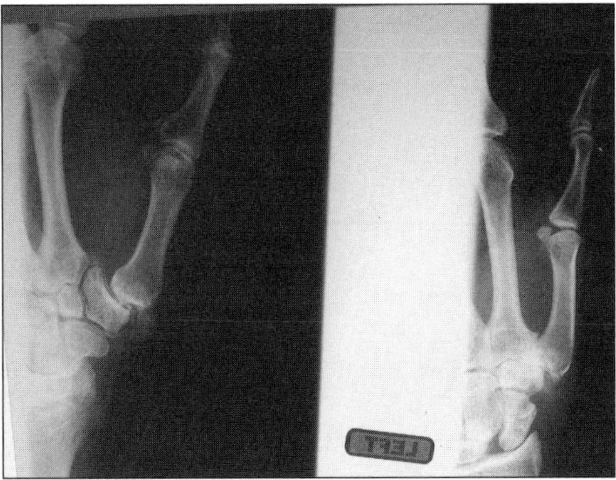

FIGURE 8.9 Anteroposterior and lateral views of advanced osteoarthritis of thumb carpometacarpal joint. Note subluxing base of thumb metacarpal, joint narrowing, and large osteophytes.

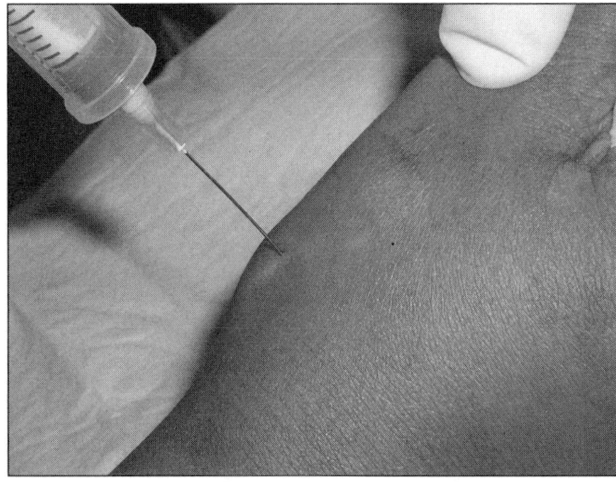

FIGURE 8.11 Injecting thumb carpometacarpal joint. Distraction is applied with one hand while injection is given with the other. May be done under fluoroscopic guidance to ensure proper placement.

the occasional subcutaneous atrophy and skin depigmentation changes seen with these injections. When surgical intervention becomes necessary, the number of options available is overwhelming (suggesting that none are perfect!) and include multiple variations of arthrodesis, joint resection, interposition, ligament reconstruction, and arthroplasty.

Surgical Interventions

Any successful surgical treatment must take into account the unique physiologic characteristics of this joint and address the specific pathological changes that occur as osteoarthritis develops and progresses.

- **Physiologic characteristics.** The thumb CMC joint has been described as reciprocal saddles oriented at 90° to each other. The dorsoradial articulation is relatively flat, offering little mechanical resistance to dorsoradial subluxation of the metacarpal, and consequently joint stability is provided by the capsule and surrounding ligaments (Eaton and Littler 1969). The anterior oblique ligament tethers the volar beak of the metacarpal to the deep intercarpal ligamentous structures (Napier 1955) and is considered the most significant stabilizer during metacarpal pronation and flexion as seen in lateral pinch and grasp (Cooney and Chao 1977; Eaton, Glickel, and Littler 1985; Pellegrini, Olcott, and Hollenberg 1993). Stresses in this joint are quite high, as well. Functional studies have shown forces 15 times those exerted at the thumb tip during pinch (Cooney and Chao 1977) and up to 120 kg during grasp (Pelligrini 1991).
- **Osteoarthritic pathological changes.** As arthritis develops and progresses, specific changes occur. The early changes include synovitis and ligamentous laxity. Since the joint stability is dependent on these ligamentous structures, subluxation becomes an early part of the disease process. Associated increased joint pressures contribute to the progressive degenerative changes affecting the metacarpal-trapezial joint and frequently extending to other articulations of the trapezoid, most notably the scaphotrapezial joint. Medial spurs push and the abductor pollicis longus pulls the base of the thumb metacarpal off the trapezium. As the base of the metacarpal subluxes dorsoradially, the metacarpal falls into an adducted posture resulting in pathologic hyperextending forces on the thumb MCP joint (Burton 1973). Any successful surgical approach, therefore, must remove the pain-generating synovitis and associated articular surfaces, provide stability from subluxation, and be able to withstand significant compressive and shear stresses, all the while, for our purposes, maintaining enough mobility and strength to allow the patient to continue high-level athletic function.

Several procedures have been described that can accomplish some of these goals but have significant drawbacks.

- **Trapeziectomy.** Trapeziectomy (Gervis 1949) is simple and effective in achieving pain relief but results in unacceptable shortening of the thumb and loss of strength and stability. Froimson (1970) proposed insertion of soft tissue to maintain length. While this procedure is somewhat effective in relieving pain, weakness and instability make it unsatisfactory for our purposes.
- **Silicone implants.** Silicone implants (multiple designs have been introduced) were better with regard to maintaining length and strength but continue to suffer from subluxation and implant failure. Silicone synovitis can be a devastating complication. A proliferative and inflammatory response to wear-generated particles results in destruction extending even to other carpal bones and ligaments (Herndon 1987; Peimer 1987). Especially for patients placing excessive strain on this implant, wear and failure would be a concern. Most authors recommend its use only in rheumatoid patients.
- **Total joint replacement.** More substantial total joint replacement implants provide good early function but are unfortunately associated with high rates of delayed loosening and failure (Cooney, Linscheid, and Askew 1987).
- **Thumb CMC joint arthrodesis.** Thumb CMC joint arthrodesis can be very successful for active patients. The development of associated arthritis in the scaphotrapezial joint appears to be quite rare even in long-term follow-up studies (Fulton and Stern 2001). Furthermore, minimal loss of functional mobility and preservation of strength make this a popular choice among many surgeons (Bamberger et al. 1992; Eaton and Littler 1969; Kvarnes and Reikeras 1985). The biggest drawback to this surgery is a high nonunion rate and prolonged healing time (Lanzetta and Foucher 1995).
- **Ligament reconstruction tendon interpositional graft.** Of all of the proposed surgical techniques in the literature, the one that we believe most predictably accomplishes the outlined goals for this patient population is the ligament reconstruction tendon interpositional graft described by Burton and Pelligrini (1986) (figure 8.12). This procedure combines several effective principles, including joint resection and interposition, but involves the use of the flexor carpi radialis tendon as a suspension system to further prevent proximal migration of the metacarpal and to recreate the stability provided by the volar oblique ligament. It has a very low failure rate and provides

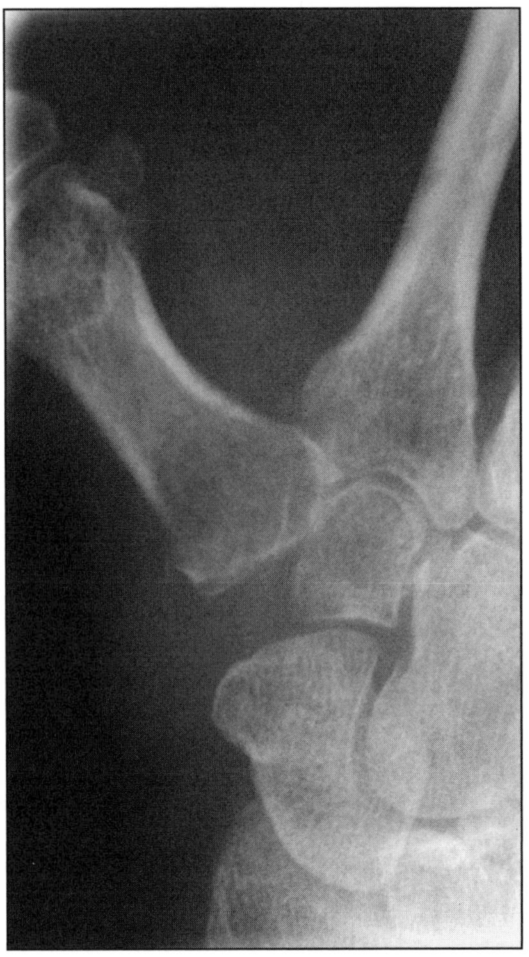

FIGURE 8.12 Following LRTI (ligament reconstruction tendon interposition) reconstruction of arthritic thumb carpometacarpal joint. The articular surface of the thumb metacarpal and the entire trapezium have been excised. The base of the metacarpal maintains its position due to the recreation of the volar oblique ligament using a slip of the flexor carpi radialis tendon. This patient had significant pain relief and improved pinch and grip strength and was able to return to playing golf.

at least as much mobility and strength as any other approach. Patient satisfaction has been reported to approach 90% in several studies (Lins et al. 1996; Nylen, Johnson, and Rosenquist 1993). Furthermore, long-term follow-up studies confirmed the longevity of these good results to at least 11 years out (Tomaino, Pellegrini, and Burton 1995). Following this surgery, patients of ours (as well as others documented in studies published by different authors) have returned to golf, tennis, and other strenuous activities. One patient from our group continues to play in professional golf tournaments (Dr. James Urbaniak personal communication).

WRIST

Radiocarpal and intercarpal arthritis can present as activity-related pain, loss of motion, swelling, and loss of grip strength. Usually related to previously treated or forgotten injuries, these arthritic patterns may take years to develop. Indeed, wrist radiographs in minimally symptomatic sedentary older individuals may show surprisingly advanced and destructive arthritic changes. In patients maintaining higher levels of activity, however, these same changes may result in pain and limitation. Two patterns warrant further discussion: radiocarpal postdegenerative arthritis and SLAC arthritis.

Scapholunate Advanced Collapse

The classic SLAC (scapholunate advanced collapse) pattern was first described by Watson and Ballet in 1984 and is considered the most common degenerative pattern in the wrist. Although the common end pathway for multiple wrist disorders, it is seen most commonly with scaphoid malrotation in association with radial malalignment, scapholunate insufficiency, or scaphoid nonunion. Watson and Weinzweig (2001) have suggested that even minor trauma can initiate a progressive deterioration resulting in carpal instability and eventually SLAC wrist.

The Degenerative Process

The SLAC process begins with scaphoid rotary subluxation. The scaphoid can be thought of as a link, maintaining the relationship between the proximal and distal carpal rows. The scaphoid's normal position is slightly flexed (mean of 47°), and as it struts across both rows, physiologic forces from the distal row assert a continuous flexion force. The lunate, on the other hand, has a natural tendency to extend (or dorsiflex). Contributing factors include the normal palmar slope of the radius (11°), the unique shape of the lunate (thinner dorsally) (Kauer 1974), and the relationship with the triquetrum (which extends via its interaction with the hamate) (Weber 1984).

Normally, the scaphoid and the lunate balance each other out—helping to maintain normal carpal relationships and sitting squarely in the corresponding fossa of the radial articulation. If, however, this balance is lost through ligamentous rupture or attenuation, the scaphoid rotates into flexion and the lunate into extension (Kleinman 2001). The scaphoid no longer sits "squarely" in its elliptical-shaped fossa, and abnormal and increased shear and compressive forces are generated (Blevens et al. 1989; Burgess 1987). Over time this results in progressive arthritis starting at the radial styloid-scaphoid articulation and extending ulnarly to eventually include the entire scaphoradial articulation (radiographic stages I and II, respectively) (figure 8.13).

Since the scaphoid can no longer effectively act as a strut between the two carpal rows, the distal row gradually collapses (moves proximally). Over time, as the capitate head wedges between the scaphoid and lunate, this caposcapholunate articulation becomes arthritic as well (stage III). Interestingly, since the lunate fossa is bowl shaped, rotation of the lunate does not seem to adversely affect shear and compressive forces, and the radiolunate articulation is spared from degenerative changes (Watson and Ballet 1984).

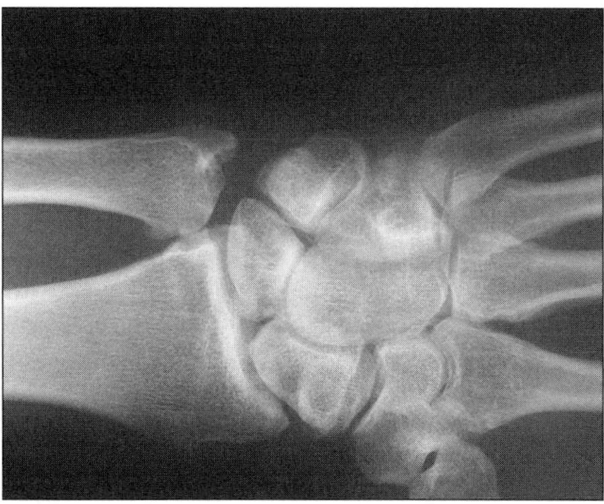

FIGURE 8.13 Stage II scapholunate advanced collapse wrist. This patient had pain with activities in which the wrist was loaded or hyperextended.

Diagnosis

Patients usually present with pain localized to the dorsal radiocarpal joint. Baseline "achiness" may intensify with activity. Forceful gripping, axial loading, and hyperextension of the wrist, all of which are necessary in most sports, seem to be especially painful. Swelling may also be noted to follow increases in activity. Weakness is probably related to the pain, while loss of motion is often a secondary complaint.

On physical exam, dorsal wrist swelling and multiplanar loss of wrist motion may be noted. The dorsal radiocarpal and especially the dorsal scapholunate intervals are often tender to palpation, with pain reproduced in these areas at the extremes of motion. Crepitus may be noted in some cases of arthritis.

A painful "clunk" can be elicited in cases of scaphoid rotary instability using the Watson clunk test (figure 8.14, *a* and *b*). In this maneuver, the examiner's thumb applies a dorsal pressure on the scaphoid tubercle. The wrist is brought from a slightly extended ulnarly deviated position into a flexed and radially deviated position. As the scaphoid tries to flex down under the influences of the trapezium and trapezoid during this motion, the examiner's thumb forces the unstable scaphoid to dorsally sublux at the radioscaphoid joint instead. This produces a painful "clunking" sensation. Although false positive "clunking" is common, the detection of associated pain improves the specificity of this provocative test (Watson, Ashmead, and Makhlouf 1988; Watson and Weinzweig 1997).

Radiographic examination of the wrist should begin with standard AP, lateral, and oblique views.

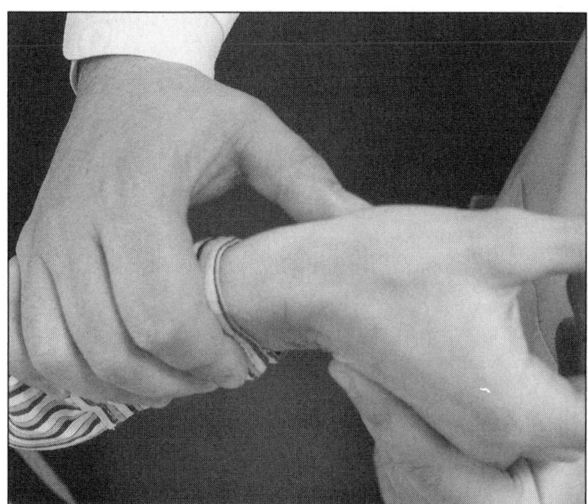

a

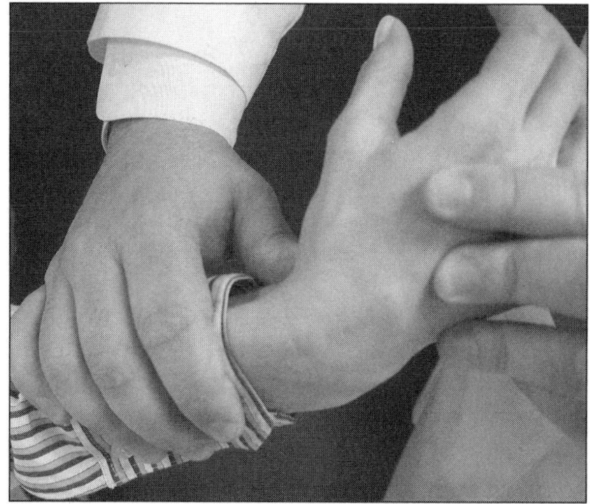

b

FIGURE 8.14 Watson's clunk test. *(a)* To begin, the wrist is placed in an ulnarly deviated slightly extended position. *(b)* Pressure is applied to the distal scaphoid pole by the examiner's thumb as the wrist is brought into a slightly flexed and radially deviated position. If the scapholunate ligament is incompetent, a painful "clunk" will be elicited during this maneuver (as the proximal pole of the scaphoid subluxes out of joint).

Subchondral sclerosis, joint narrowing, and osteophytes mark arthritic changes as in the joints previously discussed. Irregular joint surfaces and carpal alignments should be scrutinized. Any step-off in the contour of the carpal rows is abnormal (Gilula 1979). With the wrist in neutral, the relationship between the scaphoid and the lunate can be evaluated. On the AP view, the scapholunate interval should be less than 2 to 3 mm. Malrotation of the scaphoid and lunate can be seen on this view or on the lateral view as well. Special views can help bring out more subtle or earlier changes. In the clenched-fist view, the patient makes a tight fist either under fluoroscopic imaging or while an AP X-ray is obtained. If the scapholunate interval opens more than 2 to 3 mm (compared with the contralateral side), this is considered indicative of scapholunate ligament insufficiency (Kleinman 2001). Magnetic resonance imaging (MRI) (or MRI arthrogram) may have a role in evaluating this particular injury pattern, but I often have trouble interpreting the results specifically enough to alter my management.

Treatment

Treatment options basically depend on disease progression, level of symptoms, and demands placed on the wrist.

Treatment of Non-Acute Scapholunate Dissociation Injuries

We know that all patients who develop rotary subluxation of the scaphoid will eventually develop radiographically at least the characteristic carpal and arthritic changes just described (Linscheid et al. 1972; Sebald, Dobyns, and Linscheid 1974). What is not clear, however, is how long this process will take and when and whether it will become symptomatically limiting. Intuitively, the amount of activity (based on level and length of time) to which the wrist is subjected should correspond to the likelihood and degree of disability. Occasionally we have seen asymptomatic but radiographically evident chronic scapholunate dissociations misdiagnosed as "acute" with minor wrist trauma. When no symptoms have developed, however, the injury should not be regarded as acute, and conservative therapy should dominate the treatment plan. Specifically, therapy should consist of symptomatic treatment with NSAIDs and activity modification until symptoms warrant more aggressive treatment.

Treatment of Acute Scapholunate Dissociation Injuries

Acute scapholunate dissociation injuries should be treated aggressively even in the older individual if high demands will be placed on the wrist. This section describes several options and situations.

- **Direct ligament repair.** Direct ligament repair with or without capsulodesis (any Blatt variant—in which the dorsal wrist capsule is secured to the scaphoid as a "checkrein" to prevent scaphoid flexion and carpal collapse) is a reasonable approach if this situation should arise. Some loss of motion (12° in one study) is expected after a fairly lengthy recovery period, but the procedure seems to be effective in symptom relief and delay or prevention of associated arthritis (Lavernia, Cohen, and Taleisnik 1992; Wintman, Gelberman, and Katz 1995).

Treatment of Chronic Scapholunate Dissociation Injuries

When the injury is chronic, pathologic changes throughout the ligamentous architecture of the wrist prevent reduction of the carpal bones. A soft tissue repair in this situation is doomed to failure (Glickel and Millender 1984; Lavernia, Cohen, and Taleisnik 1992; Wyrick, Youse, and Kiefhaber 1998), and some form of limited arthrodesis is the most common treatment. Most commonly either a scaphocapitate or triscaphe (scaphotrapezoid-trapezium) arthrodesis is recommended (Gelberman, Cooney, and Szabo 2001). Both have their advocates, though the triscaphe seems to be technically more demanding. Loss of motion around 40% to 50% should be expected with either procedure, and significant complication rates including up to 30% incidence of nonunion need to be considered in addition to prolonged recovery times (Douglas, Peimer, and Koniuch 1987; Frykman, Af Ekenstam, and Wadin 1988; Gellman et al. 1988; Ishida and Tsai 1993; McAuliffe, Dell, and Jaffe 1993; Mih 1997; Minami et al. 1999; Watson and Hempton 1980). This clearly is a significant downside to either procedure. In the older patient who can continue to tolerate the symptoms, this downside needs to be weighed against the potential development of arthritic changes (SLAC wrist) during the patient's life span (again, when this will occur and how symptomatic it will be are not predictable).

- **Wrist denervation.** A second option to consider is wrist denervation. Although more controversial, the procedure has been used in Europe since the 1960s (Wilhelm 1966); and several large American medical centers, including the Mayo Clinic, are reporting high patient satisfaction in this exact situation. Patients with activity-limiting pain who refuse arthrodesis (because of either the associated loss of motion or prolonged recovery time) may be considered for this procedure. Berger (1998), at the Mayo Clinic, evaluates pain relief following a lidocaine injection to the posterior interosseous nerve (PIN) and the anterior interosseous nerves (AIN) before proceeding. The surgery is quite simple, consisting of a 4-cm dorsal incision just proximal to the distal radial ulnar joint with isolation and excision of 2 cm of both the PIN (on the fourth extensor compartment floor) and the AIN (just through the interosseous membrane). A high percentage of patients have been able to quickly return to their previous activities without further loss of motion. Those that fail this approach can undergo the standard salvage procedures ranging from proximal row carpectomy to total wrist fusion without further complications. Charcot joint or rapid degeneration has not been reported. We have little experience with limited wrist denervation performed as an isolated procedure, but find this approach a promising option in the older individual who is trying to maintain activity (especially activity requiring wrist motion) for a few more years.

- **Four-corner fusion and proximal row carpectomy.** If SLAC arthritic changes have already occurred, then limited intercarpal arthrodesis cannot be performed. The denervation procedure just described can still be considered, but relief may be less pronounced and a lower success rate may be expected. Certainly, this procedure can be used in conjunction with one of the salvage procedures. The two salvage procedures most commonly used are the four-corner fusion (lunocapitate-triquetrohamate arthrodesis with scaphoid excision) or the proximal row carpectomy (excision of the triquetrum, lunate, and scaphoid). Both procedures take advantage of the noted preservation of the lunate fossa in SLAC wrists. After proximal row carpectomy, the capitate head articulates with the lunate fossa (figure 8.15). With four-corner fusion, the offending scaphoradial joint is excised (scaphoid excision) and the remaining carpal bones fusion maintains the relationship between the proximal and distal rows. The lunate continues to maintain its normal relationship with the radius.

The multiple clinical studies that have been published include one directly comparing four-corner fusion and proximal row carpectomy. In stage I and II (involvement of the scaphoradial styloid joint and the entire scaphoradial joint, respectively), the two procedures seem to have equivalent results. The proximal row carpectomy is technically easier and faster and may have a faster recovery period, and so it is favored at our institution. In stage III, however, the capitate head is involved and seems to compromise results of the proximal row carpectomy. In these patients, four-corner fusion is preferred. At least 50% loss of motion compared to that of the normal contralateral wrist should be expected with relatively good preservation of strength (80% in some studies) in either procedure (Ashmead et al. 1994; Cohen and Kozin 2001; Krakauer, Bishop, and Cooney 1994; Tomaino, Delsignore, and Burton 1994; Tomaino et al. 1994; Wyrick, Stern, and Kiefhaber 1995).

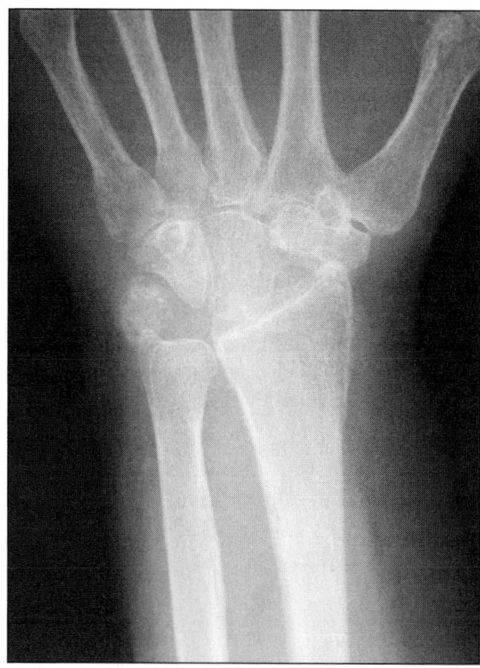

FIGURE 8.15 Wrist treated with a proximal row carpectomy. The patient has had several years of pain relief and has been able to return to moderate activities.

Radiocarpal Posttraumatic Arthritis

In patients with a history of distal radius fracture, radiocarpal posttraumatic arthritis can develop even if treatment was felt to be adequate. Knirk and Jupiter (1986) reported the predictable development of radiographic arthritic changes with just 2 mm of residual incongruence. Others have suggested that even as little as 1-mm residual step-off can result in long-term complications (Trumble et al. 1998).

Diagnosis

Even with normal posttreatment X-rays, undetected cartilage damage can lead to eventual arthritic changes. Nevertheless, as with other radiographic changes of the wrist, X-ray and clinical findings do not always correlate. Symptoms of posttraumatic radiocarpal arthritis can include activity-related pain, swelling, loss of motion, and pain.

Treatment

Conservative therapy should consist of anti-inflammatory medication, temporary immobilization as symptoms warrant, and occasional injections of cortisone into the radiocarpal joint.

If the problem is unresponsive to these interventions, the only surgical option is total wrist fusion. Pain relief and improved grip strength are expected, and risk of significant complications (nonunion rate approaches 0%) is much lower than in limited carpal arthrodesis (Hastings, Weiss, and Strickland 1993; Weiss and Hastings 1995). However, the complete loss of flexion, extension, and radial and ulnar deviation needs to be considered. Figure 8.16, *a* through *c*, shows the wrist of a 57-year-old steel worker who was unable to continue working due to pain and loss of grip. He was not financially able to retire and needed to continue working for several more years. Apparently he had experienced a scapholunate dissociation years ago and now had developed a SLAC wrist. At surgery, we found that the lunate fossa of the distal radius showed significant changes, and we proceeded to a total wrist fusion. Following recovery from surgery, the patient was able to return to work with improved grip and decreased pain.

A recent clinical series showed that patients are able to function quite well following wrist arthrodesis, frequently returning to work and recreational activities (including golf, softball, pool, hunting, and fishing). Patients seem to have problems using the hand in tight spaces where they cannot compensate for the lost motion with the elbow and shoulder (Weiss et al. 1995). Before settling on surgery, however, we usually put patients in a low-profile cast or splint so they can evaluate the potential pain relief and their function in any desired activities with a "stiff" wrist. Depending on the patient's specific needs, we usually fuse the wrist in slight extension and ulnar deviation (position of power grip). Certainly, overall function (including athletic activity) may improve, as wrist stiffness seems to be a reasonable trade-off for decreased pain and improved grip strength.

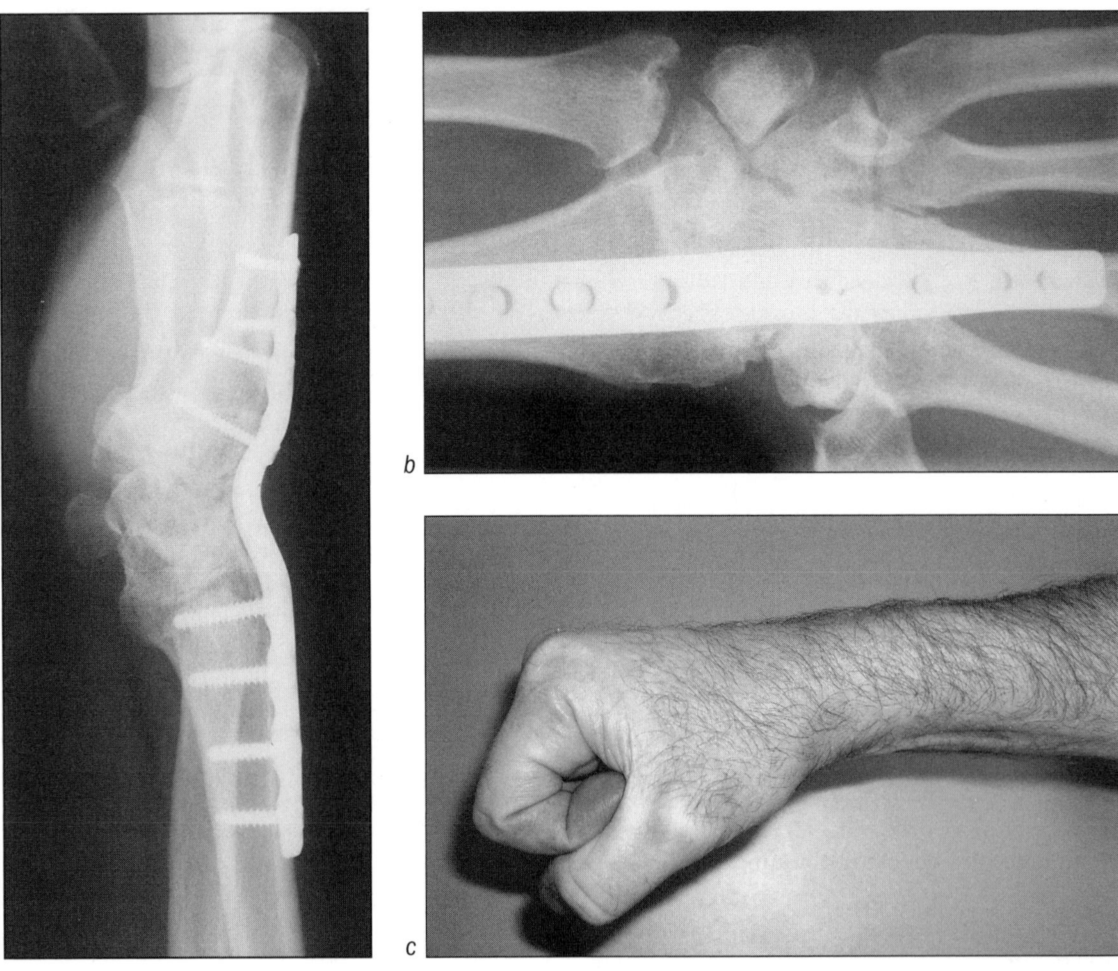

FIGURE 8.16 Total wrist arthrodesis of a 57-year-old steel worker: *(a)* lateral radiograph showing side view of plate and screws; *(b)* anteroposterior radiograph showing only the metal plate; *(c)* demonstration of his power grip after the successful surgery.

Carpal Tunnel Syndrome

Carpal tunnel syndrome describes a myriad of symptoms related to compression on the median nerve as it traverses the space created by the arch of carpal bones dorsally and the transverse carpal ligament volarly. It deserves mention in this chapter because its incidence increases with age (Phalen 1966; Yamaguchi, Lipscomb, and Soule 1965) and because the treatment algorithm may need to be adjusted in the older athlete.

Diagnosis

Patients often present complaining of insidious onset of episodes of tingling or altered sensation in their fingers. Classically, the thumb, index, and middle fingers are primarily involved (the main distribution of the median nerve); but frequently all five digits are affected. Characteristic activities—gripping the steering wheel, talking on the phone, holding a coffee cup—are often associated with these episodes. Additionally, many patients are awoken by the uncomfortable sensation in their fingers at night (Phalen 1972; Phalen and Kendrick 1957). "Shaking the hands out" is commonly reported to help resolve the episode. Even when not having overt tingling, many patients drop things and feel that they are losing grip strength. Pain is not usually associated with this disorder, though discomfort in the wrist and even radiating up the forearm is not uncommon. Loss of grip strength and dexterity, in addition to uncomfortable tingling, is a distressing symptom in any patient but has amplified negative implications for the athlete.

Several physical findings can support the diagnosis of CTS. Sensation and strength may be normal in mild and early cases. Decreased sensation, when it occurs, can be assessed subjectively by lightly touching the digits or, more objectively, using calibrated pressure monofilaments (Semmes-Weinstein, Gillis W. Long Hansens Disease Center, Carville, LA) (Gellman et al. 1986; Levin, Pearsell, and Ruderman 1978) or controlled two-point discrimination. Normal two-point discrimination is 6 mm or less. When evaluating a deficit, there often is a clear demarcation between the median nerve distribution (abnormal) and the ulnar nerve distribution (normal). In later stages, motor weakness in the median innervated thenar muscles can be elicited by checking thumb abduction and opposition strength during palpation of the thenar muscles to confirm contraction (Szabo 1991). A tingle or "electric buzz" either at the wrist or radiating into the fingers may be associated with percussing over the carpal tunnel and is referred to as a percussion (or Tinel's) sign (Tinel 1915). Two provocative tests are also helpful. The carpal tunnel compression test is considered positive if firm pressure over the median nerve at the carpal canal reproduces tingling or numbness in the digits (Durkan 1991). Phalen's test looks for the same response to the holding of the wrist in a gentle flexed position (1966). Both the tests should produce symptoms in less than 60 s. If the presentation and exam are straightforward, no further testing is necessary. However, in less clear cases, a nerve conduction study can help confirm the diagnosis. Radiographs are necessary only if accompanying wrist pathology is suspected.

Treatment

Treatment may be dictated by the severity of symptoms. In severe cases, surgical decompression of the median nerve should be performed. In milder cases, conservative treatment may be tried.

Conservative Treatment

Wrist splints, to be worn primarily at night, may be helpful especially if night symptoms are a prominent complaint. Cortisone injections into the carpal canal may alleviate symptoms at least temporarily. Although these rarely offer permanent relief, they may "buy time" until surgery can be more conveniently performed (Gelberman, Aronson, and Weisman 1980; Weiss, Sachar, and Gendreau 1994). Furthermore, there is a strong correlation between even temporary relief from an injection and permanent relief after a subsequent surgical decompression (Green 1984). To perform this injection, the volar wrist should be sterilely prepped. A 20- or 22-gauge needle can be introduced at a 45° angle to the skin at the distal wrist flexion crease. Injection sites both immediately radial and immediately ulnar to the palmaris longus ligament have been described, but the key is to recognize inadvertent contact with the median nerve. This is usually not too difficult, since the patient experiences sharp pain radiating into the fingers. An intraneural injection could cause permanent and severe injury. Once the needle "pops" through the transverse ligament, around 3 cc of anesthetic and cortisone can be introduced into the canal. Numbness in a median nerve distribution is expected but will resolve in several hours.

Surgical Intervention

If symptoms are initially severe or if conservative treatment fails, formal median nerve decompression is in order. Surgical release of the transverse carpal ligament effectively accomplishes this. Multiple open, limited open, and endoscopic techniques have been described. Limited open and endoscopic techniques require smaller incisions and have the theoretical advantage of decreased incisional pain (Brown et al. 1993; Chow

1990). This is especially important since the "classic" incision is right in the palm and can be quite bothersome during gripping of a golf club or tennis racket. Unfortunately, limiting the skin incision has not fully alleviated pain over the carpal tunnel or pillar pain (which is pain in the hypothenar or thenar areas that can develop after carpal tunnel release) (Szabo 1993). The actual benefit, as assessed by return to work or activities and patient satisfaction, is controversial and probably minimal at best (Bande, De Smet, and Fabry 1994; Jacobsen and Rahme 1996). Furthermore, presumably related to compromised visibility with use of the limited open or endoscopic approaches, there is an increased potential for incomplete release and neurovascular injury (Nath, Mackinnon, and Weeks 1993; Van Heest et al. 1995). The advantage of avoiding an incision in the palm may be worth this compromise in the patient desiring rapid return to sport, but careful consideration should be given to the increased risks.

SUMMARY

The successful treatment of hand and wrist problems in the aging athlete requires consideration of the patient's physiologic as well as chronological age. By allowing this increased flexibility in the traditional treatment paradigm, we can maximize patient satisfaction while continuing to practice sound, predictable principles.

CHAPTER

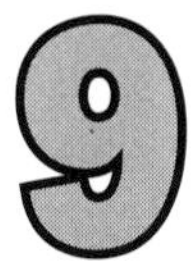

Spine Problems

Joshua D. Rittenberg, MD
Joel M. Press, MD
Amy E. Ross, MPT
Venu Akuthota, MD

The lifetime incidence of low back pain has been estimated to be as high as 90% (Frymoyer 1988), with a one-month prevalence as high as 43% of the population (Papageorgiou et al. 1995). In fact, only the common cold prompts a visit to the primary care physician more frequently (Cypress 1983). While the prognosis for recovery from a low back injury is favorable, those who have had back pain can expect recurrent episodes at a rate of 70% to 90% (Bergquist-Ullman and Larsson 1977; Von Korff et al. 1993). Spine injuries are the most common injuries reported by professional and amateur golfers (Fischer and Watkins 1996; McCarroll 1996). Back pain also occurs frequently with tennis, swimming, baseball, running, and many other sports (Matheson et al. 1988; Weinstein et al. 1998; Young et al. 1997).

Age-related changes in skeletal and neuromuscular function place the older athlete at an increased risk to sustain injury. Given this, it is probable that individuals pursuing competitive or recreational athletics into their 60s and beyond will experience a back injury at some point in their careers. The effects of injury, inactivity, and resultant deconditioning are likely to have more harmful consequences in the elderly than among younger individuals (Bortz 1982). With an accurate diagnosis, prompt initiation of treatment, attention to biomechanical factors, and an individualized approach to rehabilitation, people can achieve continued competitive participation.

ANATOMY AND BIOMECHANICS

An understanding of normal anatomy and biomechanics and of the normal and pathologic changes that occur with aging is crucial for the clinician treating the older person presenting with a spine injury.

Bony Anatomy

Segmental motion of the spine occurs via a three-joint complex consisting of an intervertebral disc between two vertebral bodies, and two obliquely aligned zygapophysial joints (z-joints or facets) posteriorly (Kirkaldy-Willis et al. 1978). The three-joint complex allows for motion along three cardinal planes: sagittal (flexion/extension), frontal or coronal (side-bending), and transverse (horizontal rotation or torsion).

The vertebral bodies, shaped like blocks, have a design well suited to resisting axial loads (Bogduk 1997). The cortical bone layer acts as a shell, containing a cancellous core arranged as vertically and horizontally aligned trabeculae. This complex internal architecture allows maximum load-bearing ability and shock absorption while maintaining a lightweight structure (Bogduk 1997).

The young, normal intervertebral disc consists of the annulus fibrosus, made up of collagen fibers, surrounding the gelatinous nucleus pulposus. The cartilaginous vertebral endplates form the top and bottom boundaries of the disc, separating it from the vertebral bodies. The disc functions to allow segmental movement and to act as a shock absorber between the vertebral bodies. The posterior elements consist of the articular processes, laminae, and spinous processes. The inferior articular process projects downward to form a synovial zygapophysial joint (z-joint) with the superior articular process of the vertebra below. With an oblique orientation, the main function of this joint is to resist sliding and twisting movements of the vertebral bodies (Kirkaldy-Willis et al. 1978). The lumbar z-joints also provide 18% of the axial weight bearing of the spinal three-joint complex (Nachemson 1960). This percentage rises in extension and falls in flexion. Furthermore, in an arthritic facet joint, the percentage of weight bearing has been measured as high as 47% (Yang and King 1984). It is estimated that 15% of chronic low back pain patients have z-joint-mediated pain (Schwarzer et al. 1994).

The sacroiliac joint (SIJ) is a C-shaped joint, with hyaline cartilage lining both the sacral and iliac surfaces, held together by bony interlocking mechanisms and strong binding ligaments (Bogduk 1997). Its function is to transmit and buffer forces between the vertebral column and the lower limbs during weight bearing.

Innervation, Blood Supply, and Muscles

The outer one-third of the annulus is innervated whereas the rest of the disc including the nucleus pulposus is not. The sinuvertebral nerve supplies the outer one-third of the posterior annulus, the posterior longitudinal ligament, and the ventral dura (Bogduk 1997). The anterior longitudinal ligament and lateral aspect of the disc are innervated by ventral rami and gray rami communicantes. The zygapophysial joints, interspinous ligaments, and multifidi are innervated by medial branches from the dorsal rami. The innervation of the SIJ remains controversial but is thought to be via the anterior and posterior rami of L4-S4 (Bernard and Cassidy 1997). It has been argued that because there is such limited range of motion, 4° of movement and 1.6 mm of total translation (Sturesson et al. 1989), the SIJ is not a likely pain source. However, injection studies have confirmed the SIJ as a potential pain generator (Schwarzer et al. 1995). In fact, the SIJ is thought to be responsible for as much as 30% of chronic low back pain (Schwarzer et al. 1995).

The vertebral body (periosteum), outer annulus, z-joints, spinal nerve root, ligaments, and muscles should all be considered potential pain generators (Bogduk 1997).

The vertebral bodies receive their blood supply via branches from the lumbar artery and veins, while the spinal nerve roots are supplied by vessels from the conus medullaris and radicular branches from the lumbar arteries. The outermost surface of the annulus fibrosus receives small arterial branches; however, the rest of the intervertebral disc is avascular and dependent on diffusion from loading for nutrition and waste removal (Bogduk 1997).

The Core

The core is composed of the back and abdominal muscles, diaphragm, pelvic floor, and even gluteal and lower limb muscles (figure 9.1). Proper muscle function and coordination are necessary to maintain spinal stability and prevent injury.

Potential Pain Generators

- Vertebral body
  -Periosteum
- Spinal nerve root
  -Anterior dura
- Intervertebral disc
  -Outer 1/3 of the annulus
- Facet joint
  -Capsule and ligaments
- Sacroiliac joint
  -Capsule and ligaments
- Ligaments
- Muscles

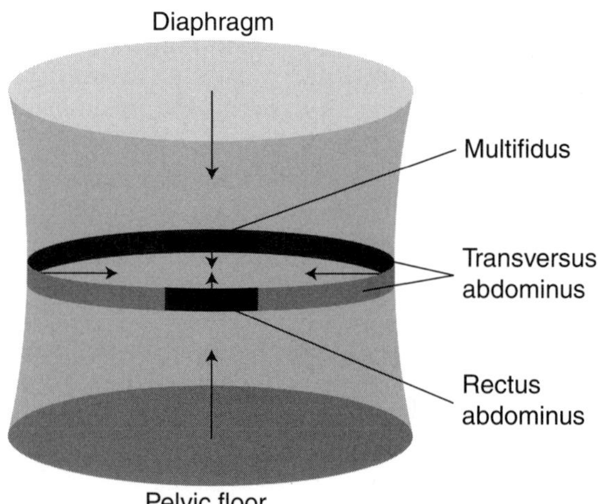

FIGURE 9.1 Schematic representation of muscles contributing to spinal and core stability.

Back and abdominal muscles control movement of the lumbar spine and provide added stability along with proprioceptive feedback. The back muscles include deep, intermediate, and superficial groups. The deep layer contains short muscles connecting adjacent spinous processes (interspinales), transverse processes (intertransversarii), and transverse processes to laminae (rotatores). These muscles have been shown to contain a large proportion of muscle spindles, suggesting that their primary role is proprioception rather than force production (McGill 2001).

The intermediate group contains polysegmental muscles (multifidus, longissimus, iliocostalis). The superficial muscles, long and polysegmental, are referred to as the erector spinae (iliocostalis, longissimus, and spinalis). The abdominal muscles include the transverse abdominis, external obliques, internal obliques, and rectus abdominis (Panjabi and White 1990).

A concept of globally and locally acting muscles has been proposed (Bergmark 1989). The global muscles insert on the pelvis and thoracic cage and act indirectly to stabilize the spine and to produce or control movements. They do not directly insert on the lumbar spine. Examples of global muscles include the rectus abdominis, external obliques, and thoracic component of the iliocostalis. The local muscle system consists of the multifidi, internal obliques, and transverse abdominis. These muscles insert directly on the lumbar spine and act segmentally, influenced locally by factors such as posture.

Lumbar spine stability has been shown to be enhanced by increased intra-abdominal pressure (Cholewicki et al. 1999). This is further enhanced by activation of abdominal muscles, particularly the transverse abdominis and obliques. Additionally, activation of the transverse abdominis occurs prior to initiation of lower limb movement, suggesting an anticipatory stabilizing role (Hodges and Richardson 1997).

McGill has described the role of coordinated coactivation of back and abdominal wall muscles in helping to provide stiffness and stability to the lumbar spine (McGill 1998, 2001).

In addition to back and abdominal muscles, imbalances or deficits in hip abductor and extensor strength have been found to be associated with the occurrence of low back pain in an athletic population (Nadler et al. 2000).

More recently, the influence of pelvic floor muscles has been described. Pubococcygeal muscle activation creates abdominal muscle co-contraction and vice versa in normal subjects; furthermore, with the position of the spine in flexion the external obliques are more active, while in extension the transverse abdominis is most active during pelvic floor muscle recruitment (Sapsford et al. 2001).

THE AGING SPINE

Disc degeneration begins as early as after the first decade in males and second decade in females. The presence of disc degeneration should be thought of as a normal process of aging ("wear and tear"), and not necessarily pathological. In a group of patients over age 60 with no history of back pain or sciatica, 93% had disc degeneration on lumbar spine magnetic resonance imaging, with an average of three levels involved. Spinal stenosis or a herniated disc was found in 57% (Boden et al. 1990).

Kirkaldy-Willis and Burton (1992) divide the progression of changes that occur in the aging spine into three phases (see figure 9.2):

- In the first phase, segmental dysfunction and joint restriction occur as the result of an initial injury. Actual tissue injury consists of z-joint synovitis and annular tearing as a result of torsional or compressive forces or both.
- The second phase is characterized by segmental instability. Degeneration of articular cartilage and z-joint laxity, along with annular bulging, tearing, and herniation of nuclear material, are seen in this stage.
- In the third stage, bony overgrowth and periarticular fibrosis restore stability but also lead to spinal stenosis (Kirkaldy-Willis and Burton 1992). People past the age of 60 are most likely to present in this stage.

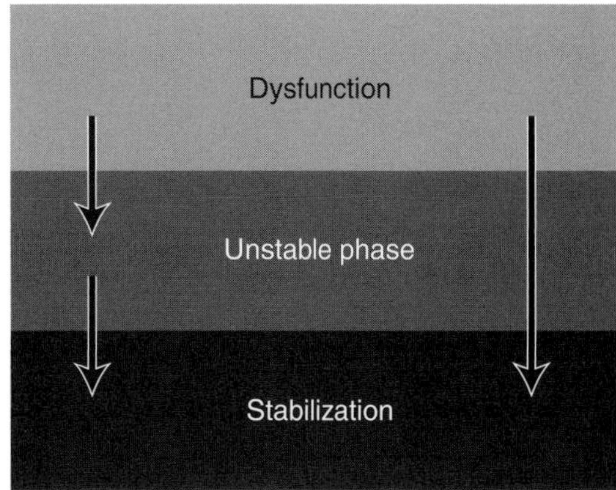

FIGURE 9.2 Three phases of the degenerative process.

Reprinted, by permission, from W.H. Kirkaldy-Willis and T.N. Bernard, 1999, *Managing low back pain*, 4th ed. (New York: Churchill Livingstone), 70.

The intervertebral disc undergoes multiple intrinsic changes with age. The vascular supply to the vertebral endplates disappears by the third decade (Cassinelli et al. 2001). As the endplates calcify, diffusion of nutrients into the disc and removal of waste slow (Bernick and Cailliet 1982; Cassinelli et al. 2001; Nachemson et al. 1970). Changes in collagen lead to increased stiffness of the annulus and increased susceptibility to mechanical failure. With age, the nucleus loses water content and becomes stiffer and fibrotic, resulting in decreased shock-absorbing ability and decreased disc height. Loss of disc height leads to upward displacement of the superior articular processes and subluxation of the z-joints (Kirkaldy-Willis et al. 1978).

Degenerative spondylolisthesis may occur, most commonly at the L4-L5 level, and can cause impingement of the traversing L5 nerve roots (Herring and Weinstein 1995). The z-joint will eventually develop erosion of articular cartilage and form osteophytes. Buckling or "hypertrophy" of the ligamentum flavum also occurs as the disc loses height.

Central spinal stenosis may occur as a result of disc degeneration and bulging or protrusion, vertebral body osteophyte formation, ligamentum flavum buckling, z-joint hypertrophy, or degenerative spondylolisthesis. Furthermore, z-joint hypertrophy, particularly of the superior articular process, and posterolateral disc protrusions may also cause lateral recess stenosis, impinging upon traversing nerve roots prior to their reaching the intervertebral foramen one level below. Stenosis of the intervertebral foramen and impingement of exiting nerve roots may result from subluxation of the superior articular facet, posterolateral vertebral body osteophytes, or a lateral disc herniation. Degenerative synovial cysts arising from the z-joint may also produce narrowing of the central canal, lateral recess, or foramen.

Lumbar extension has been shown to decrease the sagittal diameter of the central canal compared with flexion, as measured by dynamic flexion/extension myelography (Amundsen et al. 1995; Dyck and Doyle 1977). Additionally, lumbar extension decreases the intervertebral foraminal area by 15% from neutral, while flexion increases the area by 12% (Inufusa et al. 1996; Jenis and An 2000; Jenis et al. 2001). Encroachment results from vertebral body osteophytes or discs ventrally, z-joint hypertrophy laterally, and hypertrophy or buckling of the ligamentum flavum dorsally (Inufusa et al. 1996). Axial loading will also contribute to further encroachment of structures upon neural elements.

Along with changes in the spine, the entire functional kinetic chain should be considered a significant contributor to pathology in the spine. Dysfunction at distant sites such as the hip, knee, and even the foot and ankle should be assessed. Additionally, decreases in neuromuscular control, balance, and reaction time that occur with aging may also lead to increased injury susceptibility.

EVALUATION

Spending adequate face-to-face time with the patient, performing a complete history and physical exam, and obtaining diagnostic testing if indicated should yield a specific diagnosis and allow formation of an individualized treatment and rehabilitation program. Avoid vague diagnostic terminology, such as lumbar strain, lumbago, mechanical low back pain, and sciatica.

History

In the older person, accurate diagnosis is vital given the broad differential diagnosis that one needs to consider in this population. While degenerative changes are the most common etiology for back pain in the elderly, one must maintain a high index of suspicion for more serious causes, such as pathologic fracture, cancer, or infection.

A standardized questionnaire is useful for initial screening prior to the more detailed face-to-face interview. One may assess spinal pain in a systematic fashion using the OPQRST mnemonic (**O**nset, sudden vs. insidious; **P**rovoking or relieving factors; **Q**uality; **R**eferral or radiation; **S**everity; **T**ime frame, duration of symptoms). If the injury occurred during training or athletic competition, assess equipment and training history also. Use a validated functional assessment tool to assess severity of disability. Examples include the Oswestry Disability Index (Fairbank et al. 1980; Fairbank and Pynsent 2000) for low back pain and the Spinal Stenosis Scale, described by Stucki, for more condition-specific functional evaluation in lumbar spinal stenosis (Stucki et al. 1996). These and other assessment tools are readily available either via the original reference source or through organizations such as the North American Spine Society (www.spine.org).

Assess the presence of clinical "red flags," such as history of cancer, unexplained weight loss, and pain not improved with rest (Bigos et al. 1994). A retrospective study of patients diagnosed with cancer after presenting to a multidisciplinary spine center demonstrated a high likelihood for spontaneous onset of symptoms, night pain, past history of cancer, and unexplained weight loss (Slipman et al. 2003). If red flags are present, further diagnostic testing is indicated (Bigos et al. 1994). Cauda equina syndrome, characterized by lower extremity weakness and numbness, bowel/bladder dysfunction (typically urinary retention), and saddle anesthesia should be considered a surgical emergency.

Investigate history of previous lumbar spine surgery, diabetes mellitus, peripheral vascular disease, hypertension, and heart disease. Degenerative disease of the hip is found commonly in older patients and should be included in the process of forming a differential diagnosis. The presence of depression and other psychosocial stressors may negatively impact recovery and therefore should be identified and addressed. Questionnaires such as the Beck Depression Inventory or Fear Avoidance Behavior Questionnaire (FABQ) (Waddell et al. 1993) are useful for screening.

Physical Examination

The physical exam should follow and complement a thorough history. With a differential diagnosis already established, many diagnoses can be either discarded or confirmed by the exam. A systematic approach is necessary and should include an orthopedic, neurological, and functional assessment. Note even subtle abnormalities. Provocative maneuvers are an invaluable part of the spine exam.

Musculoskeletal Exam

Observation may reveal a stooped forward posture during standing or walking. Avoidance of lumbar extension is typical with spinal stenosis or with z-joint-mediated pain. An antalgic gait in the patient with back pain along with groin, thigh, or leg pain should alert the clinician to investigate for concomitant lower extremity pathology, most notably at the hip. The patient should be undressed to fully expose the spine and lower extremities. The presence of a trunk shift is frequently an indication of disc pathology (Geraci and Alleva 1997).

The palpatory exam should include assessment of bony landmarks, asymmetries, step-offs, and tender or trigger points. Tenderness over the posterior superior iliac spine or sacral sulcus is frequently present with SIJ-mediated pain (Dreyfuss et al. 1996). Pain with palpation over the spinous process should raise suspicion of disc pathology or a vertebral compression fracture. Paravertebral tenderness is generally nonspecific, but may raise suspicion for z-joint pain or myofascial pain. Marked tenderness over the sacrum should raise suspicion of a sacral insufficiency fracture in the older patient with acute low back pain.

Many provocative maneuvers have been described for assessment of the SIJ. Examples include sacral spring, posterior shear, Patrick's (figure 9.3), Gaenslen's, and Yeoman's tests (Magee 2002). Although none have been validated by scientific studies (Dreyfuss et al. 1994; Slipman et al. 1998), these maneuvers are a worthwhile part of the exam and can be helpful in the formation of a differential diagnosis and treatment plan.

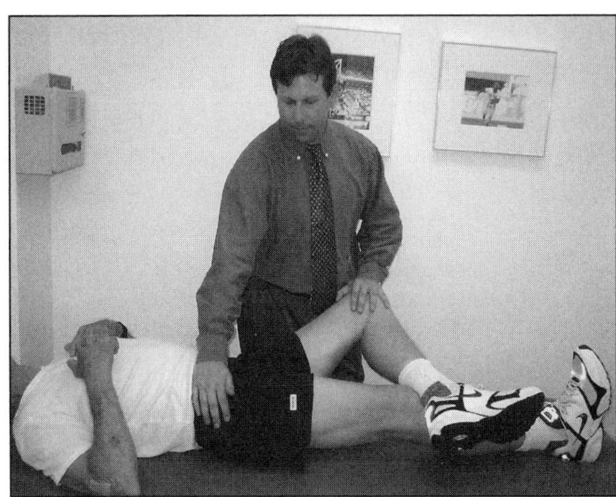

FIGURE 9.3 Patrick's test.

Lumbosacral range of motion should be assessed in all cardinal planes: sagittal (flexion and extension), coronal (side-bending), transverse (rotation), and extension/rotation. Assess directional preferences and use these to help guide a treatment program. Note segmental restrictions along with provocation of pain. Reproduction of radicular pain with ipsilateral extension/rotation is seen with lateral stenosis. Spondylolisthesis and z-joint-mediated back pain are typically worsened with extension or extension/rotation. Disc-mediated pain is more typically aggravated by flexion.

The Waddell's, or nonorganic, signs are used to evaluate for psychological distress and to help validate the rest of the exam (Waddell et al. 1980). These signs include superficial or non-anatomic distribution of tenderness, provocation of pain with sham maneuvers or distraction, inconsistencies, non-anatomic weakness/sensory loss, and overreaction. Simulated spine rotation, via rotating the entire trunk and pelvis, and axial loading with pressure over the head causing pain in the lumbar spine are examples of sham maneuvers. The presence of these signs has been shown to negatively affect surgical outcome (Akuthota et al. 2001) and return to work (Gaines and Hegmann 1999).

Evaluate distal pulses along with skin color, texture, and temperature. Investigate for peripheral vascular disease in the presence of abnormality.

Evaluation of the Nervous System

Sensory testing should assess lower extremity dermatomes and peripheral nerve distribution zones (table 9.1). The presence of bilateral distal stocking distribution sensory abnormality should alert the clinician to

TABLE 9.1 Dermatome, Myotome, and Muscle Stretch Reflex Testing Sites

Level	Dermatome	Myotome	Reflexes
L4	Distal anterolateral thigh/proximal medial lower leg	Knee extensors	Patella
L5	First web space	Extensor hallucis longus	Medial hamstring
S1	Lateral aspect of foot	Repeated toe raises	Achilles

the possibility of peripheral neuropathy, and further diagnostic testing may be warranted. A manual muscle exam should segmentally assess the lower extremity myotomes. Muscle stretch reflexes are frequently reduced in elderly persons; however, asymmetries should be noted. The presence of hyperreflexia or long tract signs should alert the clinician to investigate for upper motor neuron pathology, particularly in the patient presenting with gait disturbance.

Adverse dynamic neural tension maneuvers, also known as dural tension tests, sensitize or stretch dural tissue. The slump test, supine straight leg raise, and femoral stretch tests should all be utilized routinely, with facilitating maneuvers to increase the sensitivity of the tests if necessary.

- The slump test is performed with the patient seated in a slumped posture, hands resting behind the back, and neck flexed. The knee is slowly extended and provocation of pain is noted (figure 9.4). Facilitating maneuver: Add hip internal rotation, ankle dorsiflexion, or both (Johnson and Chiarello 1997).
- The supine straight leg raise is classically positive if reproduction of radicular pain occurs below 70°. Facilitating maneuver: Add hip internal rotation, ankle dorsiflexion, or both (Johnson and Chiarello 1997).
- The femoral stretch is performed with the subject prone by flexing the knee, with reproduction of anterior thigh pain considered a positive test. Facilitating maneuver: Add hip extension (Geraci and Alleva 1997).

Because dural tissue is irritated in cases of radicular pain, these tests can provide invaluable information by helping to identify a nerve root origin of pain. Additionally, for the treating clinician, identification of dysfunction will help to guide the treatment plan.

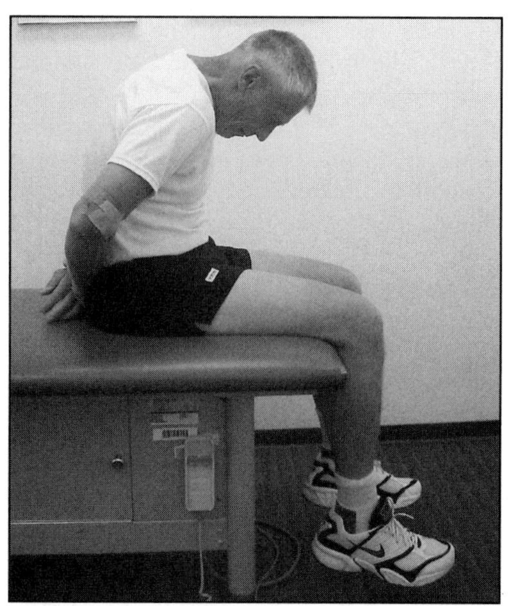
a

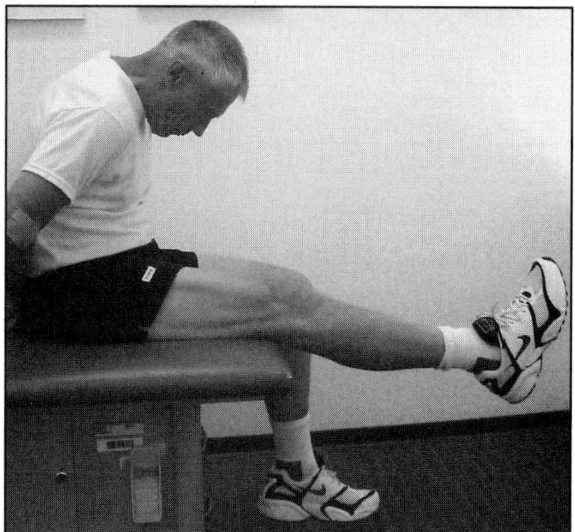
b

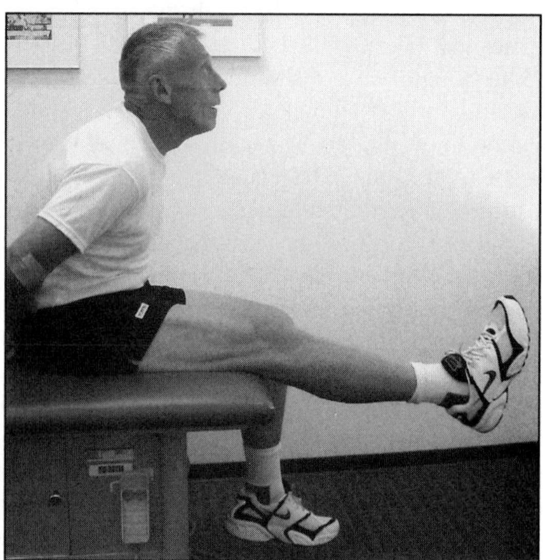
c

FIGURE 9.4 The slump test.

Further discussion of assessment and treatment of dysfunction of neural tissues is beyond the scope of this chapter; however, this subject has been written on extensively by David Butler (1991, 2000).

Biomechanical Assessment

In addition to the standard orthopedic spine exam and neurologic exam, a biomechanical assessment of the functional kinetic chain in the athlete will provide further information regarding injury pathogenesis and subsequent rehabilitation. The functional kinetic chain refers to the concept that distant or proximal structures, via their connection by joints, muscles, and fascia, may influence other kinetically linked structures (Geraci and Alleva 1997). For example, a tight iliopsoas, via attachments to the anterolateral lumbar spine, may cause an anterior pelvic tilt, leading to a compensatory increase in lumbar lordosis. Abdominal and gluteal muscle weakness may cause further increases in anterior tilt (Kaul and Herring 1998). An increase in lumbar lordosis will lead to increased weight bearing through the z-joints and decreased central canal and foraminal diameter. In the athlete, one should perform testing to assess complex and dynamic movement patterns. It is important to note segmental hypomobility, habitually poor posture, lower extremity joint restrictions, and tight or weak muscles, as they may impact overall movement quality, particularly during sports.

Perform core muscle testing in a functional manner. Static single-leg balance can provide a gross assessment of core strength. Note a drop in the opposite hemipelvis, indicating hip abductor weakness (also known as a Trendelenburg sign). Single-leg squats or performance of leg or arm reaches in multiple planes further challenges the core and neuromuscular system. In many cases, the test that has identified the dysfunction can become the treatment.

Once the exam of the spine and kinetic chain is complete, it is possible to identify potential pain generators and kinetically linked contributors.

Diagnostic Testing

Diagnostic tests are typically ordered when symptoms have been present for longer than four weeks or if strong indications, such as red flags (p. 138) or traumatic injury, are present. Other reasons for diagnostic testing include ruling out serious disease, medicolegal issues, and determining prognosis.

Imaging studies of the spine are useful for assessing abnormal anatomy but are frequently positive in asymptomatic individuals (Boden et al. 1990; Jensen et al. 1994). These studies do not determine the pain generator and must be correlated with the history, physical exam, and other diagnostic information.

Plain Radiographs

Plain radiographs provide information about alignment, bony anatomy, bone density, and disc space size. In general, plain radiographs are overused in back pain patients (Liang and Komaroff 1982). Because of the cost and radiation exposure, criteria have been proposed to establish when plain films should be ordered. The Agency for Health Care Policy and Research (AHCPR) recommends that plain X-rays should not be obtained for routine evaluation within the first month of pain unless the patient demonstrates a red flag (Bigos et al. 1994) as described previously. Fracture should be ruled out by X-ray in any patient with recent significant trauma, mild trauma in patients over age 50, history of prolonged corticosteroid use, osteoporosis, or age greater than 70. The AHCPR also recommends plain films in combination with a complete blood count and sedimentation rate for those patients in whom infection and tumor need to be ruled out.

Anteroposterior and lateral films are generally adequate for initial screening (Suarez-Almazor et al. 1997). Oblique views should be considered only when facet arthropathy is suspected, as they double the radiation exposure and cost. Coned-down lateral views of L5-S1 should not be ordered unless more detailed information is needed regarding the L5-S1 bony anatomy and disc space (Deyo 1986). Flexion/extension views should be obtained if instability is suspected.

Magnetic Resonance Imaging, Computed Tomography, and Bone Scans

Magnetic resonance imaging (MRI) and computed tomography (CT) scans offer more detailed views of spinal anatomy. Magnetic resonance imaging is the study of choice for soft tissue anatomy, while CT will delineate bony anatomy best. Both MRI and CT scans often show abnormal findings in asymptomatic subjects (Jensen et al. 1994; Wiesel et al. 1984). Advanced imaging is usually not needed urgently except in the case of cauda equina syndrome. If disc pathology is suspected, MRI is the test of choice.

Although MRI has emerged as the study of choice for evaluating spinal stenosis, CT scans can be valuable to evaluate bony stenosis. Stenosis can occur centrally, at the lateral recess, or at the intervertebral foramen. Central stenosis refers to narrowing of the central spinal canal. Lateral recess stenosis refers to narrowing of the anterolateral aspect of the central canal, bordered posteriorly by the superior articular process and ventrally by the posterolateral intervertebral disc and vertebral body (Ciric et al. 1980). Foraminal stenosis denotes narrowing of the intervertebral nerve root canal. Spinal stenosis should be designated as central, lateral recess, or foraminal.

Although some centers continue to use CT-myelography, MRI has replaced this type of study primarily because of the morbidity, expense, and insensitivity of myelography. It is common to use CT-myelography if there is a contraindication to MRI or for preoperative planning. In the past, an advantage was that this type of study also provided dynamic information with flexion/extension myelography, revealing changes not apparent with the patient in a static supine position. However, more recently, MRI open scanners have emerged that allow more choices for positioning and even axial loading.

In addition to evaluation of soft tissue anatomy, MRI will show bony edema following vertebral fracture and may be helpful in identifying an acutely injured level.

Bone scan is a test of metabolic activity used to identify areas undergoing bony changes. It is an excellent screening test when bone metastasis, fracture, or infection is suspected. It can also be used to detect pars injury, facet arthropathy, pseudarthroses, generalized bone disease, and spondyloarthropathy.

Describing Disc Pathology

Historically, disc pathology is an area in which many terms are poorly defined. Avoid nonspecific terms such as "herniated" or "ruptured" disc. A three-term classification scheme for herniated discs has been proposed to provide a clear, standardized delineation of pathology: *disc protrusion, disc extrusion,* and *disc sequestration* (Akuthota et al. 2001).

- A *disc protrusion* is a focal extension of the nucleus pulposus that is contained by the outer annular fibers and an intact posterior longitudinal ligament (PLL).
- A *disc extrusion* is a focal extension of the nucleus pulposus that is not contained by the outer annular fibers or PLL.
- A *disc sequestration* is herniated nucleus pulposus material with a noncontiguous free fragment.

Location of any of these disc pathologies should be described as central, paracentral, lateral, or far lateral. Identification of the traversing nerve root or exiting nerve root should be described when impingement is present.

Electrodiagnostic Tests

Neurophysiologic testing has a limited but valuable role in low back pain patients with radicular pain or neurogenic claudication. It should be thought of as an extension of the history and physical exam. Needle electromyography (EMG) and nerve conduction studies (NCS) provide information about nerve and muscle function, in contrast to radiographic images, which assess static anatomy and are frequently abnormal in asymptomatic individuals. Needle EMG and NCS can be utilized to confirm or refute a disputed diagnosis, such as when peripheral neuropathy is suspected in a patient with spinal stenosis. These studies are helpful for confirming presence of radiculopathy, localizing nerve lesions, and guiding surgical decision making (Press and Young 1997). Additionally, the age of an injury can be assessed, since acute and chronic lesions have distinct findings (Kraft 1990). It is important to perform EMG/NCS at least three weeks after injury or onset of symptoms to allow abnormal findings to fully develop.

Routine electrodiagnostic studies have limited sensitivity and do not identify all cases of radiculopathy. Dermatomal somatosensory-evoked potentials (DSEPs) are used in some centers because of the poor sensitivity of standard EMG/NCS and may be more sensitive for detecting neurophysiologic changes in spinal stenosis (Kraft 1998). Several studies have described the electrodiagnostic findings in spinal stenosis (Hall et al. 1985; Jacobson 1976; Kraft 1998; Seppalainen et al. 1981). The anatomically stenotic level has been correlated with EMG findings, although central canal stenosis also commonly compresses roots exiting at a lower level. The L5 nerve root is most commonly involved (Seppalainen et al. 1981). Paraspinal muscle involvement has been described as less frequent than limb muscle abnormality; however, in the experience of one of the authors this has not been the case, and testing of paraspinal muscles is integral to the needle electrode exam. Bilateral, multiradicular limb abnormalities may be found even in unilaterally symptomatic patients (Jacobson 1976).

TREATMENT

A thorough evaluation along with appropriate diagnostic studies should enable the clinician to formulate a specific diagnosis and to identify pain generators, kinetically linked contributors, and biomechanical dysfunctions to allow for a specific and individualized treatment plan.

Framing Diagnosis to Facilitate Treatment

To design a successful rehabilitation program, one must first achieve accurate diagnoses and an understanding of factors that led to injury. Kibler's model for describing musculoskeletal injuries is a useful approach to identifying primary and secondary sites of injury and dysfunction (see pp. 51) (Herring and Kibler 1998). Recall that Kibler's model can be summarized as follows:

- The tissue injury complex consists of the actual site of tissue damage.
- The clinical symptom complex refers to the clinical manifestations of injury, such as pain, weakness, numbness, decreased range of motion, swelling, and decreased athletic performance.
- The tissue overload complex refers to the tissues that have been overloaded by tensile, eccentric, or compressive forces and may be located locally or distant to the site of tissue injury.
- The functional biomechanical deficit complex refers to flexibility and strength imbalances that contribute to altered mechanics. This may be the cause, the result, or both cause and result of the patient's pain or dysfunction.
- The subclinical adaptation complex refers to compensatory patterns and motions used by the injured athlete to maintain performance.

Examples of this framework follow, along with descriptions of common accompanying diagnoses and scenarios.

Lumbar Spinal Stenosis

- Clinical symptom complex: low back pain and leg pain, worse with extension, relieved by flexion or sitting
- Tissue injury complex: mechanical or ischemic compromise of spinal nerve roots
- Tissue overload complex: lumbar paraspinal muscles and supporting ligamentous structures or vascular structures
- Functional biomechanical deficit: tight hip flexors, restricted segmental motion
- Subclinical adaptation complex: flexed posture, loss of lumbar lordosis

Z-Joint (Facet) Arthropathy With Extension-Based Pain

- Clinical symptom complex: low back pain with varying degrees of referred pain to the buttock or thigh, worse with extension, relieved by flexion
- Tissue injury complex: facet joint capsule
- Tissue overload complex: z-joint capsule and synovium, lumbar paraspinal muscles and supporting ligamentous structures
- Functional biomechanical deficit: tight hip flexors, restricted segmental motion
- Subclinical adaptation complex: flexed posture, loss of lumbar lordosis

Vertebral Compression Fracture

- Clinical symptom complex: acute, focal thoracolumbar pain with tenderness to palpation
- Tissue injury complex: vertebral body, periosteum
- Tissue overload complex: vertebral body
- Functional biomechanical deficit: segmental hypomobility, weakened extensor muscles
- Subclinical adaptation complex: increased kyphosis, loss of normal lumbopelvic rhythm

Principles of Spine Rehabilitation

In the older athlete, prompt initiation of a structured rehabilitation program can facilitate a return to athletic participation and prevent deleterious effects of inactivity. Rehabilitation of spine injuries should follow the same principles applied to other injury sites and can serve as a framework for all diagnostic subsets.

During the initial phase of treatment, relative rest or activity modification is the recommendation rather than bed rest. Patients should be educated about their injury and given reassurance from the treating physician regarding their prognosis and expected time lost from competition. Adequate analgesic control should be offered. Nonsteroidal anti-inflammatory medications may be initiated in most cases. Epidural or oral corticosteroids may be appropriate for acute radicular pain. Passive physical modalities, such as ice or electrical stimulation, may be helpful for short periods, as an adjunct, to reduce pain and muscle spasm.

Patients should be educated regarding positions to reduce symptoms and should be encouraged to "cross-train" if possible to maintain cardiovascular fitness. The patient with a flare-up of back and leg pain due to spinal stenosis may be able to tolerate more flexion-based activities (i.e., riding a stationary bike, walking in a pool backward, or exercising on a treadmill, especially uphill on an incline, or with the assistance of an unweighting harness). Bracing may provide symptomatic relief; however, its use should be limited to avoid soft tissue restriction and muscular deconditioning.

Address biomechanical deficits identified on the assessment. In the patient with extension-based pain with or without leg pain, strengthening of abdominal and gluteal muscles, along with improving flexibility of hamstrings and hip flexors and reduction in anterior pelvic tilt, will contribute to an overall reduction in lumbar lordosis and offloading of painful structures.

Stability of the spine is maintained via ligaments, which provide static resistance to movement, but more importantly by coactivation of abdominal wall and paraspinal muscles, which provide the added stability needed to perform activities of daily living in addition to sporting tasks (McGill 1998, 2001). A core strengthening program must therefore functionally train and improve endurance in these muscles, thereby providing improved dynamic stability.

Specifics of Physical Rehabilitation

A therapeutic exercise program for the older athlete should include lumbar stabilization exercises, a flexibility program aimed at increasing hip mobility, strengthening of the core (abdominal muscles, gluteals, back muscles, etc.), and cardiovascular exercise. Most patients with spinal stenosis have a flexion-based directional preference. Therefore, emphasis is typically on flexion exercises.

Patients may do basic flexion exercises in supine by actively bringing one or both knees to the chest or in sitting by simply bending forward and reaching toward their toes (figure 9.5). Standing flexion exercises are useful to alleviate symptoms brought on by walking. Patients can rest one foot on a park bench or a fire hydrant and lean forward as though tying their shoes until symptoms diminish (figure 9.6).

An assessment of flexibility may reveal decreased hip mobility due to decreased muscle length or hip capsular tightness (figure 9.7).

Triplanar (multidirectional) functional stretches are an effective and efficient means of increasing hip mobility along with improving range of motion further down the kinetic chain of the lower extremities. Figures 9.8, *a* and *b*, and 9.9 show examples of rotational hamstring and hip flexor stretches.

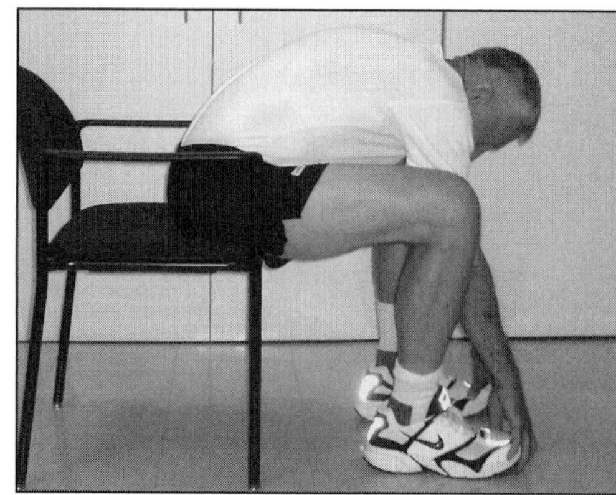

FIGURE 9.5 Seated forward bending.

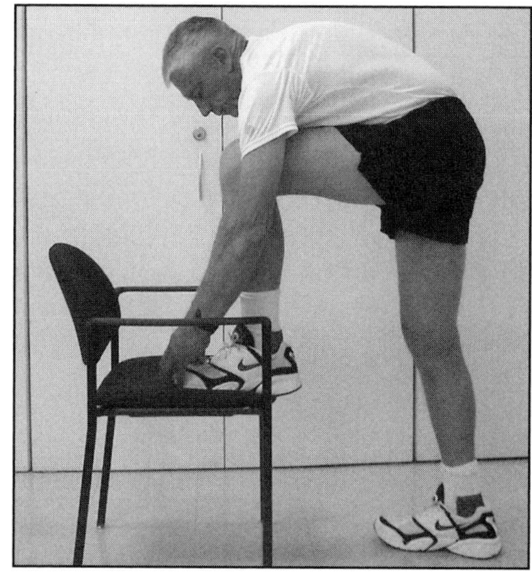

FIGURE 9.6 Standing unilateral forward bending.

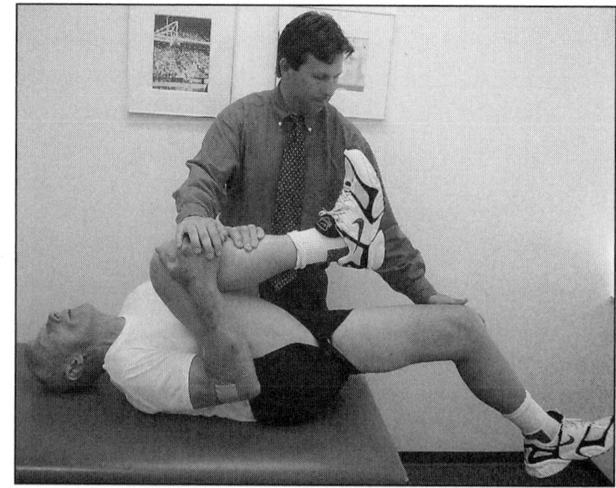

FIGURE 9.7 The modified Thomas test assesses tightness of the iliopsoas, rectus femoris, and tensor fasciae latae. In this position, a tight iliopsoas causes increased hip flexion; tight rectus femoris causes loss of knee flexion, and tight tensor fasciae latae cause the lower limb to abduct and externally rotate.

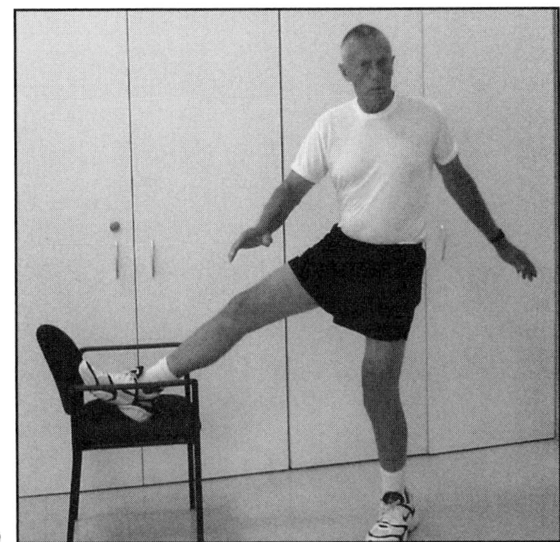
a

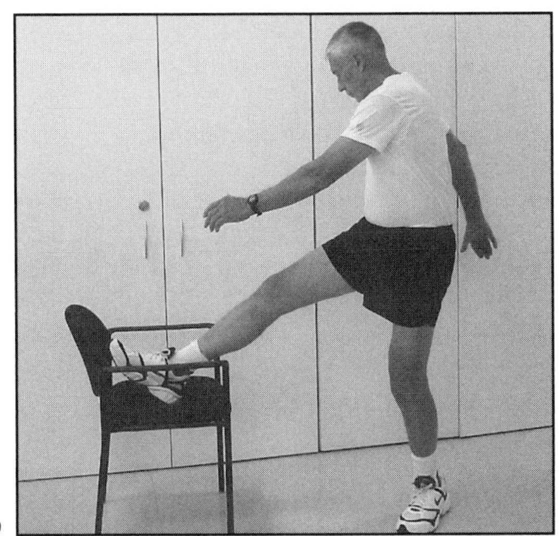
b

FIGURE 9.8 Rotational hamstring stretch.

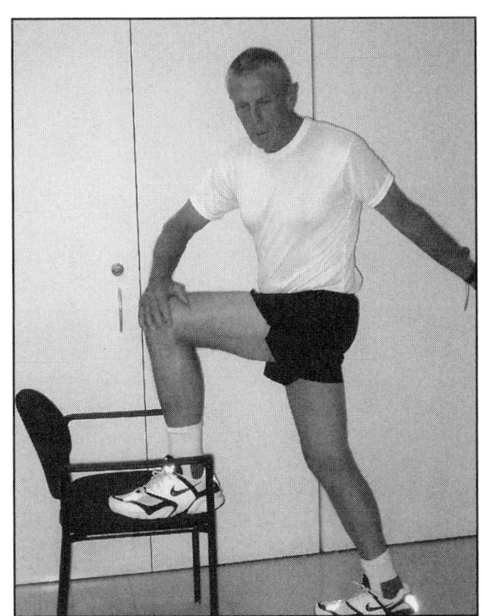

FIGURE 9.9 Rotational hip flexor stretch.

A triplanar lunge program is a useful tool to improve flexibility while increasing strength and proprioception to enhance sport performance. One can modify or advance these exercises so that they become more sport specific by changing distance and speed or by adding upper body movement or sport equipment, such as a golf club or tennis racket (figure 9.10, *a* through *c*.) Patients can further challenge their proprioceptive system by performing exercises with one eye closed,

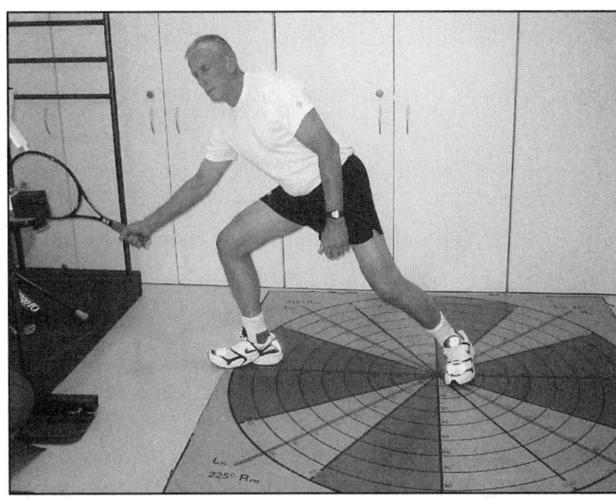
a

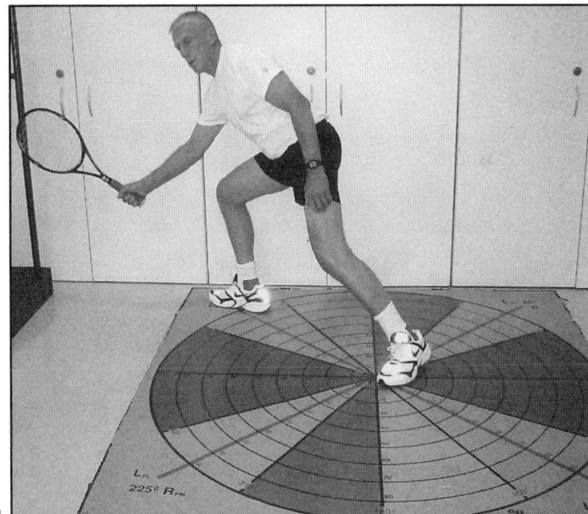
b

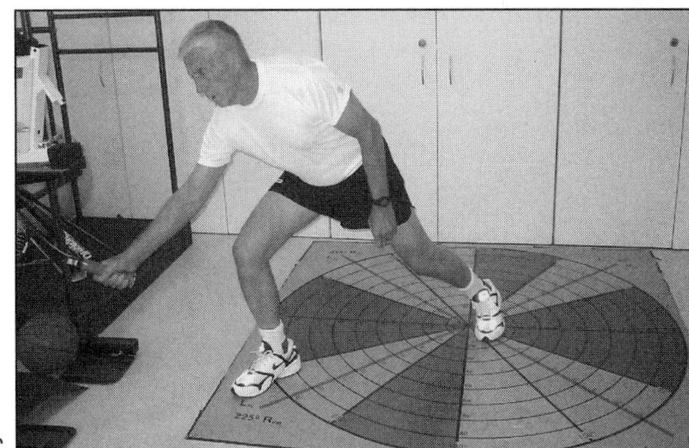
c

FIGURE 9.10 Triplanar lunges.

on variable surfaces (i.e., foam roll, wobble board, bare feet), and in single-limb stance.

Manual therapy to address capsular tightness of the hip may start with basic passive accessory joint glides with the assistance of a mobilization belt as needed. Figure 9.11 shows an example of a mobilization technique in which the patient actively lunges anteriorly as the therapist applies a mobilization force to the hip with the assistance of a belt (figure 9.11). The half-prone rectus femoris stretch can also be used to mobilize the anterior hip capsule with passive hip internal or external rotation (figure 9.12). One advantage of this technique is that the pelvis and lumbar spine are placed in a neutral to flexed position to promote opening of the lateral or central canal. Pillows should be placed under the pelvis to increase lumbar flexion if the mobilization position produces symptoms.

For older patients who are athletes, sport-specific exercises should simulate the speed, range of motion, and primary planes of movement of the activity. For example, the golfer or softball player will benefit from increased hip rotation along with strong abdominal activity during high-speed trunk rotation. Triplanar core exercises are an appropriate sport-specific exercise for these athletes. Each athlete also needs to be trained to activate the transverse abdominis with a "hollowing contraction" (McGill 1998, 2001). Because the lumbar spine has only one degree of rotation occurring at each vertebral segment (White and Panjabi 1990), the transverse plane is an ideal starting point for training the abdominal muscles while minimizing stress to the lumbar spine. Toeing-in (hip internal rotation) helps emphasize rotational movement at the hips, and holding a

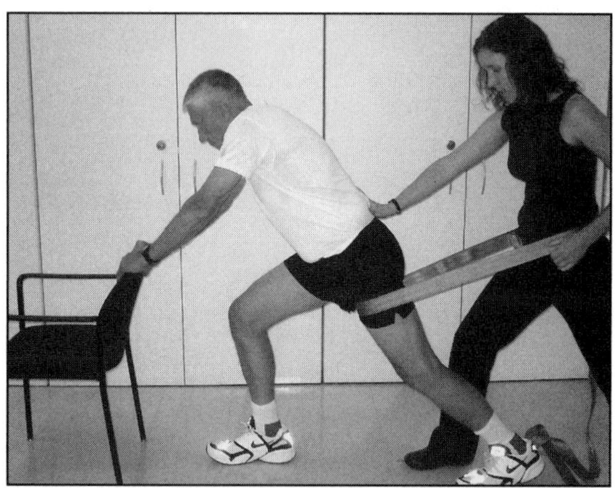

FIGURE 9.11 Standing anterior hip glide with belt.

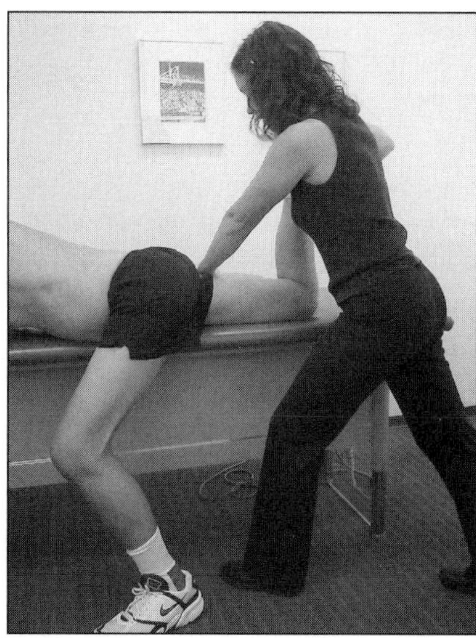

FIGURE 9.12 Prone rectus femoris stretch with anterior hip glide.

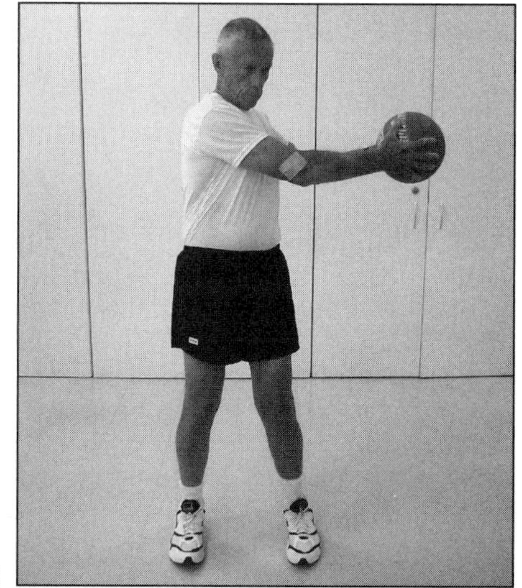

a

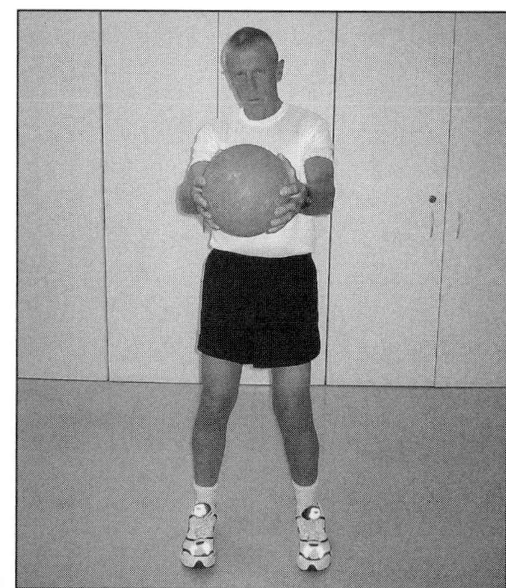

b

FIGURE 9.13 Transverse core with medicine ball.

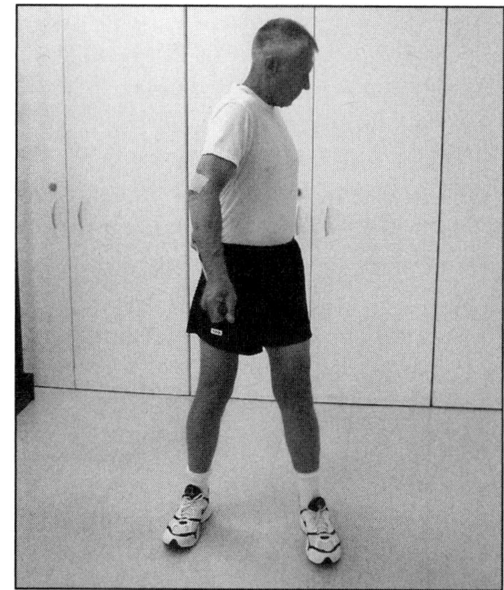
a

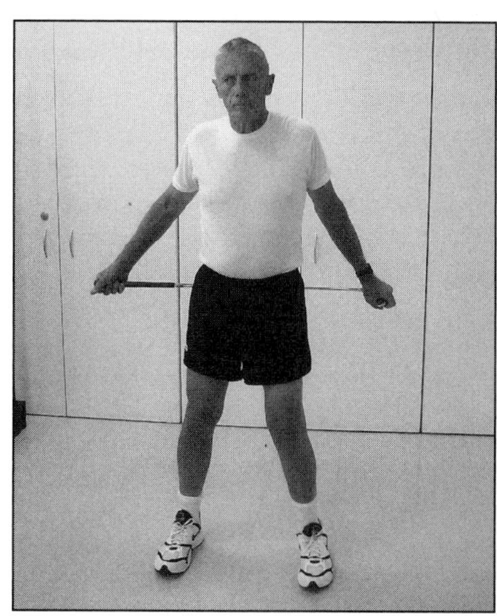
b

FIGURE 9.14 Transverse core with golf club.

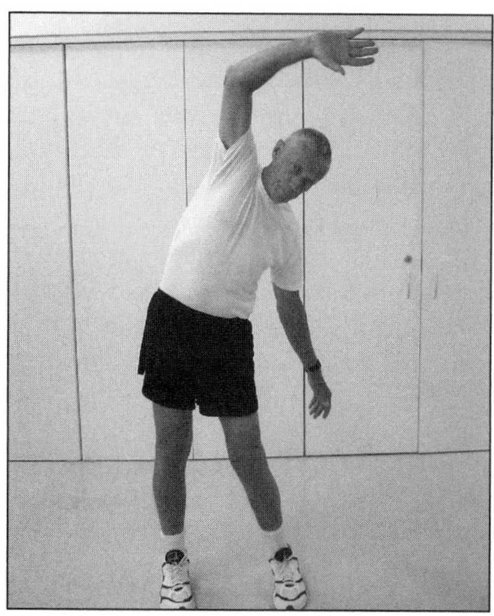

FIGURE 9.15 Frontal core.

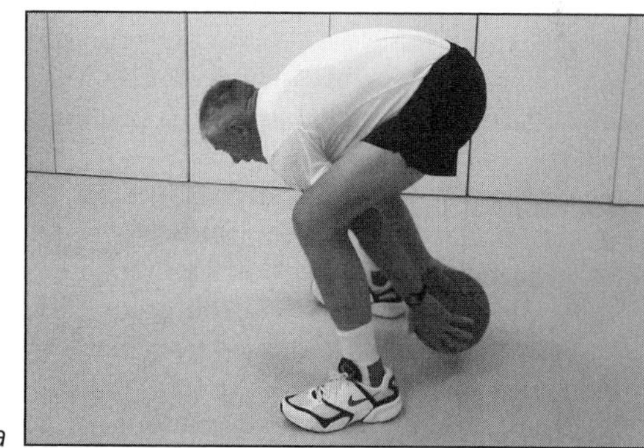
a

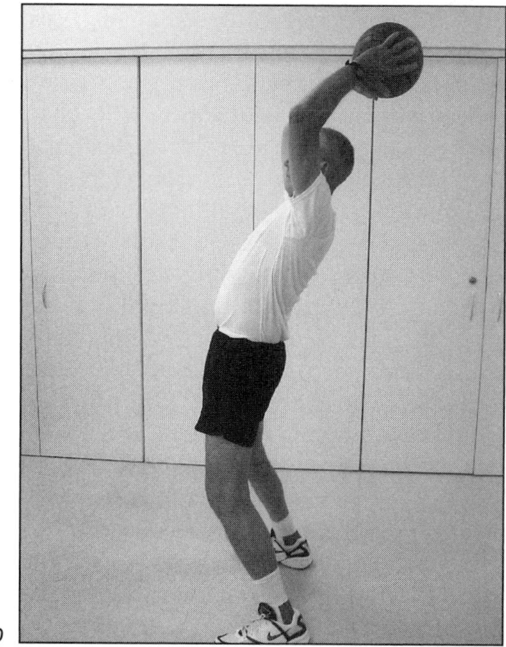
b

FIGURE 9.16 Sagittal core.

medicine ball or golf club facilitates abdominal activity (figures 9.13 and 9.14).

Eventually, the athlete needs to be able to move in all three cardinal planes. Therefore, core strengthening should also address the frontal and sagittal planes of movement (figures 9.15 and 9.16).

Most patients with spinal stenosis complain that their symptoms worsen with brisk walking or running, thereby making a cardiovascular training effect difficult to achieve. In addition to receiving formal physical therapy, these patients should be educated on the need to maintain cardiovascular fitness. Encourage patients to try a recumbent bike or an inclined treadmill, both of which place the lumbar spine in a more optimal flexed position.

Diagnosis and Treatment of Pain

Diagnostic blocks with local anesthetic may be utilized to identify a pain generator. However, it is necessary to take into consideration the significant rate of false positive responses with single blocks. The double-block paradigm, in which responses to successive injections with long- and short-acting agents are measured, is helpful to improve specificity. Medial branch blocks or intra-articular z-joint blocks are used to identify facet-mediated pain. Intra-articular SIJ injection is considered the gold standard for the diagnosis of SIJ-mediated pain; however, one should also remember that the posterior ligamentous structures of the SIJ are potential pain generators as well.

Provocative testing with discography has the potential to diagnose intrinsic disc pain but remains controversial.

The scientific basis for using epidural steroids for radicular pain caused by disc pathology is well established (Saal et al. 1990). In degenerative lumbar spinal stenosis, the role is less clear. Proposed mechanisms of action include reduction of inflammation and edema around nerve roots, alteration of local blood flow, and direct nociceptive effects.

Spinal injections are typically performed if the patient has failed to respond to standard treatment over a period of several weeks after initial presentation.

Therapeutic spinal injections with corticosteroid can be useful to reduce pain, improve tolerance for rehabilitation, and thereby facilitate a patient's subsequent return to normal function. One should always use fluoroscopic guidance to ensure proper needle location and minimize the risks for intravascular injection or dural puncture (Sullivan et al. 2000).

For patients with radicular pain, the transforaminal epidural approach is safe (Botwin et al. 2000) and effective (Lutz et al. 1998; Riew et al. 2000), delivering medication closest to the site of pathology. The caudal approach may be useful in patients who have undergone previous spinal fusion (Botwin et al. 2001). When z-joint-mediated pain is suspected, intra-articular injection or blockade of the dorsal rami medial branches may be used diagnostically. In carefully selected patients confirmed to have z-joint-mediated pain, medial branch neurotomy may provide prolonged relief of symptoms (Dreyfuss et al. 2000).

Riew and colleagues (Riew et al. 2000), in a double-blind controlled study, demonstrated the effectiveness of transforaminal epidural steroids in preventing the need for surgery in patients with compressive radiculopathy. Corticosteroid plus bupivacaine was found to be superior to bupivacaine alone. All patients were surgical candidates. Only 8 of 28 patients receiving steroid plus bupivacaine went on to surgery during an average follow-up period of 23 months after the first injection. Botwin et al. (Botwin correspondence, publication pending), in a prospective, uncontrolled study, demonstrated improvement in pain scores, tolerance for standing and walking, and subjective patient response at 2 and 12 months following transforaminal epidural injections in patients who had previously not responded to treatment with physical therapy and analgesic medications. Of 34 subjects, only 6 went on surgery. Previously published studies have refuted the effectiveness of epidural steroids for spinal stenosis (Fukusaki et al. 1998; Rivest et al. 1998).

TREATMENT OF COMMON DIAGNOSTIC SUBSETS

Degenerative Lumbar Spinal Stenosis

In the patient with degenerative lumbar spinal stenosis (DLSS), symptoms result from central, lateral recess, and intervertebral foraminal stenosis that may occur as part of the degenerative cascade. Symptoms are likely secondary to a combination of mechanical compression and nerve tissue ischemia (Porter 1996).

Diagnosis

Neurogenic claudication is the most common presenting symptom. Lower limb or buttock pain, or both, may be unilateral or bilateral, as is also the case with paresthesias and weakness. Low back pain is common but not always present. Walking, standing, and other activities involving lumbar extension are exacerbating factors. Walking downhill will be more difficult than going uphill. Bending forward, such as when pushing a shopping cart, or sitting down relieves symptoms. Patients may complain of needing to walk and stand with a stooped forward posture. Absence of pain during sitting has been found to be strongly associated with lumbar spinal stenosis (Katz et al. 1995).

The physical exam is often unremarkable (Hall et al. 1985). The bicycle test, first described by van Gelderen in 1948 (Dyck and Doyle 1977), can be used to distinguish neurogenic from vascular claudication. The subject with neurogenic claudication should be able to tolerate the exercise challenge done with the spine in a flexed and relatively unloaded position, whereas the vascular claudication patient experiences pain as the local tissue oxygen demand increases and hypoxia develops. Weakness or sensory loss most commonly affects the L5 distribution. Reduced deep tendon reflexes have been reported at the Achilles in 43% and the patella in 18% of cases (Hall et al. 1985). Diminished distal pulses should be investigated for vascular insufficiency (Spivak 1998), which may occur concomitantly and complicate the management. The straight leg raise is less commonly positive in this population compared with younger patients with disc herniations. Patients may experience reproduction of radicular pain or back pain, or both, with lumbar extension/rotation to the symptomatic side when lateral stenosis is present (Jenis et al. 2001). Sustained lumbar extension for 30 s may be a useful provocative maneuver for neurogenic claudication (Katz et al. 1995).

Progression and Treatment

The natural history of lumbar spinal stenosis is slow progression, which may or may not lead to functional decline or increased pain (Johnsson et al. 1991). Among nonsurgically treated patients, 10% to 26% worsen; ~40% improve; and ~40% stay the same (Atlas et al. 1996a, 1996b; Johnsson et al. 1992; Johnsson et al. 1991; Porter et al. 1984). Neurologic decline is rare. Surgical intervention is recommended only for progressive neurologic deterioration, cauda equina syndrome, or, most commonly, if pain becomes intolerable and significantly limits function despite a comprehensive trial of nonoperative management.

Many patients with severe symptoms are treated surgically. In general, studies looking at surgical outcome are variable, although most describe good to excellent overall results (Amundsen et al. 2000; Atlas et al. 1996a, 1996b; Fast and Robin 1985; Hall et al. 1985). Poor prognostic indicators include diabetes mellitus, previous lumbar spine surgery, hip joint pathology, and previous lumbar spine fracture (Airaksinen et al. 1997).

Conservative treatment of DLSS has received less scrutiny. Nonsurgical treatment typically consists of medications, bracing, physical therapy, therapeutic exercise, and epidural steroid injections. Pain relief has been demonstrated in a small number of patients with lumbar spinal stenosis wearing delordosing orthoses (Willner 1985).

Pharmacologic treatment typically consists of standard analgesic medications. Nonsteroidal anti-inflammatory medications and narcotic analgesics should be prescribed with caution and close monitoring to minimize complications. Calcitonin, in a double-blind placebo-controlled study, was shown to provide pain relief and improve function in this population, likely by its action on central opioid receptors (Eskola et al. 1992).

Physical therapy and therapeutic exercise regimens, emphasizing flexion exercises, should attempt to decrease lumbar lordosis and thereby increase the diameter through which compressed neural tissues pass. Manual techniques may be used initially to reduce soft tissue restriction and improve segmental motion. Stretching the hip flexors and hamstrings, mobilizing the hip capsule anteriorly, and strengthening of gluteal and abdominal muscles will also promote a decrease in the lumbar lordosis and improved stabilization. Partially unweighted treadmill walking with the use of a harness, by reducing axial compressive effects on neural structures, has been reported to successfully reduce pain and improve walking tolerance (Fardon 1997; Fritz et al. 1998; Fritz et al. 1997a, 1997b). Aquatic-based exercises are also well tolerated and should be utilized early in treatment. In a series of three patients, Whitman et al. described a manual therapy-based treatment program in combination with muscle retraining and aerobic exercise (Whitman et al. 2003). Using validated outcome measurement tools, they found significant improvements at discharge and at 18 months. Manual therapy consisted of spinal manipulation, hip mobilization, and hip flexor stretching. Flexion-based and rotational spinal mobilization exercises were utilized along with gluteal and abdominal muscle retraining.

Epidural steroid injections may serve as part of a comprehensive treatment program to facilitate progress in a functional rehabilitation program.

Simotas et al. (Simotas 2001; Simotas et al. 2000) followed a group of 49 patients for an average of 33 months utilizing a comprehensive nonoperative approach, including physical therapy, oral analgesics, and epidural steroids, finding that only 9 went on to surgery. Of the remaining 40 patients, 35 either improved or remained the same. Amundsen, in a 10-year prospective study, found that delaying surgery had no effect on postoperative outcome, even in severe patients (Amundsen et al. 2000).

Osteoporotic Vertebral Compression Fractures

Osteoporosis, the most prevalent metabolic bone disease in the United States and other developed countries (Favus 1999), is characterized by decreased density of histologically normal bone, causing bone fragility and increased susceptibility to fracture from normally benign forces. In both men and women, the rate of decline in bone mass increases with advancing age (Favus 1999). Table 9.2 lists the common causes of osteoporosis for both men and women.

Vertebral compression fractures in the setting of osteoporosis occur frequently in elderly patients, with an estimated prevalence of 20% in postmenopausal Caucasian women (Schumacher et al. 1993), and occur

TABLE 9.2 Common Causes of Osteoporosis

Women	Men
PRIMARY	
Postmenopausal (type I)	Age
Senile (type II)	Idiopathic
Idiopathic	Genetic
SECONDARY	
Nutrition	Immobilization
Vitamin C, D, calcium deficiency	Chronic disease
High caffeine, protein, or sodium intake	Respiratory, renal
Vitamin D or A overuse	Endocrine disorders
Alcoholism	Hypogonadism
Immobilization or sedentary lifestyle	Hypercalcinuria
Chronic disease (gastrointestinal, respiratory, renal)	Homocysteinuria
Endocrine disorders (hyperthyroidism, hyperparathyroidism, Cushing's)	Drugs
	Prolonged corticosteroid use
	Anticonvulsants, heparin
	Rheumatoid arthritis

in 27% of all women by age 65 (Favus 1999). In fact, approximately 750,000 vertebral compression fractures are reported annually in the United States (Ray et al. 1997; Watts 2000). Men in the United States have about half the risk for osteoporotic vertebral fracture compared with women (Favus 1999), but are clearly not spared the effects of age-related decreases in bone density.

Diagnosis

While history of trauma such as a fall commonly precedes a compression fracture, vertebral compression fractures may occur with normal daily activities, sneezing, and coughing. The golf swing produces compression loads on the spine equal to eight times body weight (Hosea et al. 1990; Hosea et al. 1994; Lindsay et al. 2000), and fractures have even been reported during the golf swing in female golfers with osteoporosis (Ekin and Sinaki 1993). The practitioner should maintain a high index of suspicion in postmenopausal women or any individual older than 70 presenting with back pain. Underlying medical problems should be ruled out as well in this population.

The vast majority of osteoporotic vertebral fractures are stable, due to sparing of the posterior elements. Radiographically, fractures can be classified as wedge, compression, or biconcave and by amount of deformity.

Treatment

Surgical intervention is typically not indicated unless neurologic or pulmonary compromise results from gross deformity (Favus 1999). Most fractures improve symptomatically within six weeks, although improvement may take several months or longer.

Traditional treatment consists of bracing, rest, and analgesics acutely. Narcotic analgesics, as always, should be prescribed with caution because of the potential for adverse side effects in older patients. Calcitonin, used in the treatment of osteoporosis, has also demonstrated efficacy in blocking nociception in vertebral fractures (Lyritis et al. 1999). Its proposed analgesic mechanisms of action include increasing blood beta-endorphin levels, inhibition of prostaglandin synthesis, hemodynamic effects, and inhibition of spinal serotonergic pathways (Eskola et al. 1992). The nasal spray is generally well tolerated and may be used in conjunction with other analgesic medications. Extension bracing for vertebral compression fractures is helpful to minimize motion and compressive forces until periosteal edema subsides (Sinaki 1993). For thoracolumbar fractures, three-point orthoses such as a Jewett brace are effective, whereas for lower lumbar fractures, one can use a wide support with elastic closures (Kaul and Herring 1998). Prevention of comorbidity associated with immobilization, such as deep venous thrombosis, pneumonia, and decubitus ulcers, should begin.

Physical therapy should start early, following the principles discussed in the previous section. In the acute phase, this may consist simply of education regarding positioning, posture, and activities of daily living (Sinaki 1993), along with passive treatments such as heat or ice. Therapeutic exercise should begin as soon as tolerable. Aquatic-based therapy, by decreasing the weight-bearing load imposed on the patient, can be helpful in the initial phases of rehabilitation. Some have advocated spinal extension exercises; however, it is important to individualize stabilization exercises and to start in the patient's pain-free range. The clinician should remember that altered spine mechanics due to compression deformity may lead to pain emanating from kinetically linked structures, such as the facet joints, ligaments, and paraspinal muscles, in addition to the fracture itself (Favus 1999).

Vertebroplasty is a relatively new treatment for recalcitrant pain due to vertebral compression fracture. The procedure involves fluoroscopically guided injection of polymethylmethacrylate cement into the vertebral body percutaneously using a transpedicular or paravertebral approach. Short-term pain relief has been reported to be as high as 70% to 100% (Barr et al. 2000; Garfin et al. 2001; Jensen et al. 1997) for compression fractures due to osteoporosis; however, long-term follow-up data are not available. Risks of the procedure are substantial and include cement pulmonary embolus and migration of cement into the spinal canal with resultant neural compression. In experienced hands and with the use of proper technique and fluoroscopic visualization, complications can be minimized (Moreland et al. 2001).

Kyphoplasty is performed in a similar manner but involves insertion and inflation of a balloon device to reduce the kyphotic compression deformity and restore vertebral body height prior to introduction of cement.

Both procedures are advancements in the treatment of patients with painful osteoporotic compression fractures. However, until long-term efficacy and safety have been proven, the procedure should be performed only in carefully selected patients who have clearly failed conservative treatment.

Prevention of Recurrence

Prevention should be addressed in all patients to minimize risks for further fracture. Promote an active lifestyle and proper nutrition. Oral bisphosphonates along with newer generation inravenous bisphosphates are used in those at increased risk for fracture.

Dual X-ray absorptiometry (DEXA) scan is the study of choice to evaluate bone density, identify those at risk for fracture, and guide treatment. The National Osteoporosis Foundation has recommended routine bone density testing for all white women age 65 and older and for younger women with risk factors (Foundation 1998; Watts 2000).

SUMMARY

Spine injuries are among the most common seen in the general and athletic populations. A thorough understanding of the normal and pathological anatomic and biomechanical changes that occur in the aging spine is necessary for an accurate evaluation of the injured athlete. The history and physical exam should provide a diagnosis and framework for treatment in most cases. Along with the standard orthopedic and neurological examination, a comprehensive musculoskeletal evaluation must analyze biomechanical factors and the entire functional kinetic chain. Radiological and electrophysiological diagnostic testing can be helpful in many cases. However, results must be correlated with the clinical evaluation, since abnormal findings on imaging studies are ubiquitous in this population. Fluoroscopically guided diagnostic injections procedures can be useful to confirm a suspected pain generator. Injections and other percutaneous interventions can be used therapeutically to help control pain and facilitate a more comprehensive functional rehabilitation program. In the active individual, a functional rehabilitation program must strive to mimic the movement patterns and loads necessary to perform the desired activity. The treatment program must be specific to the individual being treated.

CHAPTER

10

Hip Problems

Srino Bharam, MD

Utku Kandemir, MD

Marc J. Philippon, MD

Hip injuries in active athletes over 50 can lead to disabling hip pain, which can greatly affect their level of activities. These injuries result from an isolated injury, repetitive traumatic activities, and the onset of osteoarthritis. This chapter focuses on specific hip injuries involving both intra-articular and extra-articular pathology.

ANATOMY

The hip joint is considered an enarthrodial joint, which is a ball and socket joint capable of six degrees of freedom. The hip joint is surrounded by a thick capsule. The capsule and associated ligaments (iliofemoral, pubofemoral, and ischiofemoral ligaments), along with the bony architecture of the femoral head and acetabulum articulation, provide stability to the joint.

The iliofemoral ligament, also referred to as the ligament of Bigelow, is an inverted Y-shaped ligament that originates from the anterior inferior iliac spine and then splits into two arms inserting on the intertrochanteric line. This ligament, which is approximately 12 to 14 mm thick, becomes tight in extension and limits external rotation (Philippon 2001). The pubofemoral ligament originates from the pubic ramus and descends to blend with inferior fibers of the iliofemoral ligament, reinforcing the inferior and anterior capsule. Pubofemoral ligament resists extension and abduction. The ischiofemoral ligament reinforces the posterior portion of the capsule. The zona orbicularis surrounds the femoral neck in a circular pattern, which may help maintain stability of the femoral head into the acetabulum. These ligaments provide maximum stability when the hip joint is in extension. During flexion and lateral rotation of the hip, the ligaments become lax (Wasielewski 1998).

The acetabular labrum is fibrocartilage that is located around the acetabular rim to the fovea, where they blend anteriorly and posteriorly with the transverse ligament (Lage, Patel, and Villar 1996). The labrum is believed to provide stability to the hip joint. The ligamentum teres originates from both sides of the acetabular notch, with attachments from the posteroinferior portion of the cotyloid fossa, and inserts into the fovea on the medial side of the femoral head (Gray-Alistar and Villar 1997).

The bony architecture of the hip joint is formed by the articulation of the acetabulum and femoral head. The acetabulum is formed by the union of three innominate bones, the pubis, ramus, and ischium. The surface of the acetabulum is oriented 15° to 20° anteriorly and 45° caudally. The inferior portion of the acetabulum does not articulate with the femoral head (Wasielewski 1998). The articular cartilage of the acetabulum is horseshoe shaped to allow for 170° of coverage of the femoral head (Wasielewski 1998).

The labrum provides an additional 2 to 3 mm of femoral head coverage. Studies have shown free nerve endings and sensory fibers in the labrum, which may contribute to proprioception of the hip joint (Philippon 2001). The articular cartilage is thickest at the center of the femoral head.

The position of flexion, abduction, and external rotation is the maximal articular joint congruity, referred to as the loose-packed position (Wasielewski 1998).

There are 22 different muscles that exert forces on the hip to obtain large range of motion and provide dynamic hip stability. These include hip flexors (e.g., iliopsoas), innervated by femoral nerve; extensors (gluteus maximus), innervated by inferior gluteal nerve; abductors (gluteus medius), innervated by superior gluteal nerve; adductors (adductor longus), innervated by obturator nerve; and internal and external rotators. The major blood supply to the femoral head is the lateral femoral circumflex artery.

During the gait cycle, forces on the hip vary from 1.8 to 3.5 times body weight. These forces can increase up to eight times body weight with sport activities (Philippon 2003). Developmental abnormalities of the hip joint (e.g., hip dysplasia) can lead to abnormal joint forces. The shallow acetabulum seen with dysplasia leads to a decreased weight-bearing surface, which in turn may lead to arthritis.

DIAGNOSIS

Differentiating between low back pain and hip pathology can be challenging for the orthopedic surgeon. A detailed history and examination are crucial for identifying hip-related disorders and excluding other disorders that can mimic hip symptoms. Imaging studies are also useful in confirming hip pathology.

History and Physical Exam of the Hip

In assessing an elderly athlete with hip injury, one must address the level and frequency of athletic participation, type of sport, and the patient's expectations. It is necessary to evaluate the mechanism of injury and to determine whether it is an isolated traumatic event versus repetitive injury from the sport. Traumatic events can occur from a twisting injury or from a direct fall and contusions.

Details of symptoms related to the hip should include severity and frequency of pain; activity-related hip pain; pain at rest; and difficulty climbing stairs, tying shoes, arising from a seated position, and walking for more than 6 min. Associated symptoms with hip pain include locking, snapping, clicking of the hip, giving way, and loss of motion. A history of use of assistive devices and the use of nonsteroidal pain medication and its effect on pain relief should also be assessed. Previous hip surgery, hip symptoms during childhood, and family history of hip-related diseases must also be included in the evaluation.

Etiology from disabling hip pain can occur in association with both intra-articular and extra-articular pathology. Extra-articular pathology includes bursitis and tendinitis, snapping of tendons, myositis ossificans, psoas abscess, femoral or inguinal hernia, and neurologic causes and tumor. Bursitis is seen with the greater trochanter and iliopsoas tendon. Snapping of tendons can occur with the iliopsoas tendon over the brim of the pelvis and with the iliotibial tendon snapping over the greater trochanter. Tendinitis is commonly seen with the iliopsoas tendon hamstrings and piriformis tendon.

Intra-articular causes include labral tear, chondral injuries, loose bodies, ligamentum teres tear, impinging osteophytes, degenerative osteoarthritis, hip instability, synovitis, avascular necrosis, occult fractures, and stress fractures.

Examining a patient with hip injury, particularly an elderly athlete, can be complex. The history and physical exam should evaluate for pathology of the lower back, pelvis, and knee in addition to the hip.

The patient's gait cycle should be investigated to rule out abnormal gait pattern such as antalgic gait, Trendelenburg gait, pelvic obliquity, and external rotation deformity of the lower extremity. After gait evaluation, assess pain elicited with one-leg hop during weight bearing.

Normal range of motion of the hip includes 130° of hip flexion, 50° of abduction/adduction, and 30° to 40° of internal and external rotation. Motor strength testing should take place in both hips to detect side-to-side difference. Neurovascular examination of the hip involves palpating femoral, popliteal, and distal pulses and sensory and reflex exam of the lower extremity. General joint laxity should evaluate for hyperextension of the elbow and knee and thumb-to-forearm apposition.

Specific Hip Tests

With the patient in a supine position, the presence of a resting external rotation deformity of the symptomatic hip can be associated with a deficient iliofemoral ligament, presence of a labral tear, or both (figure 10.1). The Stinchfield test should be performed to assess for intra-articular hip pathology, including labral pathology, avascular necrosis, and osteoarthritis. This test is positive if pain is elicited with resistive flexion of the hip with the knee extended.

Axial distraction test (Shuck test) detecting side-to-side difference is performed to test for instability of the hip. The FABER (flexion, abduction, external rotation) test can evaluate for anterior hip pain and sacroiliac joint pathology. Pain and or snapping in the groin with flexion and neutral rotation can be attributed to snapping iliopsoas tendon. Pain with or without clicking with rotation of the hip during flexion and adduction can be related to labral pathology. The abduction external rotation test, which places the patient in the lateral decubitus position, can be associated with labral tears and anterior capsular laxity with pain elicited in the groin. The prone extension test can also elicit similar findings. Contractures of the hip joint

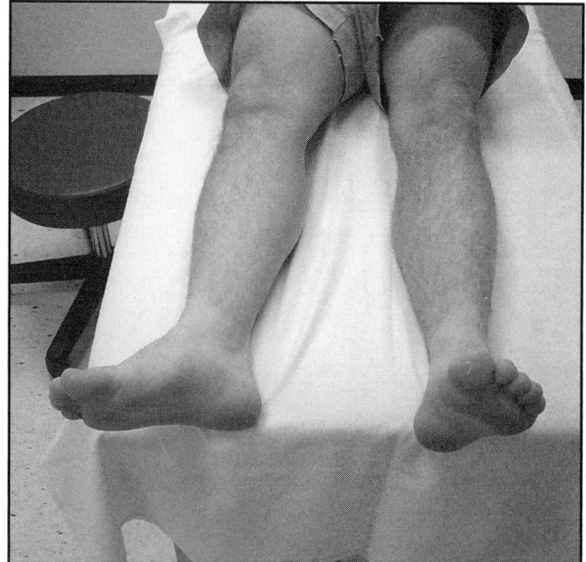

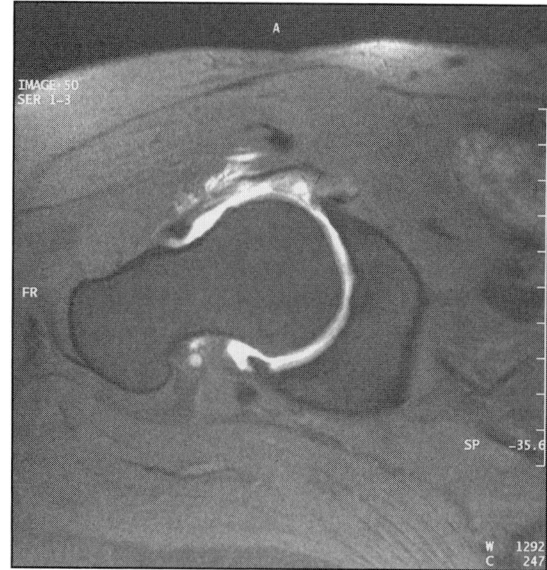

FIGURE 10.1 *(a)* Resting external rotation deformity in a patient with deficient iliofemoral ligament and *(b)* magnetic resonance arthrogram showing iliofemoral ligament tear.

can be assessed through use of the Thomas test (flexion contracture), Ober test (abduction contracture), and Ely test (extension contracture).

Examination of the hip should include palpating the greater trochanter bursa to rule out bursitis, piriformis tendon for piriformis syndrome, adductor longus tendon for pubalgia, ischial tuberosity for hamstring tendinitis, and gluteus medius tendon for tendinitis. Snapping of the iliotibial band over the greater trochanter can also be palpated in the lateral decubitus position. One can perform the piriformis test by having the hip stabilized at 60° of flexion and exerting downward pressure on the knee. This can place tension on the sciatic nerve, giving radicular symptoms and localized pain, known as piriformis syndrome.

Diagnostic Imaging

Plain radiographs should include anteroposterior pelvis and anteroposterior and lateral views of the involved hip. The pelvis X-ray allows comparison to the contralateral hip joint, assessing pelvic obliquity and SI joint pathology. The anteroposterior and lateral hip radiographs focus on the hip joint to evaluate for developmental abnormalities (e.g., Legg-Calve-Perthes disease, dysplasia), articular joint congruity, joint space narrowing, loose bodies, avulsion fractures and stress fractures, periarticular calcification of soft tissue, and subchondral collapse associated with avascular necrosis (figure 10.2). Arthritic conditions including presence of osteophytes, sourcil sclerosis, acetabular rim arthritis, cysts on both sides of the joint, and joint space narrowing are also observable. The center edge (CE) angle can be measured to determine femoral head coverage from the acetabular socket on a plain radiograph (figure 10.3). A CE angle of <20° is considered abnormal that results from a shallow acetabulum. This structural abnormality can lead to

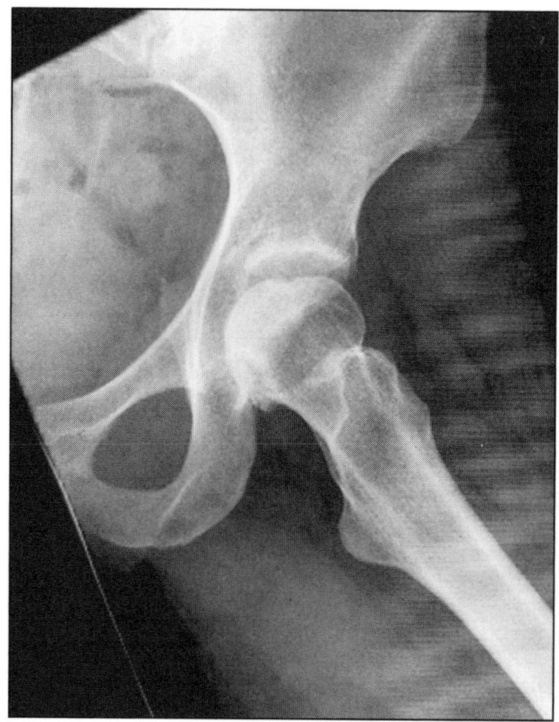

FIGURE 10.2 Subchondral collapse with avascular necrosis.

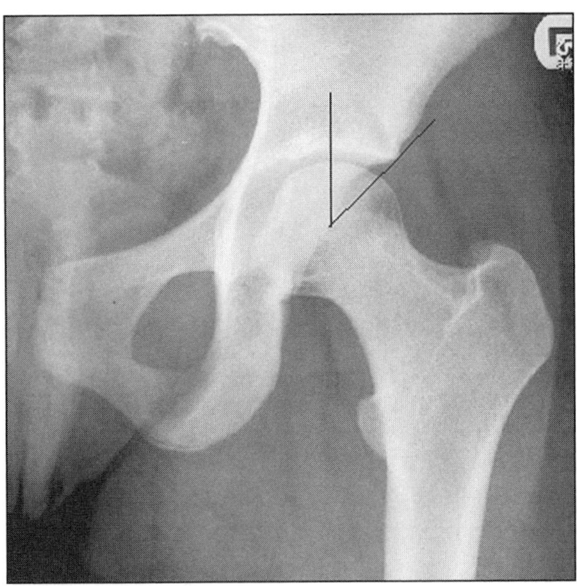

FIGURE 10.3 Center edge (CE) angle measurement of the hip.

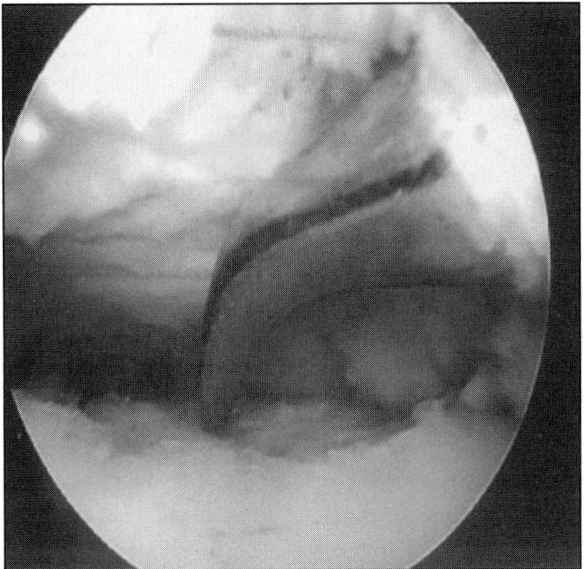

FIGURE 10.4 Arthroscopic image of loose body in the hip joint.

abnormal contact pressure in the joint and risk of intra-articular pathology. A false profile view with the patient standing in 25° internally rotated from X-ray beam can assess anterior femoral head coverage.

Plain magnetic resonance imaging (MRI) of the hip can determine the presence of avascular necrosis, stress fracture, labral pathology, hemarthrosis, tendinopathies, iliopsoas and greater trochanter bursitis, and soft tissue lesions (e.g., synovial chondromatosis, pigmented villonodular synovitis [PVNS]). However, plain MRI can detect up to only 30% of labral pathology. The use of MR arthrogram (MRA) can better delineate labral tears with 90% sensitivity (Erb 2001). Associated capsular redundancy and iliofemoral ligament deficiency and ligament teres tear can also be assessed with MRA.

Computed tomography scan is useful for evaluating loose bodies and intra-articular fractures. To determine snapping iliopsoas tendon, one can use a dynamic ultrasound test for snapping of the tendon over the pelvic brim. Other uses of ultrasound testing are for tendinopathies, muscular strain evaluation, and intra-articular effusions.

INTRA-ARTICULAR HIP PATHOLOGIES

Intra-articular hip injuries that can occur in the elderly athlete are labral tears, chondral flap injuries, loose bodies (figure 10.4), iliofemoral ligament deficiency, ligamentum teres tear, and hip instability. Intra-articular hip injuries can lead to synovitis and inflammation of the hip joint, causing disabling hip pain. These hip injuries can be isolated or found in combination, which can lead to arthritic changes of the hip joint.

Labral Tears

Labral tears are characterized by their location and their morphology. Anterosuperior tears are the most common lesions of the labrum found in athletes. Isolated posterior tears occur less frequently and in combination with anterior tears. The location of these tears has been attributed to repetitive sport-specific activities in the athlete. The morphologic types of labral tears have been classified as radial flap, radial fibrillated, and longitudinal peripheral and unstable tears (Lage, Patel, and Villar 1996). We have also found in athletes that labral tears occur as bucket-handle-type tears and delamination of the labral–chondral junction. In addition, labral tears are frequently associated with adjacent capsular laxity at the labrocapsular junction (figure 10.5). This combination of a deficient labrum and adjacent capsular laxity can lead to hip instability. Other associated labral injuries include adjacent chondral lesions (figure 10.6).

Repetitive rotational movements of the hip during athletic participation are the mechanism of injury seen in athletes (Philippon 2003). Common sport activities in elderly persons that produce these injuries include golf and tennis. Partial subluxation/dislocation injuries of the hip resulting in labral tears and their associated injuries also occur in skiers.

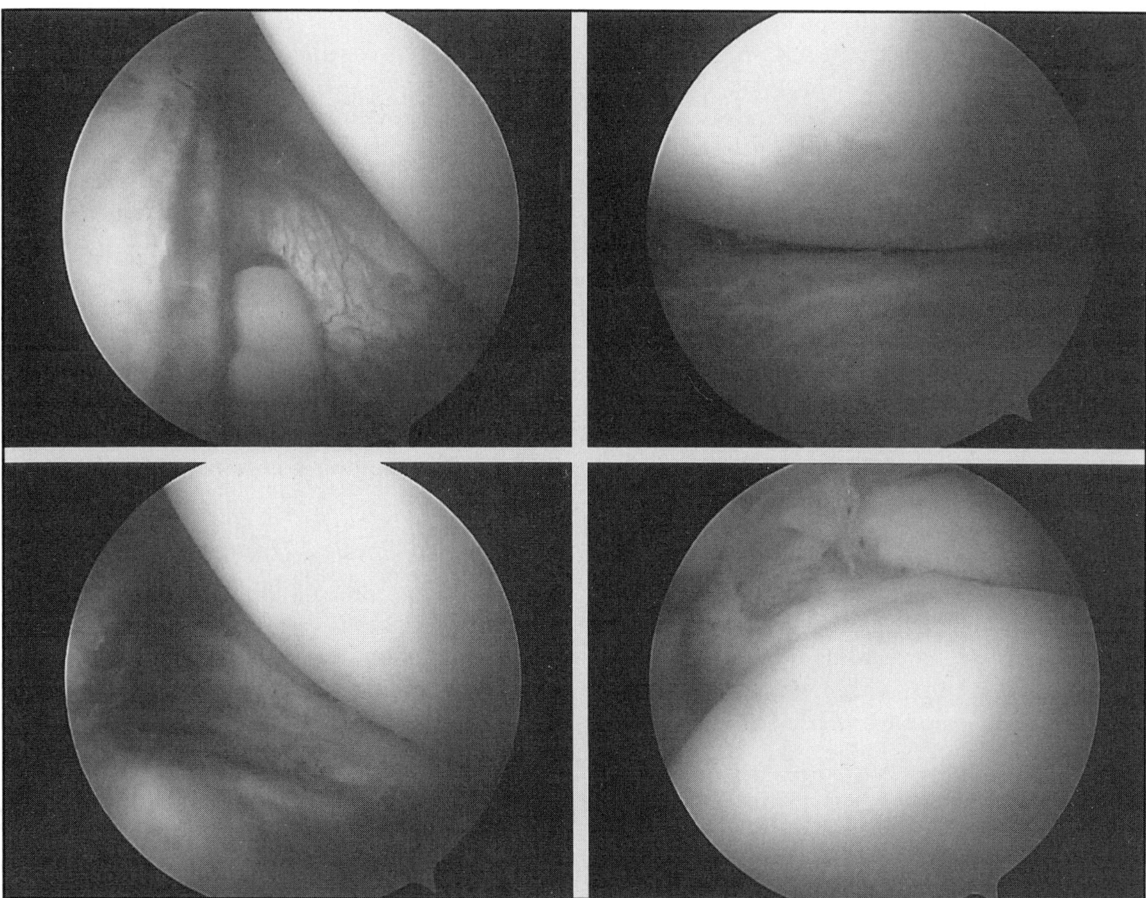

FIGURE 10.5 Arthroscopic finding of focal capsular laxity.

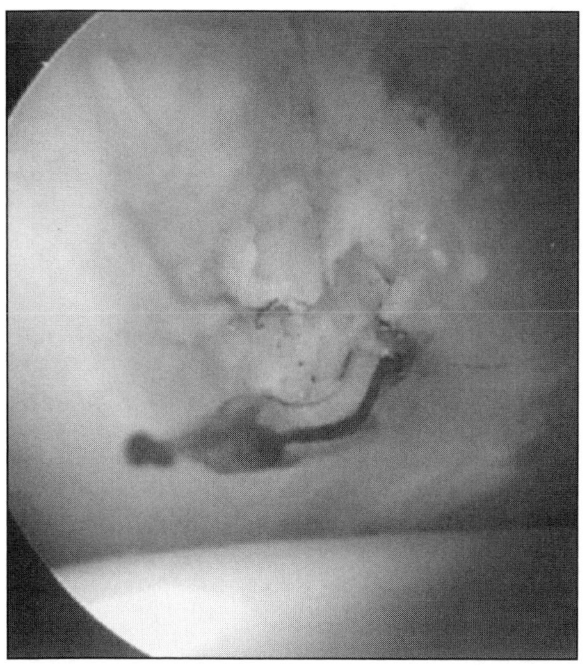

FIGURE 10.6 Chondral lesion adjacent to labral tear.

Arthritis

In elderly athletes, arthritis in the hip can affect performance, limiting what they can do and at times forcing them to discontinue their activities. Arthritis can be classified as degenerative, inflammatory, and traumatic. Degenerative osteoarthritis is the common type seen in elderly athletes. The clinician can visualize joint space narrowing, sclerosis, impinging osteophytes, and degenerative cysts on both the acetabular and femoral side of the joint on plain radiographs. Inflammatory arthritis causes a concentric loss of joint space and associated with synovitis. Acetabular fractures, hip dislocations, and fractures are causes of traumatic arthritis. Labral tears are also believed to cause traumatic arthritis (Philippon 2003).

Conservative Treatment

Conservative treatment involves activity modification and use of nonsteroidal pain medication during the acute phases of symptoms. A four- to six-week trial of physical therapy is also recommended during the acute phase for disabling hip pain. This includes stretching, isometric exercises, and range of motion exercises, avoiding painful motions. Ultrasound modalities can be a useful adjunct. As symptoms improve, implement strengthening exercises with a focus on abductor/adductor strengthening and proprioception. If there is no or little improvement, then further evaluation with the physician is needed. This would include reexamination, imaging studies, and possible steroid injections, both therapeutic and diagnostic.

Alternative therapy with chondroitin sulfate supplements may help for arthritic conditions; however, the clinical benefits have not been established.

Surgical Treatment

Mechanical symptoms such as pain with rotation, clicking, and locking of the hip caused by impinging intra-articular pathology can be addressed with arthroscopic intervention after failed conservative treatment, including a trial of at least four weeks of physical therapy. Arthroscopic capsulorrhaphy for capsular laxity leading to hip instability has also been performed by our senior author (Philippon 2003). Symptomatic loose bodies within the hip joint should be removed early if possible. Early arthritic conditions that have the mechanical type of hip pain can also be addressed with hip arthroscopy. Performing a capsulectomy can improve limited motion. Arthroscopy can remove impinging osteophytes, which limit range of motion, cause pain, and propagate labral tears. Degenerative ligamentum teres with atrophied fat pad has been associated with underlying osteoarthritis (figure 10.7).

When significant arthritic changes in the hip are present, however, it is important to address expectations of return to athletic activities. When the patient has daily, severe symptoms affecting daily activities and quality of life, consideration of a total hip replacement is in order. Return to sport can occur in low-impact activities, including golf, swimming, biking, and tennis.

Postsurgical Physical Therapy

Our post-op protocol (Philippon 2001) includes for the first two weeks early motion with the use of a CPM (continuous passive motion) machine 0° to 70° and starting immediately after surgery, 2 to 4 h a day, and the use of a stationary bicycle, seat high and no

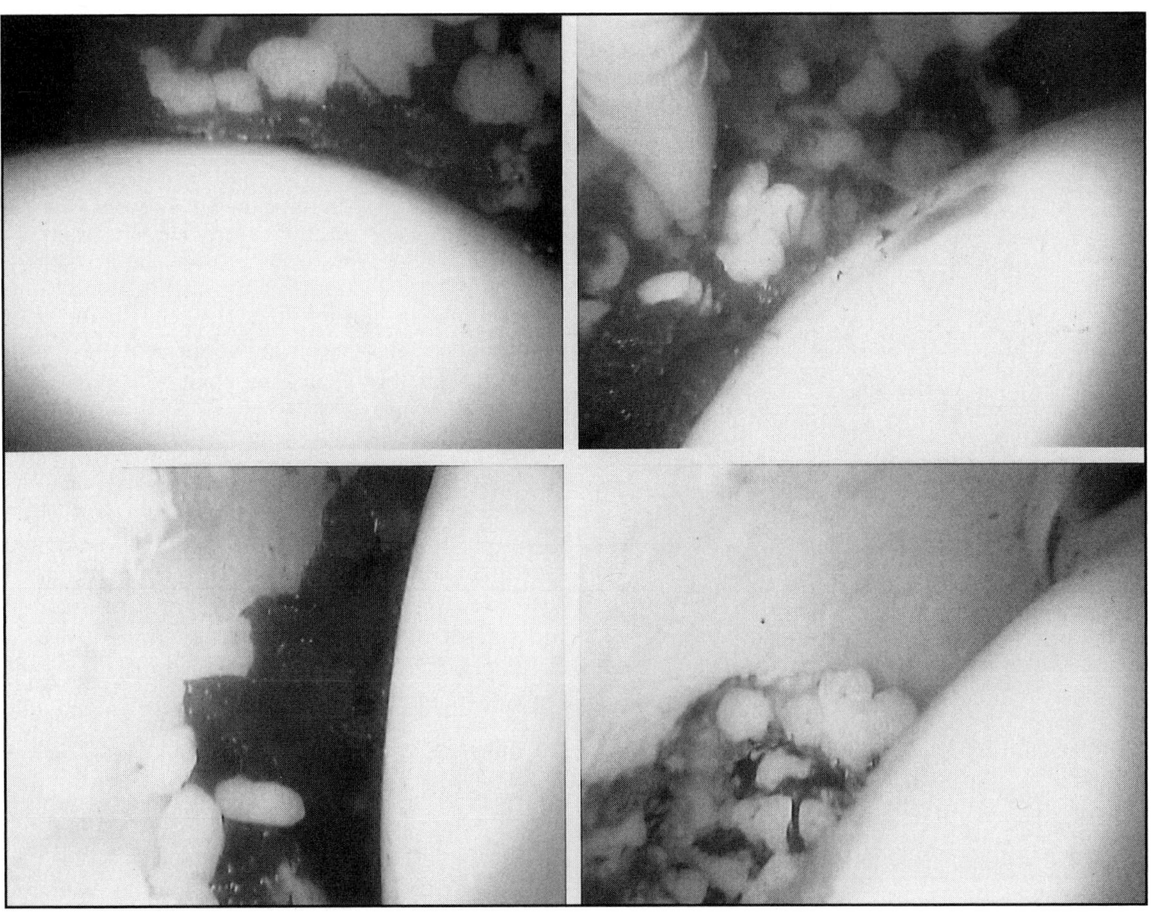

FIGURE 10.7 Arthroscopic finding of degenerative ligamentum teres with atrophied fat pad.

resistance. Rotational precautions are established for the first three weeks, particularly in patients undergoing capsulorraphy procedures. Isometric exercises are also implemented, and ultrasound modalities are recommended. Strengthening exercises begin in week 3. Week 6 to 8 is the time to address proprioception and sport-specific conditioning as tolerated.

Other Conditions

A common intra-articular hip finding in the active golfer with hip pain is labral-chondral delamination with adjacent capsular laxity. The senior author, M.J. Philippon, has treated a professional golfer on the Senior PGA Tour with arthroscopic intervention; this golfer went back to compete at preinjury level five weeks after surgery.

Loose bodies in the hip can result in locking and in clicking of the hip with pain elicited with motion. If multiple loose bodies are present in the joint, one should consider a diagnosis of synovial chondromatosis. Recently the senior author treated a retired NHL hockey player with chronic mechanical hip pain who was found to have degenerative labral tear and synovial chondromatosis (figure 10.8).

One must consider avascular necrosis (AVN) of the hip in athletes with hip pain. Risk factors for AVN include history of steroid use, alcohol abuse, and previous hip injury (dislocation and femoral neck fractures). Treatment for symptomatic AVN in early stages can include arthroscopic core decompression; for advanced stages of collapse, total hip replacement is the surgical treatment of choice.

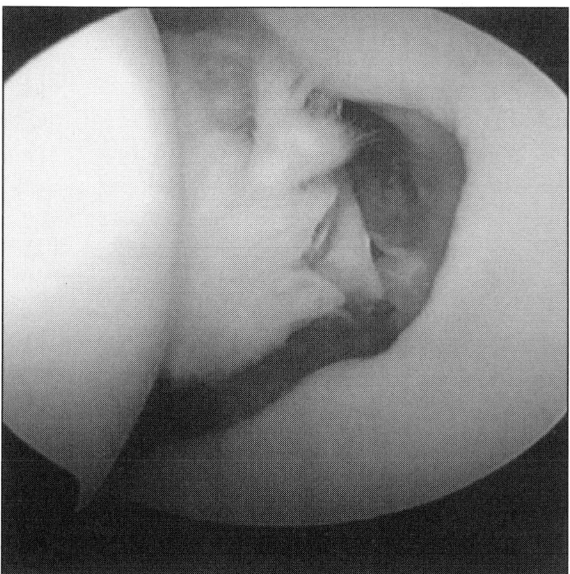

FIGURE 10.8 Loose bodies of synovial chondromatosis are shown in an arthroscopic view.

Stress fractures can occur in the femoral neck and should be evaluated for in an athlete with hip pain during activity. Stress fractures are most commonly seen in female athletes with a history of amenorrhea, eating disorder, and increased sport activities. However, these fractures can also occur in runners over 50 years old. Fractures on the compression side of the femoral neck are treated with protective weight bearing for six weeks. Repeat MRI is necessary to determine if the fracture is healed before the athlete is allowed to return to sport. Tension side fractures are potentially unstable and require internal fixation.

TENDINOPATHIES

Tendinopathy of the hip can cause disabling hip pain in the elderly athlete. The majority of these conditions improve with activity modification, anti-inflammatories, and physical therapy.

Iliotibial Band Syndrome

Iliotibial band (ITB) syndrome refers to snapping (coxa saltans) over the greater trochanter causing pain on the side of the hip. Runners commonly manifest this syndrome. Usually a component of bursitis is associated with the syndrome. One can identify the snapping of the ITB with dynamic ultrasound imaging (Pelsser et al. 2001). Snapping of the iliopsoas tendon can give symptoms of groin pain with snapping of the hip. The snapping sensation is usually a loud, audible clunking during flexion and extension of the hip. This condition is found commonly in a younger population, but can also occur with older athletes. Dynamic ultrasound testing can also confirm the diagnosis of snapping iliopsoas tendon.

Athletes with ITB perform stretching exercises (leg crossovers) involving the ITB to do in conjunction with a physical therapist for six to eight weeks. Abductor strengthening is also implemented, and ultrasound modalities to the trochanteric bursa are recommended as well.

Consider operative intervention after no improvement with therapy. Studies have described open procedures involving Z-plasty or partial excision of the ITB and bursectomy for recalcitrant bursitis (Brignall and Stainsby 1991; Zoltan, Clancy, and Keene 1986). However, arthroscopic releases and bursectomy can lead to less morbidity and earlier return to sport (figure 10.9).

Partial release with surgery for refractory snapping of the iliopsoas tendon, with good results, has been described (Jacobson and Allen 1990). Endoscopic release of the iliopsoas tendon is associated with less morbidity. Postoperative rehabilitation includes early

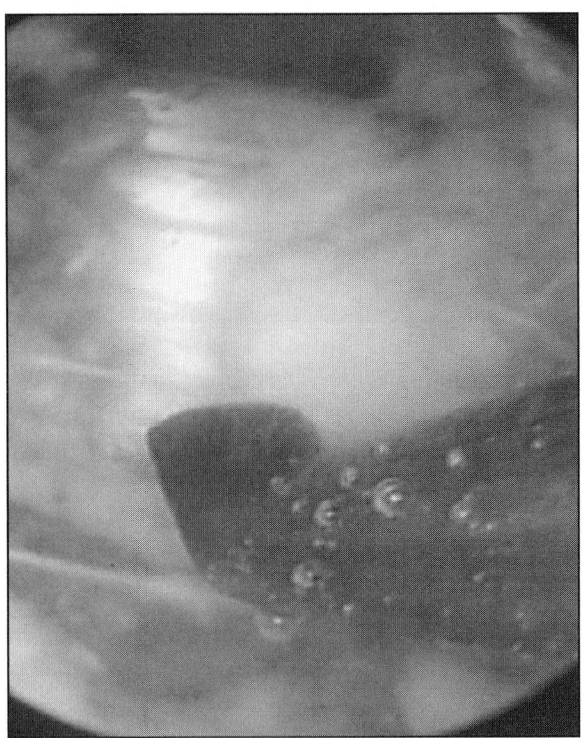

FIGURE 10.9 Arthroscopic release of iliopsoas tendon.

motion with isometric exercises and stretching exercises implemented in week 2.

Abductor Tendinitis

Tendinitis of the abductors (gluteus medius and minimus) from repetitive activities leads to pain and abductor weakness (Kagan 1999). Magnetic resonance imaging can evaluate gluteus medius tendinopathies (Kingzett-Taylor et al. 1999). Stretching exercises with abductor strengthening and anti-inflammatory medications should improve symptoms with physical therapy for six to eight weeks and activity modification. If no improvement is seen after conservative management, it is appropriate to consider surgical debridement. Endoscopic debridement of the tendon has been described by the authors (Kandemir et al. 2003).

Pubalgia

Pubalgia, also known as "sports hernia," refers to groin pain caused by adductor tendinitis during athletic activity. This injury is seen particularly in young athletes participating in soccer, hockey, rugby, and football but also occurs in older athletes. We have seen pubalgia in older-age tennis players. Treatment involves an aggressive stretching program with strengthening of the lower abdominal muscles for six to eight weeks. Steroid injections as adjunctive therapy are also a possibility. Consider surgical management only after failed conservative management. Surgery utilizing releases of the adductor tendons has been reported to be 97% successful in high-performance athletes (Meyers et al. 2000).

HIP ARTHROSCOPY

The latest development in technology has made it possible to treat aging athletes' arthritis arthroscopically. This allows the elderly athlete to return to sport with improved symptoms. In advanced cases of arthritis, hip arthroscopy can also serve as a temporizing treatment to allow athletes to perform high-impact activities that would not be possible with a total hip replacement.

Although the details of the surgery are not pertinent here, it will be useful to give some idea of what it is currently possible to do arthroscopically:

- Labral tears are debrided to a stable rim, leaving as much labrum intact as possible.
- Adjacent capsular laxity is treated with focal thermal modification utilizing flexible radiofrequency (RF) probes.
- Partially torn ligamentum teres tears can be a source of impingement and are treated with thermal shrinkage with flexible RF probes.
- Microfracture technique (Steadman et al. 1999) to stimulate a bleeding response for fibrocartilage growth can be used to treat focal grade III-IV changes of the acetabulum (figure 10.10).
- Motorized shavers are effective for removal of loose bodies.

Postoperative rehabilitation takes place immediately after advanced arthroscopic surgery. This includes early motion of the hip and protective weight bearing for the first two weeks. Strict rotation precautions for three weeks are implemented for patients undergoing focal capsulorrhaphy. Protective weight bearing is extended to six weeks after use of microfracture techniques of the cartilage. A strengthening program begins three weeks after surgery with a focus on abductor and external rotator strengthening.

ATHLETIC PARTICIPATION AFTER TOTAL HIP REPLACEMENT

Total hip replacement is one the most successful operations with respect to improving patient outcome and lifestyle. Athletes with advanced hip arthritis undergoing total hip replacement are able to participate in

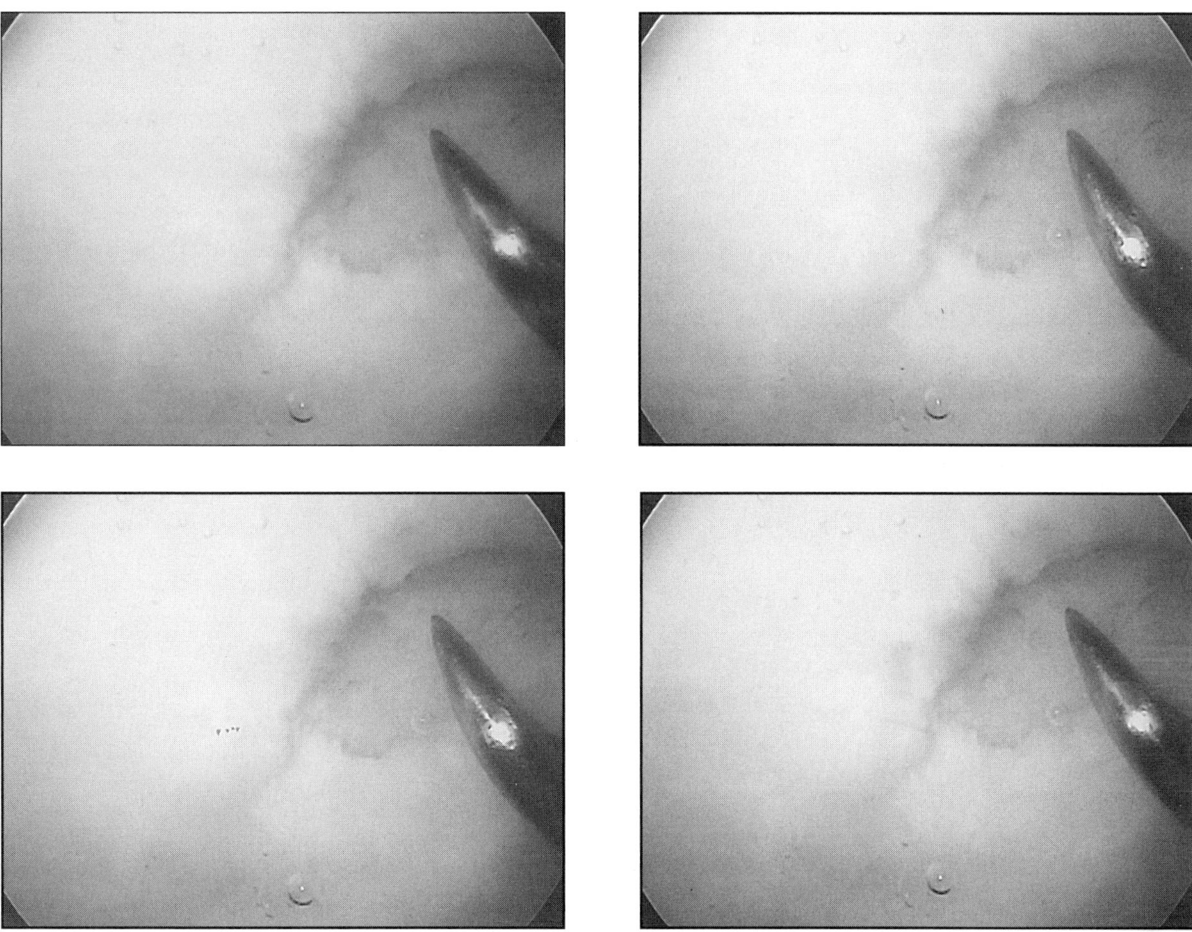

FIGURE 10.10 Microfracture performed for grade IV changes in the hip joint.

low-impact sport activities. Kilgus recommends the following sports for patients with total hip replacement: golf, hiking, bicycling, swimming, skiing without moguls, and double tennis (Kilgus et al. 1991). The 1999 Hip Society survey in addition named canoeing, horseback riding, low-impact aerobics, and bowling. A survey at a Hip Society meeting showed that 96% of 47 Hip Society surgeons allowed their total hip patients to play golf (Healy, Iorio, and Lemos 2001). Mallon and Callaghan (1992) found no clinical and no radiographic difference between cemented versus non-cemented hip replacements for golfers. Another study looked at 58 competitive tennis players with 75 hip replacements and return to competing at preoperative levels (Mont et al. 1999).

Minimally invasive total hip replacement utilizing a small incision (3 to 3.5 in.), minimizing soft tissue exposure and avoiding cutting muscles, is gaining popularity among surgeons and patients. This procedure decreases hospital stay, shortens the recovery time, and allows athletic patients to return to low-impact sports earlier.

SUMMARY

Disabling hip pain in the athlete over 50 can occur from repetitive rotational injuries, as in a golf swing or in tennis; overuse injuries; and direct trauma. Determining the source of hip pain and whether the pathology is intra-articular versus extra-articular can be diagnostically challenging. The use of imaging and arthroscopic intervention has improved our understanding of treating these injuries. In both the conservative and postoperative contexts, the role of physical therapy is crucial in the management of disabling hip pain and in returning to sport activity.

CHAPTER

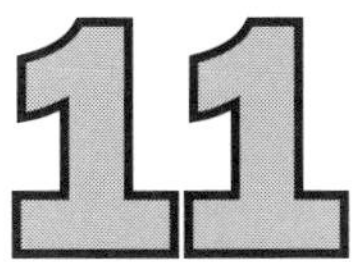

Knee Problems

Douglas J. Martini, MD
Lauren A. Carlson, MPH

The context in which we approach treatment of the older active patient is truly a relevant and challenging problem. In our time as caregivers we have seen an evolution of technologies and expertise in both operative and nonoperative techniques. As recently as the early 1980s, anterior cruciate ligament (ACL) reconstruction on patients over 35 was generally frowned upon, the common sentiment being that these individuals were past their peak of athletic activity and beyond the reach of treatments whose assets were outweighed by their liabilities. The progression to the present era released physicians from artificial restrictions as to how and when a surgical procedure should be performed, introducing tremendous freedom and increase in technological advancement, but also requiring additional cautionary measures.

Any treatment must acknowledge that in its primary stages, osteoarthritis (OA) is a disease solely affecting the articular cartilage. As it advances, the entire joint becomes affected. The challenge that remains is not mastering the surgical procedure, but making an informed decision about the appropriate and rational application of each treatment to attain the ideal correlation between a patient's symptoms and a physician's response. One should incorporate into the treatment algorithm all attempts at conservative care, including physical therapy, bracing, and judicious use of medications, before considering surgery. If the patient's functional limitations persist despite these interventions, then surgical options may be explored.

Decreased mobility associated with knee pain and dysfunction is more considerable than with OA in other joints. Older athletes consider activity restriction due to knee pain and dysfunction monumental. The challenge of our generation is to keep these athletes "in the game."

When considering OA, we recognize that 4.2 million Americans exhibit some involvement of the knee. The tremendous expense incurred by patients and their insurance companies, in addition to socioeconomic factors like work absenteeism and high rates of workers' compensation, will only become more problematic in the coming years as the nation's Baby Boomers gradually progress into their 60s and beyond. The increasing number of adults over 60, coupled with a continual increase in average life expectancy, will present a unique challenge to physicians, who can, with proper knowledge and understanding, guide their patients toward appropriate treatment and the ability to remain physically active and fit longer than has ever been possible.

OSTEOARTHRITIS OF THE KNEE

Treatment of the active senior, based on an understanding of the pathophysiology of OA, can be separated into three categories: those that control symptoms, those that modify the disease, and those that represent a disease cure. In the past, therapies dealt only with the symptoms, having little or no effect on the disease process. Recent treatments, based on a more thorough understanding of hyaline cartilage, have shifted the focus toward altering the progressive pathological cascade. The basic science of hyaline cartilage serves as a central theme for the education of patients on how treatments may, with the help of new technologies, modify the disease process. As the caretakers of both bone and joint of the graying athlete we are committed to extracting those therapies that are curative.

Osteoarthritis is not an inevitable consequence of aging. Normal aging involves superficial fibrillation of the central medial tibial plateau that is seen almost universally in elderly patients. Despite these significant changes, biochemical analysis of the hyaline cartilage showed only minimal changes. The authors concluded that the aging of articular cartilage is not a form of early OA.

While the involvement of articular cartilage is a primary factor in a diagnosis of OA, secondary to that diagnosis is the eventual degeneration of the entire periarticular environment, including subchondral bone, synovium, muscle, capsule, and ligaments, as referenced in figure 11.1. A comprehensive treatment program must address the entire periarticular environment. Early intervention and treatment may not alter the course of articular cartilage damage, but may help to maintain the integrity of the periarticular capsule, ligaments, muscle, and tendinous structures. This may be invaluable to the functional outcome of any therapy.

The pathophysiology of pain associated with OA is multifactorial, with each of the periarticular structures contributing individually. Potential factors include subchondral bone microfracture, osteophyte-induced impingement or irritation of the synovial nerve endings, periarticular muscle spasm, and synovial inflammation from debris particles.

History and Physical Examination

The basics of history and physical examination for the active senior are no different than for any other patient but require acumen at distinguishing symptoms of arthrosis from those of instability. Cases featuring pure instability or pure arthritis are clear-cut, but the area between these extremes requires the greatest skill in determining and outlining the appropriate treatment. That is, for the older athlete, restricting his or her options to a single treatment modality is insufficient. The physician's plan must feature a fully inclusive progression from simple to complex therapies, in which each step can act as a substitute for the preceding one if the more conservative treatment option is unsuccessful.

History

Essential to an accurate diagnosis of OA in the active senior is a thorough and accurate history, detailing both distant events and circumstances, such as remote trauma and surgical procedures, and more recent matters involving the patient's symptoms. Outlining a course of treatment and planning further surgical procedures require that the exact nature of prior interventions be ascertained. When the patient is unable to recall the details of those procedures, it is helpful to request all operative notes. Reviewing the patient's records requires some effort, but is justified and appropriate based on the value of knowing the full extent of anatomical involvement.

The onset of symptoms is quite important. Symptoms of OA are insidious in onset with gradual progression in severity, and are aggravated by weight-bearing activities. Knee pain with a mechanical origin occurs more suddenly, is sharp and stabbing, and is more often associated with changes in position such as twisting. Attention should be given to the extent to which these knee symptoms affect the patient's activities. Having to quit a round of golf halfway through because of sharp, stabbing knee pain is very different from having increased knee pain in the evening after completion of a round of golf. In failing to understand how the patient's knee pain affects his or her life, one misses the opportunity to be able to identify the best course of treatment.

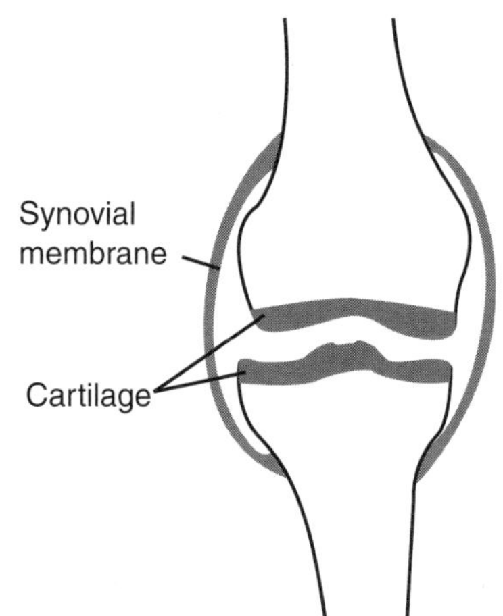

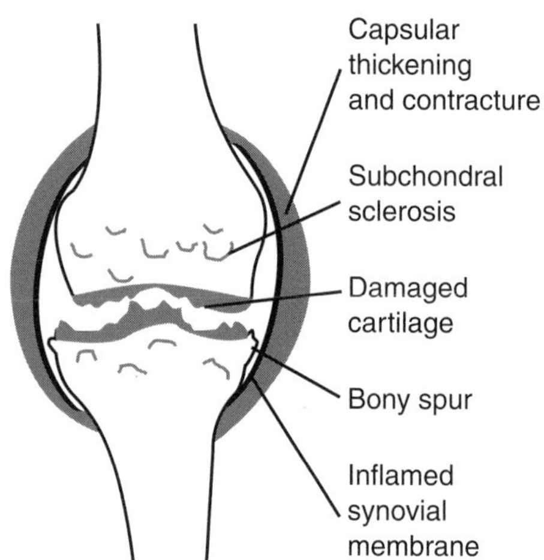

FIGURE 11.1 Differences between a healthy knee and an osteoarthritic knee.

Physical Exam

The physician examining the older athlete can maximize effectiveness of the examination by physically inspecting the knee, palpating, measuring range of motion, assessing muscle strength, and testing meniscal and ligament strength. The inspection should identify any mild varus or valgus deformity and asymmetry of the quadriceps muscle, so the patient should wear shorts or a gown. It is inappropriate to perform an exam with the lower extremities covered. It is important to observe the patient's gait and his or her manner of rising from a chair and moving to the examining table.

With the patient supine, a range of motion exam is performed. This must include extension measured in terms of that which exceeds neutral and also compared to the contralateral side. Simply noting that extension is full is insufficient. Average extension in adults is 3° to 6° of hyperextension. Such concrete guidelines to not apply to measures of flexion, which must take into account the patient's stature. A tall, thin person may be able to achieve 145° of flexion quite easily, whereas for a short, stout person 125° represents terminal flexion. A common way to note range of motion of 3° of hyperextension to 140° of flexion is 3-0-140°. Similarly, a 6° flexion contracture would be labeled 0-6-140°. Even small decreases in extension can have clinical significance. In an article on classifying and treating arthrofibrosis, Shelbourne, Patel, and Martini (1996) observed a parallel in the symptoms of type I arthrofibrosis (which is an extension loss only) and more severe types of arthrofibrosis. It is also worth noting that when this extension was restored, symptoms resolved predictably.

Manual muscle testing, although quantitatively not accurate, is sufficient for establishing the extent of muscle weakness. In the acutely inflamed knee, the extent of muscle weakness may be overstated by reflex inhibition. In these cases, more aggressive strengthening without addressing the pain usually fails.

The menisci and ligaments are tested by established methods such as Lockman, McMurray, anterior drawer, and pivot shift. In the chronic ACL tear with unicompartmental arthrosis, sometimes objective instability becomes very difficult to identify. This subset of patients has been referred to as arthritically stable. A high index of suspicion based on historical information describing previous instability-related events can often lead to the correct diagnosis. With a thorough understanding of ligament stability, the physician is prepared to identify both the primary pathology and the most appropriate treatment option.

The physician treating the older athlete should understand the significance of patellofemoral symptoms. As the incidence of patellofemoral symptoms increases with age and is often a component of the overall symptoms of this population, one should obtain a history of anterior knee pain, considering the "movie sign" and additional pain during ambulation up and down inclines. Physical findings relevant to the diagnosis include retropatellar crepitation, patellar grind, medial and lateral mobility, and retinacular tenderness. Awareness of underlying patellofemoral symptoms should always be incorporated into a physical therapy (PT) prescription.

Radiographic Examination

The radiographic examination of the knee is an important means for diagnosis (figure 11.2). At least 50% to 75% of people older than 65 exhibit some radiographic evidence of OA on plain X-ray films. In the population over 75 years, this number approaches 100%. Only 40% to 60% of these people, however, may be clinically symptomatic. Knee pain is not a predictor of radiographically evident disease, and no strong correlation exists between the clinical outcome and its radiographic appearance. Therefore, to assume that changes observed on X-ray represent the current cause of a patient's symptoms would be naive. In making treatment decisions, it is important to treat the patient rather than his or her X-ray—considering the clinical picture in the background of the X-ray.

The standard radiographic series in diagnosing OA includes posteroanterior 45° weight-bearing, sunrise, and lateral views. Measuring mechanical malalignment requires a bilateral weight-bearing X-ray. Several authors have noted that single-leg weight-bearing films accurately represent the extent of mechanical deformity, believing that this more accurately represents the mechanical environment of the single-leg stance during normal ambulation. How to apply this information to corrective procedures such as osteotomy and arthroplasty has yet to be determined.

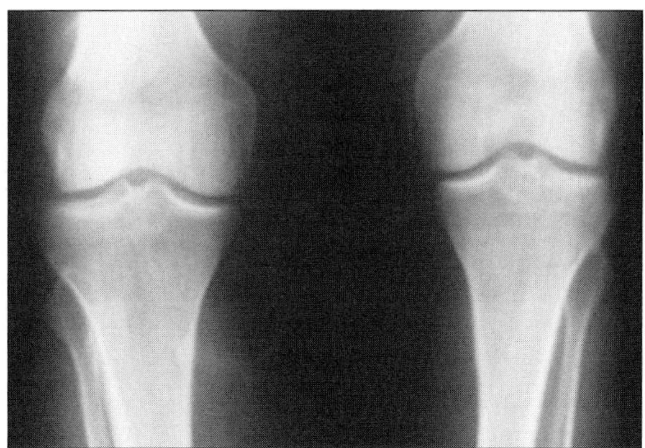

FIGURE 11.2 Normal knee.

Of note in these radiographic studies are joint space narrowing, subchondral sclerosis, osteophytes, and bone remodeling in each compartment. It is widely believed that a diagnosis of OA requires identification of at least a 40% decrease in articular height on X-ray. Therefore, it is important to remember that absence of joint space narrowing on plain films does not exclude the possibility of arthritis, especially with a full-thickness cartilage lesion. Lysholm, Hamberg, and Gillquist (1987) experienced difficulty in predicting cartilage damage based on plain films. In this arthroscopic study, they routinely found Outerbridge II and III changes with only a minimal difference in radiographic appearance. Radiographic evidence of joint space narrowing is also not an absolute predictor of cartilage health. Fife et al. (1991) identified 33% of 161 patients with X-ray evidence of narrowing whose cartilage was normal in appearance at the time of arthroscopy.

No classification system is completely accurate. Therefore, it is appropriate to use a system that is reproducible and that the examiner is comfortable with. The Fairbanks classification seems to be a reasonable system.

Routine use of magnetic resonance imaging (MRI) and computed tomography (CT) scans is not recommended due to the overuse of MRI in diagnosing the painful knee. When used discriminately, these tests can be very helpful in diagnosis and treatment in well-defined situations, but it is important that they remain an adjunct to an accurate history and a thorough physical examination. Operating on the results of an MRI-diagnosed degenerative meniscal tear with concomitant arthritis can be injudicious, as this test often produces a very strong false positive. In deciding whether to use an auxiliary test, consider how these findings will alter the course of treatment. For example, if a 55-year-old male presents with a large tense effusion and 20° flexion contracture and is unable to straighten his leg, an MRI study would probably contribute significantly to deciding to proceed with arthroscopy.

TREATMENT

Treatment of OA in the older active patient should begin with proven conservative therapies such as PT, bracing, and medication. When the patient's pain and impairment exceed the scope of these therapies, more invasive measures may be considered. As with the overall treatment algorithm, the definitive procedures, including arthroplasty, must be delayed until the more conservative surgical interventions have been implemented and proven ineffective.

Physical Therapy

At the core of treatment of the active aging patient is PT. Although subject to limitations, including a limited ability to cure, PT finds its importance in the reality that the patient's condition will never worsen given an appropriately designed program. Factors of importance include the intensity and delivery of these programs, as the active senior may respond differently than his or her younger counterpart.

Appropriate Physical Therapy Goals

One must understand the entire periarticular environment when addressing PT for the older athlete. The impairment in these patients may be multifactorial to include joint pain, instability, decreased range of motion, proprioceptive defects, and muscle weakness. Minor et al. (1989) outlined the following goals of a PT regimen:

- Reduction of impairment and improvement of function; that is, reduction of joint pain, increases in range of motion (ROM) and strength, normalization of gait, and facilitation of the performance of daily activities
- Protection of the OA joint from further damage through reducing stress on the joint, attenuating joint forces, and improving biomechanics
- Prevention of disability and poor health secondary to inactivity through increasing the daily level of physical activity and improving physical fitness

When considering a therapy regimen, one should not underestimate the importance of the latter point. Active seniors are, by definition, not sedentary; but their inability to participate in activities of choice due to knee pain can affect their entire sense of well-being. Setting up a well-structured rehab regimen empowers the patient to take control of a problem. It is worth reiterating that the goals of PT need to be reasonable and obtainable, and also individualized to reflect the patient's level of physical activity.

A functional progression should be the initial aim of a PT regimen, helping the patient reduce the impairment and prepare for a return to activity. Since this patient is more aerobically fit than a sedentary counterpart, one must remember the level of aerobic fitness when applying a PT program. Compliance with any therapy regimen will decrease if the program causes more pain, so aggressive strengthening or advancing a functional progression is never prudent in an actively inflamed knee.

Some Basic Principles

Although it is beyond the scope of this chapter to include every nuance of managing the older active patient, several ideas should be thoroughly understood:

• First, **simple improvements in terminal extension can make significant functional improvements.** In personal communication, Shelbourne noted that in the aging athlete, functional score can be drastically improved with increased extension from a strict regimen with an extension board (figure 11.3). This progress may be related to existing arthrosis as a "flexion disease." In this case, any weight bearing with a flexion contracture actually loads the worn portion of the joint. Terminal extension may allow weight bearing on more normal cartilage (figure 11.4). Also, a flexion deformity encourages pericapsular adhesions and muscle atrophy from ineffective quadriceps contraction.

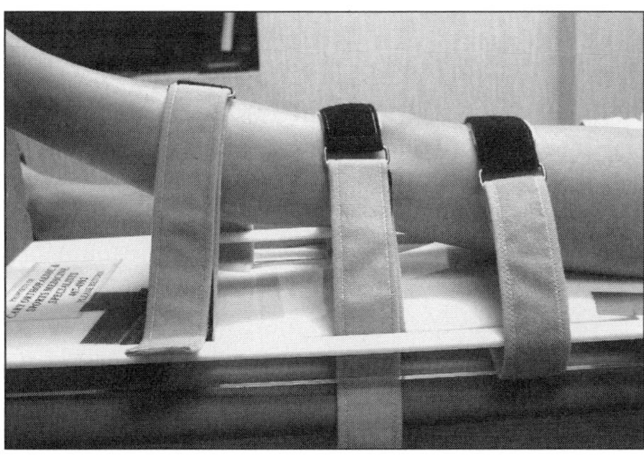

FIGURE 11.3 An extension board can be used to maintain terminal extension in an acutely inflamed knee.

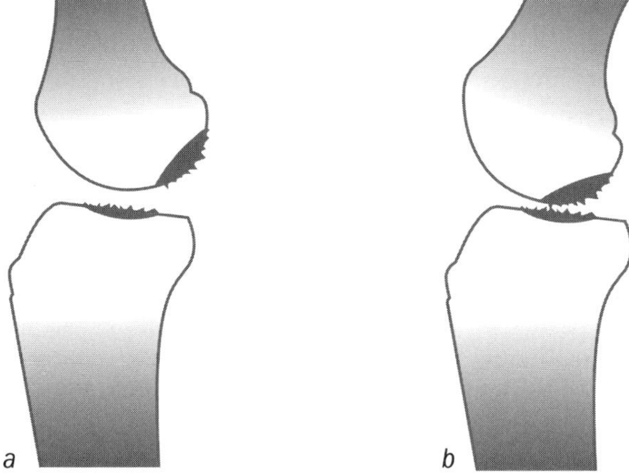

FIGURE 11.4 *(a)* In terminal extension there is less contact area between the chondral damage of the femoral and tibial surfaces. *(b)* A flexion contracture increases the contact area between damaged areas.

• Second, **weight bearing is healthy for the joint.** Once the acute phase of inflammation is under control, advancing the weight-bearing activity can be tolerated well. Activities such as water therapy, stair steppers, elliptical trainers, and cycling all have much lower joint loading profiles than walking or running to increase levels of fitness and therefore have tremendous value in managing arthrosis in the active senior. Numerous studies have demonstrated that certain weight-bearing exercises increase functional outcome but do not increase the arthrosis patient's level of pain. A pilot study at Boston City Hospital (unpublished data) involved two groups of OA patients. One group used a stationary bike under the supervision of a physical therapist for up to 20 min, three times a week, and could use acetaminophen as needed; the other was limited to a therapeutic regimen of ibuprofen. At the study's conclusion, the stationary bike group reported greater reduction of pain and improved functional status.

• Third, **periarticular muscle strength must be improved to increase muscle function.** Fisher et al. (1993) proved the benefit of such a regimen. They focused on the quantitative effects of PT on muscular function and endurance in 40 individuals with OA. Physical therapy was performed three times a week for three months in a single outpatient PT center. Significant improvements were noted in muscle strength and endurance and in the functional abilities to climb stairs, rise from a chair, and walk. The majority of these improvements occurred during the first month of therapy. Deyle et al. (2000) designed a randomized clinical study to evaluate the effectiveness of manual PT and exercise in treating OA of the knee. At eight weeks, distance walked over a certain time period had improved by 95% over that seen in a control group. The treatment group maintained improvements at one year; and only 5% of those treated required arthroplasty, compared with 20% of the control group. Clearly the individuals involved in these studies are not identical to the population we are discussing. These study groups cited OA as their primary complaint and were much more sedentary than the active senior; but the same principles apply, showing support for the value of PT in treating active patients.

Nontraditional Regimens

Some nontraditional therapeutic regimens can be helpful in individual cases. In some communities, water therapy is becoming increasingly available, and this can be extremely valuable as an intermediate step in reconditioning the knee and managing its acute flares. This modality remains most effective when coupled with traditional-level therapy. In the fragile or significantly deconditioned patient, Pilates therapy proves itself very successful based on its lower impact and strong neuromuscular and proprioceptive element. The exact indication for these types of therapies has not been clearly delineated, but patient experience identifies them as effective supplements.

Bracing

Bracing as an option for treatment of the middle-aged athlete has become much more attractive (figure 11.5). Historically, these appliances seemed to be cumbersome and poorly tolerated, but new designs and lighter materials allow for a positive correlation between braces and effective therapy. A host of literature affirms that certain body types, especially those with short, obese legs, remain a difficult match and are probably not ideal for unloader bracing. Patient education about the goals and expected outcomes is important: This is not a cure for the early degenerative knee, but it can be a powerful adjunct to comprehensive treatment. It is also very effective at keeping the older athlete "in the game," which is perhaps its greatest utility in our specific patient population.

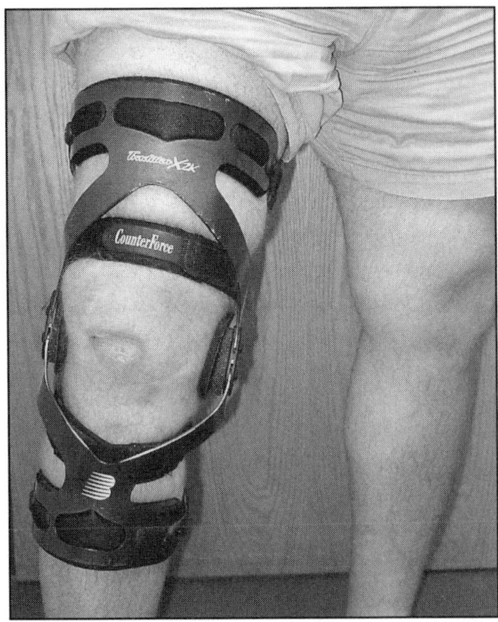

FIGURE 11.5 A 52-year-old male with end stage medial compartment osteoarthritis. Medial unloader brace immediately decreased pain. Patient wished to consider more definitive procedures but not until he had more symptoms while wearing the brace.

Recently, the lack of information about how these braces work and questions about their clinical efficacy have been replaced by well-designed studies demonstrating their usefulness. Kirkley et al. (1999) performed a prospective randomized study evaluating the efficacy of bracing on varus gonarthrosis. The unloader brace and neoprene sleeve groups showed a strong tendency toward clinical improvements in disease-specific quality of life. The authors concluded that the use of a knee brace in addition to medical treatment provided significant benefit and that on average, the unloader brace was more effective than the neoprene sleeve.

Using an analysis of gait symmetry, Draper et al. (2000) demonstrated improvement in function after varus bracing of the knee. This study provided an objective measurement of function in 30 consecutive patients via gait analysis on four different occasions: immediately before and after fitting, then at three months with the brace on and off. After the brace was fitted, all patients reported immediate improvement, and consistent improvement was also noted during stance and swing phases of gait. Improved indices of symmetry correspond to a significant increase in the Hospital for Special Surgery knee score from 69.9 to 82.0 (p = .001). The patients felt that the unloader brace immediately enhanced the knee's function.

An in vivo analysis of the effectiveness of an unloader brace during heel strike was performed by Dennis et al. (1999). Forty patients, all with marked unicompartmental arthritis, walked on a treadmill and were monitored with fluoroscopic surveillance in the frontal plane. The procedure was repeated after patients were fitted with an unloader brace. The fluoroscopic images were downloaded to a computer and digitalized, and the captured heel strike images were analyzed. Concomitant with this analysis, a questionnaire measured the subjective reduction of pain during wearing of the brace. Eighty-five percent of the patients said that the brace was effective in decreasing pain; 15% experienced no change in knee pain; and 78% demonstrated increased tibial-femoral height, which was on average 1.7 mm. An average 2.0° change in the tibial-femoral angle occurred in 78% of the participants. The authors concluded that articular offloading with unloader braces can be achieved and correlates with relief of knee pain. They also question the effectiveness of unloader braces in obese patients, as all participants who felt they had no improvement were obese.

Studies such as these support the use of unloader braces. Active seniors may benefit more than the general population; active people tend to present earlier in the disease process because the knee pain hinders participation in activities. Thus the brace may allow continued athletic involvement for years before a more definitive procedure is considered. A second benefit is the diagnostic aspect: Pain relief with application of an unloader brace is a good prognostic finding when one is considering a high tibial osteotomy (HTO) or unicompartmental arthroplasty.

Medical Therapies

The OA patient has a pharmacoepia of medicines available. Mass media are replete with advertisements for these new and superior medications. Acetaminophen and nonsteroidal anti-inflammatory drug (NSAID) use will remain a mainstay of management of joint pain although only part of a comprehensive treatment plan. Several new options for the pharmacological management of OA symptoms require discussion.

Chondroitin and Glucosamine

Despite the lack of evidence-based data to support their use, chondroitin and glucosamine have become popular supplements to traditional therapeutic regimes. A recent periodical indicated that over 100 combinations of these products exist, and an AltaVista Internet search for the term glucosamine returned over 34,000 sites (Delafuente 2000). Delafuente points out that the majority of these sites provided anecdotal, unsubstantiated reports of product benefits. He concludes that recent enthusiasm for chondroitin and glucosamine supplementation stems from several factors: the publicity surrounding the book *The Arthritis Cure*, which encourages chondroitin and glucosamine use; the passage of the 1994 Dietary Supplementation and Health Education Act—legislation that severely limited regulatory powers of the federal government in regard to dietary supplements, allowing their production and sale without any testing for efficacy, safety, or uniform industry standard on manufacturing; and finally, the high prevalence of arthritis and lack of effective drug therapy void of side effects.

Much of the product literature refers to chondroitin and glucosamine as a cure for arthritis, and although it is clear that these statements are not substantiated, there is a reasonable basis in science for their use.

Chondroitin sulfate is one of many glycosaminoglycans (GAGs) that compose cartilage's extracellular matrix. Researchers are unsure whether the 10% of the supplement that the body absorbs is absorbed intact or after being metabolized. Chondroitin is believed to stimulate the integration of sulfur into cartilage, which has a major stabilizing effect on the extracellular matrix, and in vitro studies suggest that it increases the synthesis of hyaluronan via chondrocyte-derived fibroblast cells. Another proposed effect includes initiation of a mild anti-inflammatory response and chondroprotective effect through limiting the release of liposomal enzymes.

Glucosamine is an aminosaccharide important for the synthesis of glycolipids, glycoproteins, GAGs, hyaluronan, and proteoglycans. These cellular entities are the building blocks of many structures of mesenchymal origin. Oral glucosamine is water soluble and quickly absorbed by the gastrointestinal tract, where it is rapidly incorporated into GAGs by chondrocytes. The presence of glucosamine activates core protein synthesis, leading to an increase in proteoglycan concentration in the intracellular ground substance. This potential mechanism is appropriate for the treatment of OA, because concurrent with OA is the decreased proteoglycan synthesis that allows production levels to fall below levels of proteoglycan loss, resulting in a net cartilage matrix loss (Pelletier and Martel-Pelletier 1993). Glucosamine in a negative feedback loop decreases proteoglycan degradation. It also appears that glucosamine may stabilize cell membranes, play a role in stimulating the regeneration of cartilage, and act as a selective COX-2 inhibitor, thereby contributing a mild anti-inflammatory effect.

Studies on Chondroitin and Glucosamine Supplementation

Chondroitin is most often sold in conjunction with glucosamine, but there are few evidence-based studies to confirm the efficacy of this combination. Das and Hammad (2000) performed a randomized, placebo-controlled study to evaluate the efficacy of the combination in treating OA of the knee. The Lequesne Index of Severity of OA of the Knee (ISK) was the primary outcome measurement. When taking the combination of supplements, patients with mild to moderate OA showed significant improvement in ISK scores at four and six months ($p = .003$ and $p = .04$, respectively). The improvement in response rate was 52% in the medicine group and 28% in the placebo group. Unfortunately, patients in the treatment group who had advanced radiographic OA were not subject to these improvements. The study concluded that the glucosamine-chondroitin combination was effective in treating radiographically mild to moderate OA as measured by the ISK.

Studies on Chondroitin Alone

A few studies evaluate the efficacy of chondroitin alone versus treatment with placebo or diclofenac sodium. These studies have design problems, including small numbers and short duration; but despite these limitations, it appears that chondroitin therapy is beneficial in treating OA. Mazieres et al. (1992) quantitated the value of chondroitin sulfate in a placebo-controlled study, giving chondroitin for three months over a total study period of five months. Concomitant use of NSAIDs was recorded. At study completion, all parameters (visual analog pain scale, Visual Analog Scale, and patient and physician global assessment) significantly improved ($p \leq .05$), in addition to a noteworthy decrease in use of NSAIDs over the placebo group. Others have performed similar studies with similar outcomes (Fleisch et al. 1997).

Morreale et al. (1985) evaluated oral chondroitin sulfate and diclofenac over six months. One group received 400 mg chondroitin, three times a day for three months, followed by three months without treatment; another group received 50 mg diclofenac once a day for one month, followed by five months without treatment. The Lequesne index at three months decreased by 78% from baseline in the chondroitin group and 62% in the diclofenac group. At six months follow-up, the Lequesne index was 64.4% lower in the chondroitin group and only 29.7% lower in the diclofenac group. The authors concluded that chondroitin is effective in treating OA and that its effects last longer than those of diclofenac.

Verbruggen, Goemaere, and Veys (1997) examined chondroitin's chondroprotective effect by noting the extent to which it halts radiographic changes associated with OA. Evaluation of hand radiographs performed annually for three years in a chondroitin-treated group compared to a non-chondroitin treatment group showed a significant decrease in the number of patients with erosive OA. Patients on chondroitin had an 8.8% incidence of new joint involvement versus the placebo group at 29.4%. It is important that further scientific investigation continue so that the medical community may more precisely define the usefulness of this treatment.

Studies on Glucosamine Alone

Several clinical studies on treatment with glucosamine are worth noting. Pujalte, Llavore, and Ylescupidez (1980) conducted a randomized, double-blind placebo-controlled study using oral glucosamine, three times a day for six to eight weeks, and measured articular pain, tenderness, swelling, and ROM. The treatment group showed statistically significant reductions in pain scores and joint tenderness and swelling. Concluding physician assessments rated the treatment group as 100% successful, the placebo group as only 60% successful. These findings support the use of glucosamine in treating OA.

Drovanti et al. (1980) performed a double-blind placebo-controlled trial using 500 mg oral glucosamine three times a day for 30 days and measured pain, tenderness, swelling, and restricted motion weekly. All measured parameters improved over time. At three weeks, all parameters improved by about 50%. Interestingly, in addition to finding glucosamine helpful in treating OA, the authors concluded that the effect of glucosamine on pain may reflect a direct action on cartilage rather than a change in cartilage metabolism, because of the rapid onset of action.

Vaz (1982) was the first to perform a double-blind study comparing glucosamine sulfate to ibuprofen. In this eight-week study the glucosamine group received 500 mg three times a day and the control group received 400 mg of ibuprofen three times a day. Objective parameters were noted by the physician and subjective decrease in pain was recorded by the subjects. Significant pain relief was not observed until after week 2 in the glucosamine group, reflecting a longer period than for the ibuprofen group. At eight weeks, the glucosamine group reported pain substantially less than did the ibuprofen group. At the end of the study period, physician judgments of subjects' overall improvement indicated a good response in 44% of the glucosamine group and in 15% of the ibuprofen group. The authors suggested that glucosamine was at least as good as ibuprofen in treating OA. The validity of the study is impaired by the dosage of ibuprofen given, and the question remains whether a larger dose would have proven more therapeutic.

Recommended Glucosamine and Chondroitin Dosage

Although recommended doses vary among preparations, there is general agreement that the most acceptable initial dose of glucosamine is 1,500 mg/day and for chondroitin is 1,200 mg/day. This regimen continues for six to eight weeks, at which point the dose decreases to 1,000 mg/day and 800 mg/day, respectively. Although the effects of these preparations take longer to become apparent, they have also been known to last longer after cessation of the therapy.

Unfortunately, as a result of the plethora of Web sites unsanctioned by the medical community and the numerous possible combinations of chondroitin and glucosamine that they promote, there is a great deal of hype regarding the efficacy of these supplements. Moreover, the few well-done clinical studies have been overshadowed by the abundance of poorly designed studies and false claims sponsored by manufacturers of these products.

To resolve some of the controversy, the NIH is currently funding a multicenter scientific study to evaluate the efficacy and long-term benefits of these supplements. Nondocumented qualitative patient observation reveals that over 50% of those who opt for this treatment modality report positive results. The concern remains that patients may overlook established and confirmed therapies in favor of those that have potential but whose absolute value remains unproven. In general, it is probably reasonable to leave the decision to take these supplements up to the patient but to strongly discourage their use as the only treatment modality.

Hyaluronic Acid

Viscosupplementation appears to be useful in treating the active senior who has early to moderate OA. Hyaluronic acid (HA), a polysaccharide chain secreted by synoviocytes and chondrocytes, is found abundantly in the synovial fluid and ground substances of chondrocytes. Its several important functions are maintaining viscoelasticity of the synovial fluid, reducing inflammation, and acting as an autoregulatory agent. Its usefulness in treating OA lies in its anti-inflammatory, viscoelastic, analgesic, and chondroprotective properties.

Originally it was hoped that, as suggested by in vitro studies, HA may favorably alter the natural history of the disease. To date, this therapy has been shown to decrease pain in OA, but any favorable effects on articular cartilage have not been proven. Some controversy still exists regarding the efficacy of HA, mainly because numerous studies have produced a broad spectrum of results. Table 11.1 presents a review and summary of these studies.

Possible Modes of Action

Viscoelasticity of HA is an important contributor to normal joint function. Balazs and Denlinger (1993) have demonstrated the importance of this function. When mechanical forces move the joint slowly, HA is viscous; however, with greater energy transmission or increased rate of movement, the synovial fluid becomes more elastic and absorbs energy more efficiently, thus improving the performance of the joint (Simon 1999). High molecular weight HA has been shown to increase the endogenous synthesis of HA (Altman and Moskowitz et al. 1998). It is widely known that as the cascade of OA progresses, the HA concentration can decrease as much as 50%. Additionally, the remaining HA is of a poorer quality. Because exogenous HA diminishes rapidly and within 48 h is no longer present at all, the stimulation of endogenous HA may account for the prolonged pain relief provided by viscosupplementation as compared with other treatments.

Hyaluronic acid has been observed to have a nocioceptive effect in the normal knee (Weiss and Band 1999). It has been suggested that the decrease in HA associated with progressive OA is related to the decreased capacity of HA to provide nocioceptive protection. Exogenous and endogenous HA may restore and perhaps enhance these nocioceptive properties. In vitro, when added to chondrocytes in culture, HA enhances proteoglycan synthesis. This may serve as a chondroprotective or chondroreparative mechanism of action. Some animal models of OA show that the addition of HA slows the progression of cartilage damage (Corrado et al. 1995). Finally, other studies have shown that intra-articular HA has a direct anti-inflammatory effect on synoviocytes by inhibiting arachidonic acid release or by blocking prostaglandin-E_2 production. This mechanism can also explain the lasting effect of HA (Pelletier and Martel-Pelletier 1993).

Studies on Hyaluronic Acid

Many of the initial study protocols failed to demonstrate substantial difference in HA over other treatments, especially when the control was a placebo injection. It seems that quite often the placebo group had a positive response. The explanation is not entirely clear, but some investigators have concluded that HA is no better than placebo. However, it is important to consider the time period of these studies and to ask about benefits of HA that extend past the time of improvement in the control group. Dougados et al. (1993) performed a one-year randomized, placebo-controlled trial including parameters measuring pain, function (as assessed by the Lequesne index), and synovial effusion. Physician and subject global assessments were obtained. At week 4, a statistical difference was observed in only one of the measured parameters, pain after exercise, which improved markedly in the treatment group ($p = .026$). At week 49, the treatment group showed a significant improvement in function ($p = .046$) over the placebo group. According to the final physician assessment, 77% of the HA group but only 54% of the placebo group improved substantially. The global improvement percentage of 77% is impressive, but seems to be overshadowed by the 54% global improvement in the control group.

In a similar study design, Corrado et al. (1995) evaluated the synovial fluid of the two study groups to examine the biological effect of HA versus placebo. All patients received five weekly injections and were followed for two months. At day 35, there was no difference in pain during active motion between the two groups; however, pain intensity was down by 50% in the treatment group and 29% in the placebo group. From day 35 to day 60, the HA group had a progressive decrease in pain as measured by visual analog scale (VAS), while the placebo group experienced no change in VAS score. Synovial fluid cell counts at the end of the study actually decreased in the treatment group and increased in the control group.

Altman and Moskowitz et al. (1998) studied groups receiving HA, placebo injection, or naproxen. The active treatment group fared better than the placebo group but responded similarly to the naproxen group.

TABLE 11.1 Randomized Trials Evaluating Hyaluronic Acid vs. Placebo in Treatment of Osteoarthritis of the Knee*

Study	Active treatment	No. of patients	Patient characteristics	Study design	Outcome measures	Results favoring hyaluronate
Wobig et al. 1998	Hyland G-F 20, 3 injections	110	Mean age 62 yr; K-L 1-3; VAS pain >70	Multicenter, double-blind, 12 wk, 26-wk phone follow-up	VAS pain and function	VAS pain and function
Lohmander et al. 1996	Artzal, 5 injections	240	Mean age 58 yr; Lequesne index ≥4	Multicenter, double-blind, 20 wk	VAS pain, Activity level, Lequesne index	None
Adams et al. 1995	Hyland G-F 20, 3 injections	102	Mean age 61 yr; K-L 1-3; VAS pain >50	Multicenter, double-blind, 12 wk, 26-wk phone follow-up	VAS pain, MD global	None
Scale et al. 1994	Hyland G-F 20, 2 vs. 3 injections	80	Mean age 59 yr; Larson score 2-4; VAS pain >40	Single center, double-blind, 12 wk, 26-wk phone follow-up	VAS pain and function, Pt/MD global	VAS pain and function, Pt/MD global
Dahlberg et al. 1994	Hyaluronic acid, 5 injections	52	Mean age 45 yr; normal X-ray; arthroscopic evidence of osteoarthritis; VAS pain >40	Single center, double-blind 52 wk	Knee function, VAS pain, ROM, Activity level, Lysholm scale	None
Henderson et al. 1994	Hyalgan, 5 injections	84	Mean age 67 yr; VAS pain >30	Single center, double-blind, 20 wk	VAS pain, RRM, Function	RRM (one subgroup)
Puhl et al. 1993	Hyaluronic acid, 5 injections	195	Mean age 61 yr; VAS pain >50	Multicenter, double-blind, 14 wk, 18-wk phone follow-up	Lequesne index, RRM, VAS pain, Pt/MD global	Lequesne index, VAS pain
Dougados et al. 1993	Hyalgan, 4 injections	110	Mean age 68 yr; VAS pain >40	Multicenter, single-blind, 52 wk	VAS pain, Lequesne index	VAS pain, Lequesne index
Dixon et al. 1988	Hylauronic acid, up to 11 injections	63	Mean age 69 yr	Multicenter, double-blind, 25 wk	VAS pain, ADL assessment	VAS rest and pain

*Abbreviations: ADL = activities of daily living; K-L = Kellegren-Lawrence (or equivalent) radiographic grade (1= minimal or no changes; 2 = questionable formation of osteophytes or joint-space narrowing; 3 = osteophytosis and joint-space narrowing; 4 = end stage, with bone-to-bone interface); ROM = range of motion; RRM = return to rescue medication (NSAID or analgesia); VAS = visual analog scale (×100).

Reprinted, by permission, from J.R. Watterson and J.M. Esdaile, 2000, "Viscosupplementation: Therapeutic mechanisms and clinical potential in osteoarthritis of the knee," *Journal of the American Academy of Orthopedic Surgeons* 8(5): 277-284.

The authors concluded that HA was as effective as naproxen therapy with fewer side effects.

Adams et al. (1995) used three groups to compare HA only, HA plus NSAID, and NSAID only. Treatment of the NSAID-only group was supplemented with weekly arthrocentesis of the knee for three weeks. Joint pain and function were evaluated by an blinded observer. At week 12, analysis of joint pain and function demonstrated significant improvement in the HA-only versus the NSAID-only group (p = .05). A telephone interview at week 26 indicated that both the HA-only and HA-NSAID groups had less knee pain than did the NSAID-only group. This is perhaps the most interesting study design in that the NSAID-only group also received arthrocentesis treatments. Serial aspiration alone is a known treatment, and this recognition adds strength to the study.

Patient Selection for Hyaluronic Acid Supplementation

Patient selection is an important feature of viscosupplementation, although its exact role in a treatment algorithm of the active senior is unclear. Perhaps it should be second-line treatment, after a thorough PT regimen and course with NSAIDs. In vitro studies created great enthusiasm about this treatment option and a hope that it may be disease altering; but to date, no study has demonstrated this to be the case. Since the effects seem to be real but temporary, it appears that this therapy simply delays further intervention. Whether viscosupplementation can be effectively combined with other therapies is unknown. The orthopedic community awaits studies that compare the efficacy of the unloader brace with that of the unloader brace and viscosupplementation. Unfortunately, one can make no clear, informed specific recommendation on the use of viscosupplementation. In executing any given treatment, the physician should use good judgment and have reasonable expectations about its outcome and should clearly articulate this information to the patient.

Surgical Treatment

When considering operative intervention for this active group, one needs to consider several parameters, including

- the clinical results or survivorship associated with a given procedure,
- its morbidity and attendant complications,
- the difficulty of eventual conversion to a total knee arthroplasty (TKA), and
- the effect of a given procedure on the outcome of a TKA (Engh and McAuley 1999).

A primary goal of treatment is to allow this group of patients to remain active; however, simpler or less invasive procedures should not be chosen in place of the most appropriate procedure if the simpler procedure offers little hope of improvement. Similarly, definite procedures should not be performed if the accompanying activity restrictions are unacceptable to the patient. Variables Used for Selection of the Surgical Procedure lists the factors that one must consider when deciding on a surgical procedure (Hanssen et al. 2000).

Surgical options for the athlete over 50 cover a broad spectrum from simple to complex. These choices include arthroscopic partial meniscectomy, arthroscopic lavage and debridement, arthroscopic chondroplasty, realignment osteotomy, unicompartmental arthroplasty, and TKA.

Variables Used for Selection of the Surgical Procedure

Historical

- Age (chronological, physiological)
- Activity level
- Pain (severity, location, character)
- Mechanical symptoms
- Systemic inflammatory disease
- Prior joint infection
- Prior meniscectomy

Physical examination

- Range of motion (total arc, flexion contracture)
- Ligamentous deficiencies
- Gait (adductor thrust)
- Malalignment (magnitude, direction)
- Body habitus
- Patellofemoral findings (pain, stability)

Radiographic

- Alignment (mechanical, anatomical)
- Arthritic involvement (location, severity)
- Joint-line obliquity
- Periarticular deformity

Miscellaneous

- Durability of results
- Patient expectations
- Surgeon capabilities
- Potential complications
- Postoperative recovery
- Effect on subsequent total knee arthroplasty

Arthroscopy

Arthroscopy is a valuable tool in the treatment of the older athlete yet has the potential to be one of the most abused. Its most attractive features—minimal invasiveness and ease of performance—are the same factors that lead to abuse. The complication rate remains low, but the incidence of complications increases in patients over 50 years (Rodeo, Forster, and Weiland 1993) and it becomes increasingly important to clearly define the treatment goals. The greatest utility of arthroscopy may be in treating mechanical symptoms of short duration both in the absence of radiographic evidence of arthritis and in patients with concomitant arthritis. The technical application of arthroscopy does have its limitations; therefore, real caution and discretion in patient selection are warranted. Patients who present with early arthritis and deep, aching pain that is non-activity related and is associated with a feeling of stiffness may derive a more concrete benefit from a treatment geared toward the degenerative condition. In the same patients, however, arthroscopy may be perfectly acceptable if they recognize that it is only a palliative measure, understanding that it can be a reasonable intermediate treatment that buys time until the more definitive procedure becomes necessary. As Jack Houston stated, there is no surgical procedure that can't make the patient's condition worse. This is an important concept to embrace in choosing the most appropriate treatment for the older active patient.

Arthroscopic Partial Meniscectomy

Classic meniscal signs in the absence of OA should be treated just as in the younger active patient (figure 11.6). Degenerative tears increase in frequency in the 40s, 50s, and 60s; and increased athleticism in the active senior as compared to more sedentary counterparts affords no extra protection from this process. Therefore, the first presentation of acute knee pain, swelling, and joint line tenderness with or without mechanical symptoms must be managed appropriately. Surgical intervention is not necessary in all of these cases, nor will conservative measures be sufficient for every case. As a tangible influence of managed care on this patient population, the patient has often been treated by a primary care doctor for more than six months and presents with a painful, swollen knee and medial joint line tenderness. Findings at the time of arthroscopy may include kissing grade IV lesion with a large meniscal tear. Would more timely arthroscopic intervention have prevented the chondral damage? Unfortunately, there is at this time no literature predicting the frequency with which a degenerative medial meniscal tear will proceed to concomitant OA.

The physician's approach to the active senior presenting with isolated meniscal signs, normal or near-normal X-rays, and normal alignment should consider arthroscopy if there is little or no improvement during the patient's use of a compression sleeve, use trial of NSAIDs, or involvement in a supervised PT regimen. Usually this is a period of three to four weeks. If mechanical symptoms exist or develop during this time, the merits of conservative treatment have not become evident and it should be deemed unsuccessful.

Arthroscopic Lavage and Debridement

The outcome of arthroscopy when significant chondral damage exists (figure 11.7) is quite unpredictable, and the role of arthroscopy in the knee with concomitant arthrosis remains controversial. Its use in patients with arthrosis and malalignment, whose weight-bearing axis crosses the affected compart-

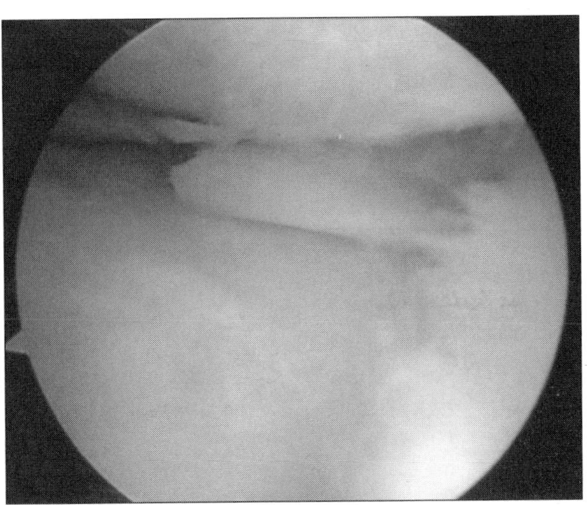

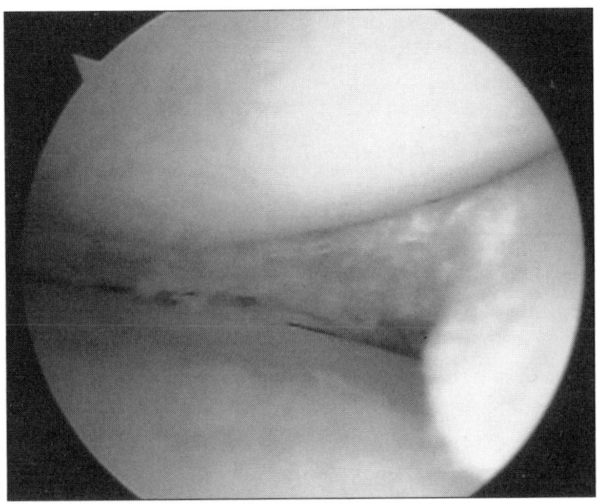

FIGURE 11.6 Isolated degenerative medial meniscal tear in 64-year-old recreational golfer with normal radiographs and alignment. Patient returned to full activity after one month.

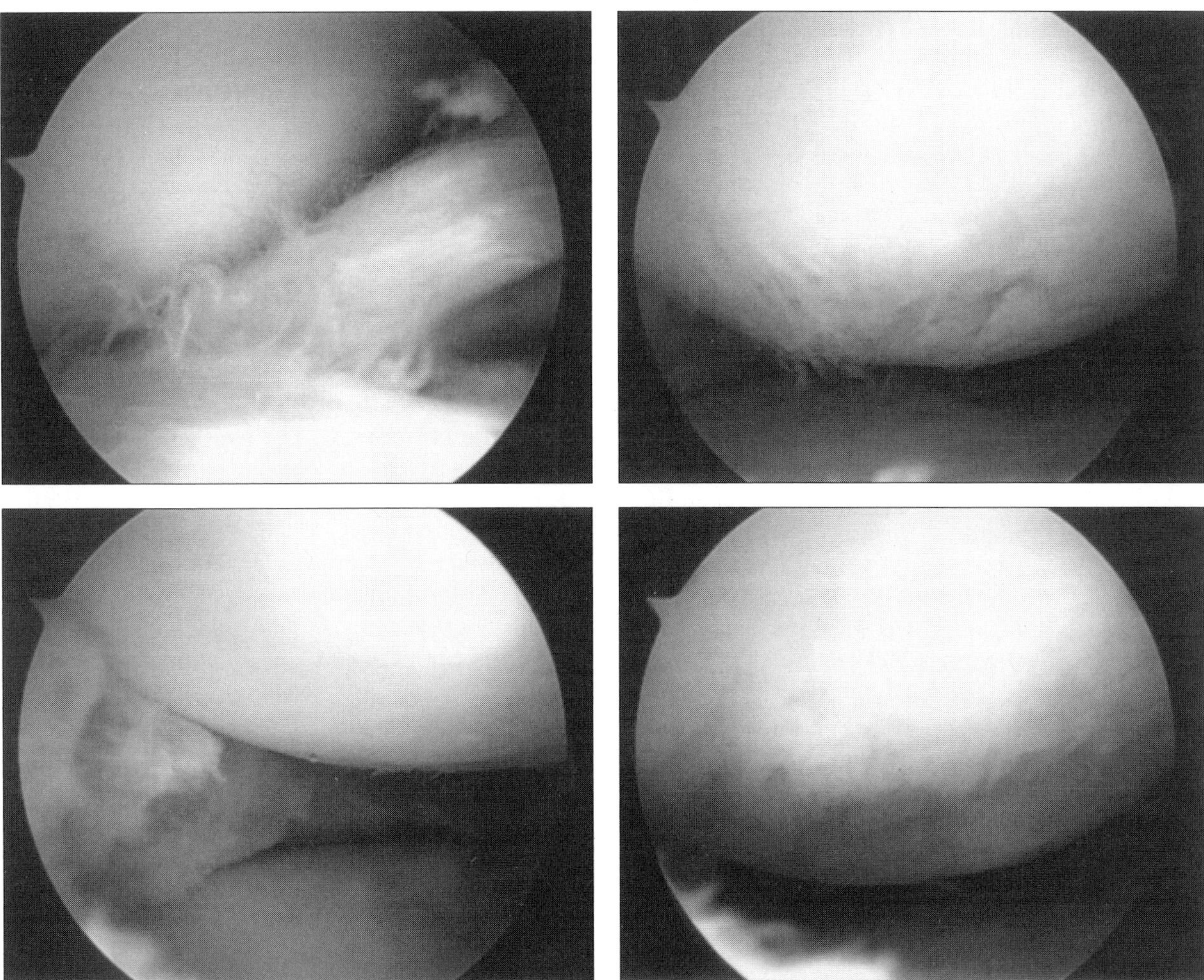

FIGURE 11.7 A 64-year-old female avid golfer and tennis player with a degenerative medial meniscal tear and CdeIV chondral defect. Partial meniscectomy and simple debridement of the unstable margins was performed. Patient used an unloader brace postoperatively and discontinued its use after four months, having no pain or swelling.

ment, should be discouraged (Baumgaertner et al. 1990). Salisbury, Nottage, and Gardner (1985) felt that patients with genu varum and medial knee pain are poor candidates for debridement because only 32% of patients with genu varum undergoing arthroscopic debridement had good clinical results, while 94% of those with normally aligned knees experienced a good result. Preoperative radiographs have a predictive value in the outcome of arthroscopic debridement in patients over 50. Anderson and Goldstein (1991) performed a retrospective review of clinical outcome of arthroscopic debridement including considerations of preoperative X-rays. Whereas 68% of the patients with ≥1 mm of tibiofemoral joint space had a good clinical outcome after debridement, only 29% of those with tibiofemoral joint space ≤1 mm considered their surgery successful. This study supports what is clinically intuitive: The more radiographically advanced OA appears to be, the less likely arthroscopic debridement will be successful.

Jackson, Silver, and Marans (1986) noted that among active older patients (average 53 years), arthroscopy on those with no chondral damage had a success rate of 95% (results reported as excellent or good) at 2.5 years. When chondral damage was present, the success rate dropped to 80% during the study period. Clinically identifying those patients with chondral damage is challenging. Lysholm, Hamberg, and Gillquist (1987) had difficulty correlating pre-op X-rays with operative findings. Often, grade II and III changes were found intraoperatively with normal pre-op X-rays. Radiographic changes more consistently corresponded to advanced outerbridge changes on both sides of the joint surface. Magnetic resonance imaging scan sequences have become more sensitive to changes in articular cartilage, but it is impractical to perform MRIs on the knees of all older athletes. No method is entirely reliable or practical in predicting the presence or absence of articular surface damage in the active senior. With this in mind, it is important to provide and document careful preoperative counseling to inform the patient about the possibility of finding significant chondral damage at the time of arthroscopy.

Using arthroscopy as a tool to clean out and debride the knee is not a new idea. Magnuson (1941) stated that a thorough rework of all mechanical irritation products of joint degeneration will render the patient symptom free. Despite performing this as an open procedure with all the inherent morbidity, he proved it to be useful. With the development of advanced arthroscopic techniques we can perform the entire procedure arthroscopically. However, the greater ease—from the point of view of both the surgeon and the patient—should not be confused with better performance. Is turning a wet knee into a dry knee beneficial to the patient? What can the older athlete hope to expect?

Table 11.2 outlines the results of numerous arthroscopic debridement studies. As shown, each study group had 24% to 48% poor results, and many of these studies noted that the individuals in the poor outcome group often observed an acceleration in the severity of their symptoms after this procedure.

Despite objections such as those just mentioned, arthroscopic debridement can be useful as a means for treatment of the older athlete with localized unicompartmental symptoms and mild to moderate OA. It is less invasive than other options (i.e., HTO and unicompartmental arthroplasty), but it is necessary to explain clearly that the results are unpredictable and may actually worsen the patient's condition and that a positive outcome may deteriorate with time. With this disclosure, arthroscopic lavage and debridement remains an excellent surgical option for the appropriate patient.

Arthroscopic Chondroplasty

Management of diffuse chondral injury in the active older patient presents a challenge to the physician. Chondroplasty is differentiated from debridement in that the former attempts to induce a reparative response to damaged cartilage. One must be careful when extracting data from treatment of isolated well-contained focal full-thickness lesions in the younger population (less than 45 years). Applying the results of these procedures to the older athlete is like comparing apples to oranges and often leads to the injudicious use of chondroplasty in the older active population.

Bone marrow stimulation promotes the formation of fibrocartilage (figure 11.8) (Salter et al. 1980). The mechanical qualities of fibrocartilage have demonstrated wear resistance inferior to that of hyaline cartilage (Mankin 1982). Therefore, one must ask whether the palliative effect of this procedure is predictable enough to justify considering it an option in treating

TABLE 11.2 Arthroscopic Debridement Studies

			RESULTS	
Author	Year	Follow-up (mo)	Good (%)	Poor (%)
Sprague	1981	14	74	26
Shahriaree	1982	26	76	24
Jackson et al.	1986	39	68	32
Bert and Maschka	1989	60	66	34
Baumgaertner et al.	1990	33	52	48
Gross et al.	1991	24	72	28
Ogilvie-Harris and Fitsialos	1991	49	68	32
Rand	1991	60	67	33
Average		38	68	32

Adapted, with permission, from R.A. Gambardella, 1994, Arthroscopic treatment of degenerative joint disease, 1113-1121. In F.H. Fu, C.D. Harner, and K.G. Vince, eds., *Knee surgery*, vol. II. (Baltimore, MD: Williams & Wilkins).

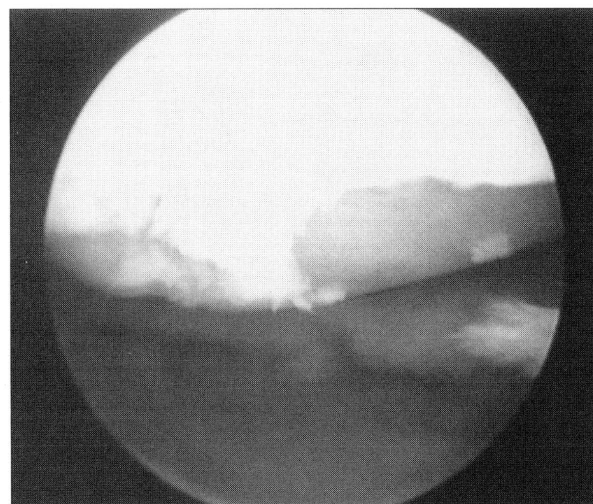

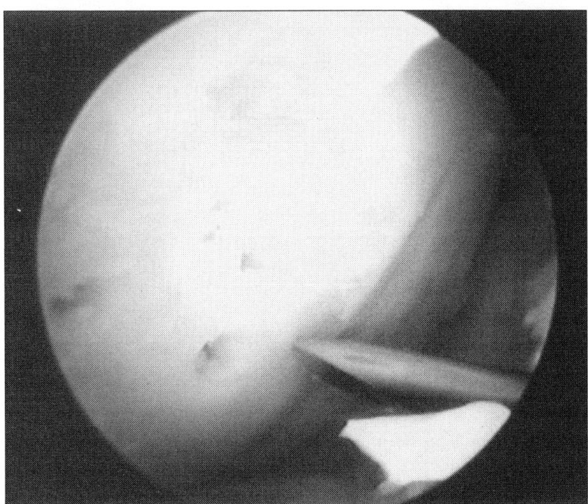

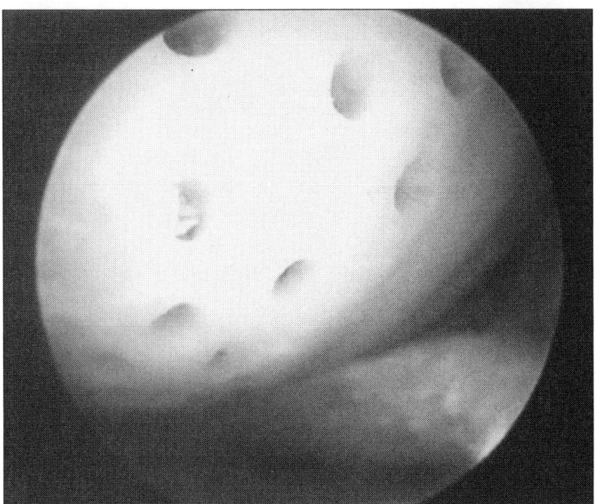

FIGURE 11.8 A 76-year-old male with known advanced medial compartment arthritis with sudden onset of pain, swelling, and mechanical symptoms. Although a degenerative medial meniscal tear was present and formal drilling chondroplasty performed, the patient had acceleration of symptoms requiring a total knee arthroplasty within six months.

the older active patient. Johnson (1986) subjectively evaluated the efficacy of arthroscopic abrasion chondroplasty in a study with a two-year minimal follow-up focused on strict adherence to surgical technique and restricted weight bearing for a minimum of six months; 78% of the patients reported an improvement in their condition, but 16% reported a deterioration in their condition subsequent to the procedure. The literature as a whole seems to indicate that the modest success of chondroplasty in this group is offset by the alarming number of patients whose symptoms accelerated afterward (Rand 1991).

The results of abrasion chondroplasty remain unpredictable at best. There once was widespread enthusiasm for this procedure in the aging athlete. Those investigators who obtained the best results also used the most restrictive weight-bearing regimen (up to six months). The cumbersome weight-restrictive program coupled with uncertain results makes arthroscopic abrasion chondroplasty difficult to support as a treatment for the active senior. Furthermore, in the context of increasing cost consciousness, the socioeconomic consequences of prolonged enforced continuous passive motion and non-weight-bearing activities are difficult to present to both patients and their insurance companies. When faced with an unanticipated grade IV lesion at the time of arthroscopy, it is acceptable to debride the chondral margins to a stable articular rim; however, this treatment is not highly efficient when used solely to stimulate the marrow.

Ligamentous Instability and Reconstruction

Ligamentous instability in an aging athlete produces as much dysfunction as in a younger athlete. Chronological age is not a contraindication to ligamentous reconstruction, but physiological age is a strong factor. The patient's current level of physical fitness and activity is an important consideration when one is addressing the treatment of functional instability. Many active 50- to 60-year-olds are ideal candidates for ligament reconstruction, but many more are probably not. Making this assessment requires skill on the part of the physician, who must also discuss realistic expectations about the procedure's outcome with the patient.

Anterior Instability With Normal Alignment and Radiographs

Anterior instability with normal alignment and normal radiographs is not a complex condition. The physician must determine whether or not the patient will accept activity modification in order to lower the risk of giving-way episodes. Derotational braces can be quite helpful if the person has a sense of instability at low levels of activity. If the patient is unwilling to alter his or her level of activity and has repeated episodes of instability, reconstruction becomes an option. The reconstruction is no different than in the younger active patient: Although some surgeons feel that allograft ACL reconstruction is a better choice in the older athlete because it decreases the comorbidity associated with graft harvest, ultimately the graft source should be at the surgeon's discretion. Principles of rehabilitation should not change, but the program's intensity must reflect the patient's overall level of strength and condition. It must be stressed that the decision to proceed with ACL reconstruction in this group needs to individualized.

Anterior Instability, Normal Alignment, and Unicompartmental Arthritis

The second scenario, that of the patient with anterior instability, normal alignment, and unicompartmental arthritis, is not as straightforward as the first. These patients are often active and complain of pain and secondary instability. They are physiologically young and will often not consider procedures that require significant activity restrictions. Activities in which these patients participate prevent them from being good candidates for unicompartmental arthroplasty.

Shelbourne and Stube (1997) discussed their experience with this clinical situation in a slightly younger age group. They concluded that an isolated ACL reconstruction can provide long-term stability and symptomatic pain relief in patients with instability and arthrosis. The procedure has low morbidity and was not found to compromise future success of tibial osteotomy or total knee replacement. It is important to be careful in applying these results to the older active patient. The study does illustrate an important point, however: Addressing the long-standing ligamentous instability can effectively and predictably increase the functional capacity of the active senior, in addition to providing lasting subjective improvement.

Ligamentous Instability, Unicompartmental Arthritis, and Malalignment

The final scenario is even more complex: that of the older athlete with ligamentous instability, unicompartmental arthritis, and malalignment. Trial use of an unloader brace can be helpful in that it can effectively eliminate pain associated with activities. If the athlete exhibits signs of instability when using the brace, further intervention may be required. These are difficult cases and require good judgment. An isolated ACL reconstruction with malalignment may not address all the components of tibiofemoral laxity, as Noyes, Barber, and Simon (1993) demonstrated increased incidence of posterolateral laxity and increased recurvatum (figures 11.9 and 11.10).

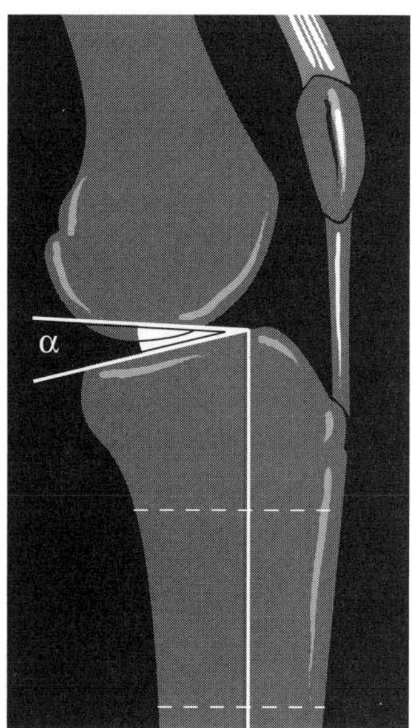

FIGURE 11.9 Measurement of tibial slope.

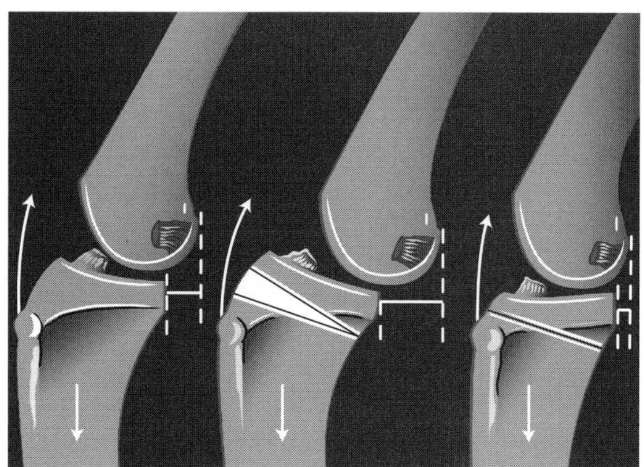

FIGURE 11.10 Relationship between tibial slope and anterior translation associated with anterior cruciate ligament (ACL) tear. Increasing the tibial slope increases the effect of ACL tear; decreasing the tibial slope decreases the effect of ACL tear.

In younger patients (including those in their 40s and 50s), several studies have produced good results in support of the use of a combination of HTO and ACL reconstruction (Dejour et al. 1994). There is no literature supporting this in the older active patient, yet no upper age limit has been established for the combined procedure. The patient must clearly understand that this is an extensive surgery and is considered a salvage procedure. As the physician considers the patient's physiologic age, activity level, and pattern of ligamentous instability, it remains a possibility.

Treating ligamentous instability in the older athlete is challenging. The decision to proceed with reconstruction, which must not come before a thorough course of more conservative treatment, should not be based on age alone. Rather it must be based on a synthesis of many factors—physiological age, activity level, quadriceps strength, range of motion, and impairment caused by the instability. The physician must account for all patholaxity—the extent of radiographic arthritis and the degree of malalignment—before the correct operative intervention is decided upon. Additionally, to attain a comprehensive understanding, the physician must recognize the procedure's effect on TKA, and the patient must be aware that TKA may be the definitive procedure. It is perhaps these complex knee instability and arthrosis cases that push the outer limits of sports medicine.

Osteotomy

The ideal candidate for consideration of an osteotomy is a physiologically young, more active, heavier person whose desired level of activity or work requirements would be perceived as too high for prosthetic replacements. Interestingly, the activity level that is considered too high has become debatable as more and more total joint surgeons are allowing higher levels of activity. Although the most favorable activity levels are not carved in stone, more concrete evidence supporting osteotomy for this population comes from biomechanical studies demonstrating that certain activities, especially running and jumping, create surface loads that exceed the limits of polyethylene. Nagel, Insall, and Scuderi (1996) showed that post-osteotomy levels of activity can include physical activity such as tennis, skiing, and running. They concluded that osteotomy is appropriate for patients under 60 years with varus deformity who have high levels of physical activity preoperatively and wish to participate in the same activities postoperatively. They also stressed that "the best" level of post-op activity to be expected was no better than that obtained preoperatively, and that in general, the average postoperative level of activity decreased.

Patients who are potential candidates for a realignment osteotomy must be carefully counseled before committing to the procedure. It is important for patients to understand that osteotomy is not intended to make the knee joint normal, that there are certain risks accompanying the surgery, and that the success of the procedure tends to decrease over time. With these considerations in mind, the proximal realignment osteotomy remains a viable option for the older athlete.

Risks of surgery include peroneal nerve injury, intra-articular fracture, loss of function, compartment syndrome, stiffness, and infection. Newer, more rigid forms of fixation have allowed more aggressive rehabilitation regimens that include immediate weight bearing and ROM.

Medial Compartment Osteoarthritis

Realignment osteotomy (or HTO) has long been a palliative intervention used in the treatment of unicompartmental OA. The objective is to transfer the weight-bearing line away from the arthritic medial compartment to the healthy compartment (figure 11.11). Requisite for use of the procedure are a lower extremity angular deformity and a healthy contralateral compartment. The debate regarding the extent of patellofemoral disease that can be present without interfering with expected positive results has been resolved; it appears that mild to moderate patellofemoral disease does not adversely affect the outcome. Literature also exists to support use of this procedure

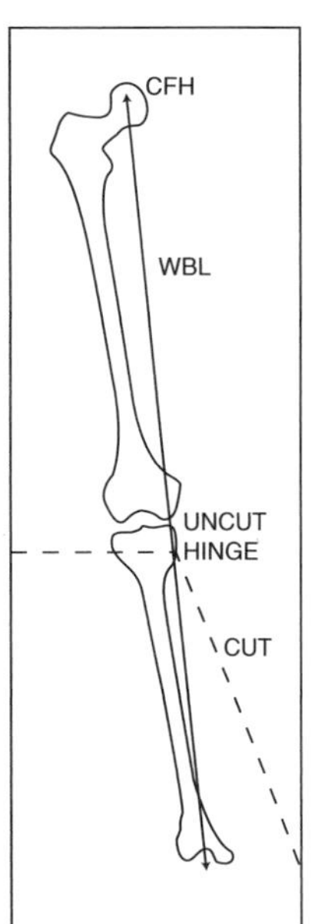

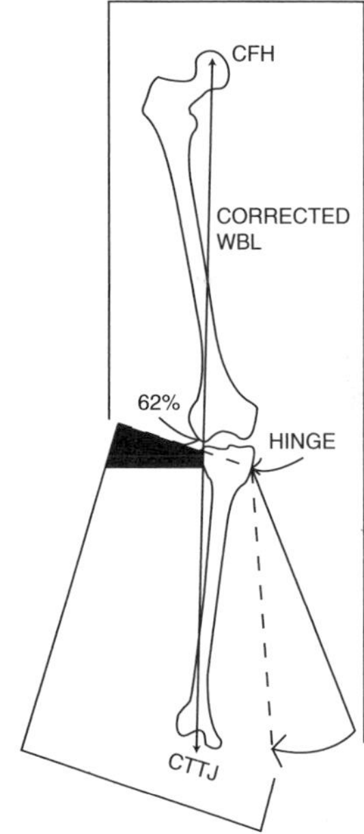

FIGURE 11.11 Noyes has demonstrated a reliable method or preoperative planning for an osteotomy. A line from the center of the femoral head (CFH) is fashioned to intersect the 62% coordinate (with medial = 0; lateral = 100%). The size of the osteotomy is determined by making the bony cut that will allow the tibia to rotate to the 62% coordinate. CITJ = center of the tibiotalar joint; WBL = weight-bearing line.

in treating chronic instabilities of the anterior and posterior cruciate ligaments.

Many surgeons may be reluctant to perform this procedure based on a perceived suboptimal outcome of HTO and the extended survivorship of TKA. One must look at the literature with a discerning eye. Some early studies used imprecise pre-op planning, less rigid fixation, and prolonged post-op immobilization, and no consensus exists as to the degree of connection required to obtain an optimal result.

Lateral Compartment Osteoarthritis

Although lateral compartment OA occurs with a lesser frequency, it will be encountered in the older athlete. It is most likely to be seen in posttraumatic patients after a lateral tibial plateau fracture and remotely after an open lateral meniscectomy. As with the HTO for medial compartment OA, success rates have been variable. Unlike what happens with medial compartment HTO, though, if clinical improvement is achieved it is likely to be maintained (Hanssen et al. 2000).

One remaining issue of realignment osteotomy is the ease of conversion to a TKA. Katz et al. (1987) quantified the difference between primary TKA and revision of HTO to a TKA. The 21 members of each group had an average age of 62 years. In the revision osteotomy group, the average length of time between osteotomy and TKA was 48 months, with a range of 7 months to 12 years. The results of this study are important, considering that most HTOs are eventually converted to a TKA, and reinforce the notion that prior surgical intervention complicates the TKA. Of the 21 individuals in the revision osteotomy group, 48% reported excellent results, 33% reported good results, and 19% reported results as only fair. Excellent results occurred in 86% and good results in 14% of the primary TKAs. The average arc of motion was 103° for the primary TKA group and 95° for the revision osteotomy group. The authors also noted some technical challenges that complicate the revision of HTOs to TKAs, including an average increased operating time of 30 min in the revision osteotomy group; the group's observed shortened distance from tubercle to joint; and—posing the least threat to the surgeon—the retained staples, which can actually be left in place.

Unicompartmental Knee Arthroplasty

The indications for unicompartmental knee arthroplasty (UKA) have expanded tremendously over the past several years. Once reserved for older, sedentary patients with unicompartmental disease, UKA now has a much broader patient base of individuals with noninflammatory arthritis, mild varus or valgus deformity, and predominantly unicompartmental involvement, without ligamentous instability or morbid obesity. This development is due in part to new designs with minimum bone resection and the ease of conversion to a TKA, and possibly to a changing perception within the community most affected by the results, including physicians and patients.

As the TKA has evolved into a reproducibly successful procedure, the indications for its use may have changed. Although this change is not quantifiable, it certainly exists: In the 1970s and 1980s, pain and serious impairment were the most significant motivation for proceeding with TKA, whereas decreasing function is now an acceptable rationale. This, combined with an increased life expectancy for older patients and their desire to be significantly more active than previous generations, creates a unique opportunity to consider UKA with its advantages over the TKA. Multiple factors make UKA more appealing. It is not highly invasive and requires minimal bone resection, does not require autologous blood donation, involves only a 23-h observation, and requires no inpatient rehabilitation. In fact, the PT requirements are quite modest.

Clinical Rationale for Unicompartmental Knee Arthroplasty

Clinical rationale for proceeding with UKA is founded mostly upon the understanding that OA of the knee is a segmental disease and becomes bi- or tricompartmental only very late in the process. Additionally, the active senior seeks medical attention earlier in the disease process because the knee pain interferes with remaining active—as opposed to the more sedentary patient who eventually seeks treatment after a prolonged inability to put on shoes and socks or rise from a chair without extreme difficulty. Reformation of UKA to require only minimal bone resection has facilitated TKA to the extent that conversion of a UKA to a TKA is reported to be no more difficult than a primary TKA. This is quite a contrast to the days when revision could be a difficult procedure requiring bone grafting and long stems. Recent studies have also demonstrated excellent clinical outcome and prosthesis survivorship.

As the life expectancy of the older athlete increases and it remains clinically advantageous to have only one TKA, is the UKA therefore classified as an intermediate procedure? Repicci (2001) has defined the role of UKA by identifying two possible ways to increase the life of a prosthetic system. One is to eliminate the chance of failure by using biomaterials that will never fail—essentially, make the prosthesis perfect. There is no question that part of the success of present-day arthroplasty is due to the introduction of cobalt-chrome and titanium alloys, improved joint-bearing surface designs, and better understanding of polyethylene. However, the mechanical properties of the new-generation prostheses still have known limits that cannot be ignored when considering post-prosthetic activity. The second way to increase the life of a prosthetic system is to serially replace it. For the physician to embrace this concept of serial replacement, certain conditions must be met:

- A reasonable success rate
- Low morbidity
- Low cost
- High forgivability
- Non-interference with any subsequent planned procedure

Repicci (2001) considers the use of UKA an application of serial replacement, noting that this procedure has reproducible results in decreasing pain and increasing function with a 90% success rate at 10 years. The prosthetic design lends itself to easy removal, which allows UKA to be converted to TKA without affecting the bone cuts. "The combined functional life of the UKA in conjunction with the future TKA can increase the functional capacity of the entire system by 20 to 30 years." The active senior is an ideal candidate for UKA as defined earlier: A procedure that is minimally invasive, has low morbidity, and a predictable length of prosthetic survivorship is ideally suited for a busy and active lifestyle. But can we extrapolate the results from the existing literature to our population, which is decidedly more active than the general population?

Unicompartmental Knee Arthroplasty in the Older Athlete

The exact role of UKA in the older athlete is currently being defined. Examining the appropriateness of this procedure requires comparison to its alternatives. There is clinical overlap between the UKA and HTO. Broughton, Newman, and Baily (1986) performed a retrospective review comparing patients who had an HTO or UKA, with an average follow-up between 5 and 10 years. The average age was 71 years for the UKA group and 63 years for the HTO group. The operation's success was measured by the Bailey knee assessment scale. Seventy-six percent of the UKAs were rated as having had good results, as were 43% of HTOs. The end of the study presented a significant difference ($p = .001$) in levels of pain: In the UKA group, 62% of the individuals rated themselves as pain free, as compared with 19% of the HTO group. The UKA group also scored better in areas of function and movement, but these findings were not quantitated or detailed in the article. During the follow-up period, revision was required in 3 of the 32 UKAs (9.4%); among the 21 HTOs, 10 (47.6%) required revision. No radiographic signs of late deterioration were seen in the UKA group at completion of the study. It should be noted that in this particular study, the HTOs were placed in a cast postoperatively for six weeks, which is now rarely done. Despite all the inherent faults of a retrospective study, the preceding data strongly suggest consideration of a UKA when HTO is an option.

Considerable clinical overlap exists between UKA and TKA. Arriving at the appropriate treatment decision requires that the physician take all variables into account. The UKA is far less invasive than is the TKA, affording an easier initial postoperative course. Some surgeons have reported performing the UKA as an outpatient procedure, but the majority prefer a 23-h observation. Review of several physicians' postoperative protocols indicates only moderate narcotic use after a UKA (figure 11.12).

No studies compare narcotic use after these two procedures, but personal experience supports the idea that patients who undergo a UKA experience significantly less pain than those undergoing TKAs. Intraoperatively there is less blood loss; there is no need for inpatient rehabilitation; and most people report driving a car independently at two weeks (Repicci 2001). Additionally, the incidence of infection, arthrofibrosis, and deep vein thrombosis is lower in UKA than in TKA. The UKA, by preserving the ACL, posterior cruciate ligament, and patellofemoral joint, offers more proprioceptive feedback; and postoperatively, the knee feels more like a normal knee (Parker, Dimeff, and Kolczun 2001). This may be an important factor as physicians and therapists assign a more important role to proprioceptive function in ensuring the athlete's safe return to sport. The orthopedic community awaits a study documenting the change in proprioception preoperatively to postoperatively and defining the significance of these changes. The UKA would be a much more attractive procedure if it were proven that these findings had clinical significance. Finally, newer prosthetic designs with onlay technique make a UKA revision to a TKA much easier than a revision TKA.

Cost of the procedures, although not of clinical significance, must also be taken into account. Repicci (2001) performed cost analysis showing UKA patient expenses, including hospital, surgeon, and all ancillary services, for 100 cases, also including the cost of converting the anticipated 10 failures at 10 years to TKA. The analysis showed that the cost of UKA is approximately one-half that of a primary total knee replacement. Unfortunately, one cannot ignore these cost comparisons when considering the aggregate cost of treating OA in the health care system. Data have

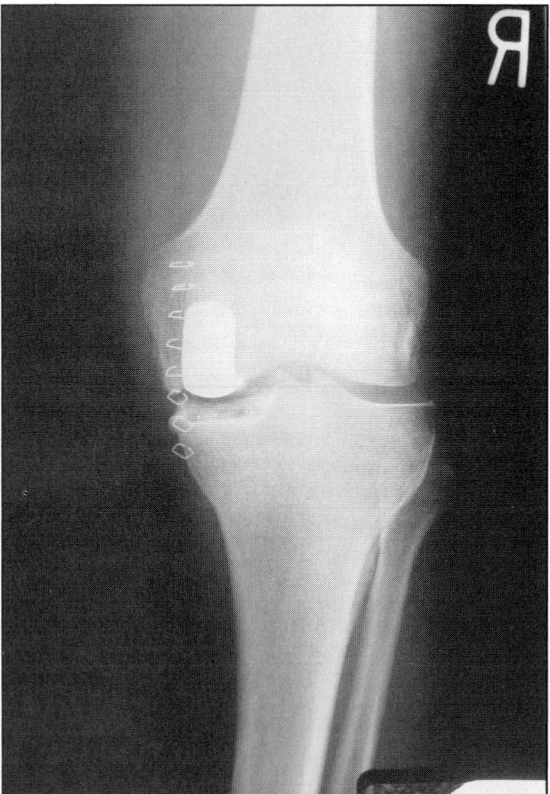

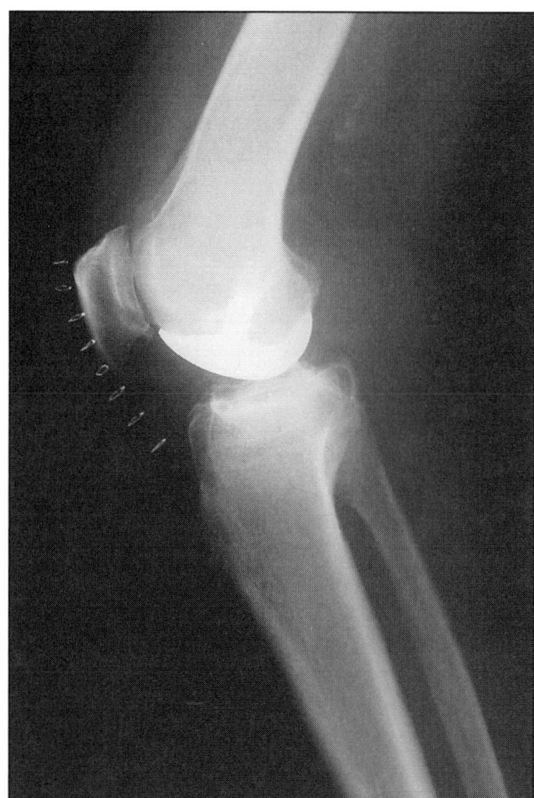

FIGURE 11.12 A 65-year-old female with isolated medial compartment osteoarthritis who enjoyed gardening. Patient underwent a unicompartmental arthroplasty and returned to clinic at one week postoperatively with 97° of flexion and minimal use of a walker. She felt that formal physical therapy was unnecessary.

shown TKA to be cost-effective and associated with significant improvements in quality of life. If such data become available for the UKA, this could represent billions of dollars of savings for the health care industry and society.

In conclusion, evidence-based data imply a significant role for the UKA in managing degeneration in the older active patient. As with the TKA, patients are not permitted to return to running or other high-impact activities. There is an upper weight limit that restricts prediction of a good outcome to certain individuals. For the younger, heavier individual who engages in heavy labor or physical activity, the HTO probably has an advantage. The older athlete with unicompartmental disease who is involved in moderate activities such as walking, golfing, or cycling is a more appropriate candidate for UKA. The perioperative course is much easier than for a TKA with an earlier return to ambulatory and recreational activities. Careful patient education must include continued activity modifications and an expected survivorship of 80% at 10 years (Engh and McAuley 1999). One must also clearly explain to the patient that the procedure may be only an extended temporary solution that is most often followed by a TKA.

Total Knee Arthroplasty

Total knee arthroplasty is the definitive treatment for tricompartmental arthritis. The procedure has stood the test of time and remains durable with predictable and reproducible outcomes. Intermediate procedures or treatments for the active senior should consider the effect on the eventual outcome of TKA, as these procedures may eventually be converted to a TKA. Additionally, great care is necessary when one is choosing to proceed with TKA in the over-50 active population, especially the younger subset of this group, as revision TKA can be associated with larger bone resections and poorer long-term outcomes.

Postoperative Physical Activity

Healy, Iorio, and Lemos (2001) noted that patients with high-level skills prior to surgery are felt to have the best chance of safely resuming those activities after surgery, and did not recommend initiating participation in sports that the patients were not involved in prior to arthroplasty. Increased physical activity is associated with increased joint-bearing surface wear (Schmalzried, Shepherd, and Dorey 2000). Particle formation as a reflection of bone cement and polyethylene wear has been associated with periarticular osteolysis. Patients who are more active are more likely to develop particulate-induced osteolysis as a direct result of their increased physical activity. Increased athletic participation increases the exposure to risk of periprosthetic fracture. Fortunately, this is rare (<1%), but its consequences are devastating (Ayers et al. 1997). Healy and colleagues (2001) compiled the responses of 48 members of the Knee Society regarding recommendations about levels of physical activity after TKA (table 11.3). Certain activities contribute to the active senior's rehabilitation following TKA, including low-impact activities such as walking, swimming, bowling, golf, and stationary bicycling. Those with experience in moderate-intensity exercises like road bicycling, tennis, hiking, and canoeing are encouraged to continue participating in those activities within the confines of their own limitations. High-impact activities such as jogging, soccer, volleyball, basketball, and football are to be avoided following TKA.

The results of TKA are impressive—it can enhance the functional status and improve the quality of life of individuals who require it (figure 11.13). Because the material properties of the components in a TKA are finite, one must be careful not to assign this pro-

TABLE 11.3 Activity After Total Knee Arthroplasty[†]

Recommended/ allowed	Allowed with experience	Not recommended	No conclusion
Low-impact aerobics	Road bicycling	Raquetball	Fencing
Stationary bicycling	Canoeing	Squash	Inline skating
Bowling	Hiking	Rock climbing	Downhill skiing
Golf	Rowing	Soccer	Weightlifting
Dancing	Cross-country skiing	Singles tennis	
Horseback riding	Stationary skiing*	Volleyball	
Croquet	Speed walking	Football	
Walking	Tennis	Gymnastics	
Swimming	Weight machine	Lacrosse	
Shooting	Ice skating	Hockey	
Shuffleboard		Basketball	
Horseshoes		Jogging	
		Handball	

*NordicTrack.
[†]1999 Knee Society Survey.

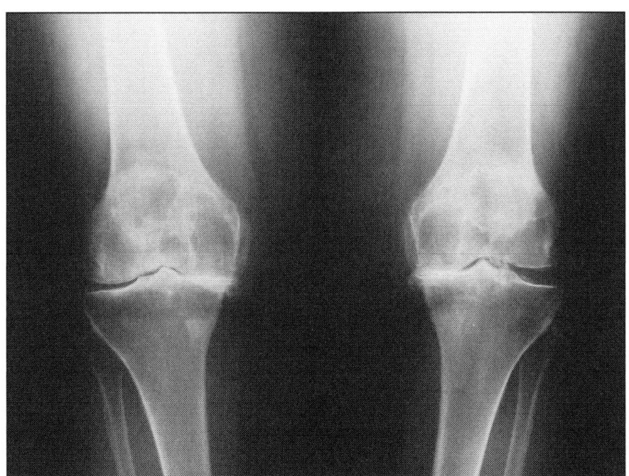

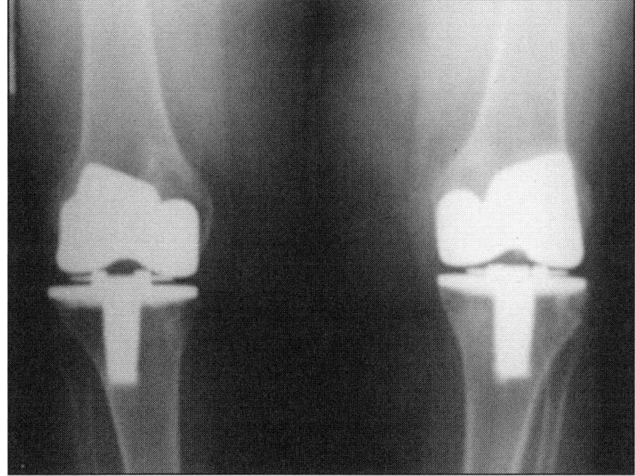

FIGURE 11.13 A 71-year-old retired teacher with increasing pain during a walking program. Based on level of activity and existing pain, bilateral total knee arthroplasty represented the best clinical choice.

cedure too quickly to active patients in their 50s or 60s. All reasonable intermediate procedures should be examined and discussed with the patient. In those circumstances in which TKA is the only reasonable option, the possibility of eventual revision needs to be outlined in detail. Long-term studies for this specific population will ultimately define the success of the TKA in the active older patient.

SUMMARY

Diagnosing and treating OA in the older active patient has evolved into a manageable and promising undertaking. Seen with increasing frequency, each of these patients presents a unique challenge that allows the well-informed health care provider to adapt a known set of therapies to a familiar, but not necessarily predictable, condition in order to achieve the most desirable results. Modern advances in medical and surgical care, including PT, orthopedic devices, pharmaceuticals, and operative procedures and materials, offer health care professionals the opportunity to give their patients a renewed sense of youthfulness. Given proper compliance with a treatment algorithm, patients can be assured that they will be able to maintain activity levels higher than those possible in the past and can hope for an equally promising quality of life.

CHAPTER

12

Foot and Ankle Problems

Ryan W. Simovitch, MD
Mark E. Easley, MD

Sport injuries to the foot and ankle are common. The older athletic patient often has more challenges than the younger patient in recovering from injuries. For example, the younger patient may have a severe sprain, but it is generally a sprain of a relatively healthy ankle. The older athlete may have a similar ankle sprain, or even a less severe one, superimposed on an ankle that has been exposed to previous trauma. Typically, this makes the injury more complex and may delay recovery. This chapter focuses on common sport-related problems of the foot and ankle with attention to the aging athlete.

We cover injuries to the ankle, hindfoot, midfoot, and forefoot, reviewing the disease process, pathoanatomy, diagnosis, and treatment for each injury. Discussion of ankle injuries includes details of acute ankle sprains and associated neuralgias, syndesmotic injuries, anterolateral ankle impingement, subtalar instability, peroneal tendinopathy, peroneal tendinitis and tears, peroneal tendon instability, osteochondral lesions of the talus, os trigonum, symptomatic medial posterior talar process, posterior ankle impingement, flexor hallucis longus (FHL) tendinitis, and Achilles tendon pathology. In addition we focus on lateral talar process, anterior calcaneal process, and base of the fifth metatarsal fractures. Our discussion of hindfoot pathology emphasizes posterior tibial tendon insufficiency, heel fat pad atrophy, plantar fasciitis, plantar nerve compression, and calcaneal stress fractures. Topics related to the midfoot include accessory navicular, and Lisfranc injury. The section on the forefoot is a potpourri of topics including hallux valgus, hallux rigidus, sesamoid disorders, hallux metatarsophalangeal (MTP) joint sprain, capsulitis, synovitis, MTP joint instability, interdigital neuroma, Freiberg's infraction, metatarsal stress fractures, and several toenail disorders.

Many of these disease processes or injuries are common to younger athletes, but our aim was to choose those common or particularly distressing to the active senior. The many references are meant for the sport enthusiast or physician desiring more in-depth information regarding both nonoperative and operative treatment.

ACUTE ANKLE SPRAINS

The prevalence of ankle sprains is estimated at 1/10,000 people per day; ankle sprains account for 25% to 50% of injuries from running sports (Anderson and Davis 2000). Typically, patients recover from ankle sprains without much permanent impairment; but in the older population, recovery is generally more prolonged. Whereas the younger patient may recover fully within weeks, recovery may take the older patient months. An acute ankle sprain superimposed on a previous ankle problem or a history of multiple ankle sprains, which is more likely in the older athletic patient, may make a full recovery more difficult. In addition, ankle sprains in the older athlete may be superimposed on an arthritic ankle joint, leading to prolonged recovery and rehabilitation challenges. Often termed weekend warriors, older recreational athletes sometimes lack the dynamic ankle stabilizers essential to prevent recurrent sprains and rehabilitate an acute sprain. Generally, proprioception as well as strength declines with age. Both of these variables are essential to preventing recurrent ankle sprains.

Anatomy and Pathophysiology

The lateral ankle ligament complex comprises the (1) anterior talofibular ligament (ATFL), (2) calcaneofibular ligament (CFL), and (3) posterior talofibular ligament (PTFL) (figure 12.1). The ATFL provides primary restraint to anterior translation of the talus within the ankle mortise and secondary restraint to inversion of the talus. The CFL resists inversion of the talus within the ankle mortise. The PTFL augments the lateral ankle support provided by the ATFL and CFL. While this ligament complex provides static support to the lateral ankle, the peroneal tendons offer dynamic stability. Medial stability is provided by the deltoid ligament (Clanton 1999; Schon 2000; Scioli 2000).

Ankle sprains are graded according to the degree of ligament disruption and resulting instability. Lateral ankle sprains are far more common than medial ankle sprains. They are graded according to compromise of the ATFL and CFL (table 12.1) (Clanton 1999; Schon 2000; Scioli 2000).

Ankle sprains compromise the static support to the lateral ankle. Although scar tissue typically forms to maintain continuity of these lateral ankle ligaments, they are attenuated. However, with intact peroneal tendons, dynamic stability is maintained and can usually compensate for the loss of static restraint (Clanton 1999; Schon 2000; Scioli 2000).

Evaluation

The clinical presentation of an acute ankle sprain in an older athlete closely resembles that in a younger patient but is worth reviewing. Patients usually do not complain of pain unless they invert the ankle. They report instability. The clinical exam includes the anterior drawer and inversion tests (figure 12.2). It should be noted that in the setting of degenerative joint disease, altered joint conformity may yield negative results for these tests. Radiographs are generally normal unless multiple sprains have developed a fixed varus deformity, which is more common in an adult

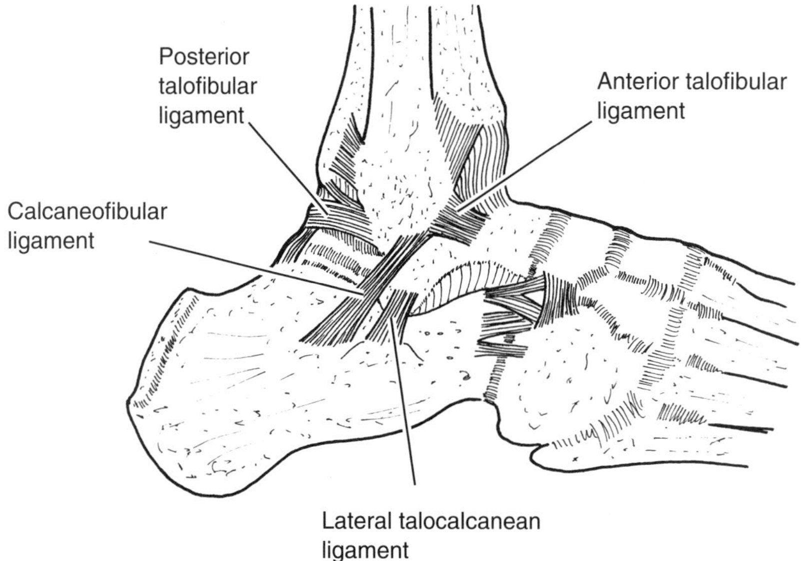

FIGURE 12.1 Lateral ankle ligament complex.

Reprinted, by permission, from J. Watkins, 1999, *The structure and function of the musculoskeletal system* (Champaign, IL: Human Kinetics), 210.

TABLE 12.1 Grading of Lateral Ankle Sprains

Grade	Injury	Exam
I	Partially torn anterior talofibular ligament (ATFL)	Normal drawer sign and talar tilt
II	Torn ATFL; intact calcaneo-fibular ligament (CFL)	Drawer sign 2+ (<5 mm) Mild talar tilt (<10)
III	Torn ATFL and CFL	Drawer sign 3+ (>10 mm) Talar tilt 3+ (>15)

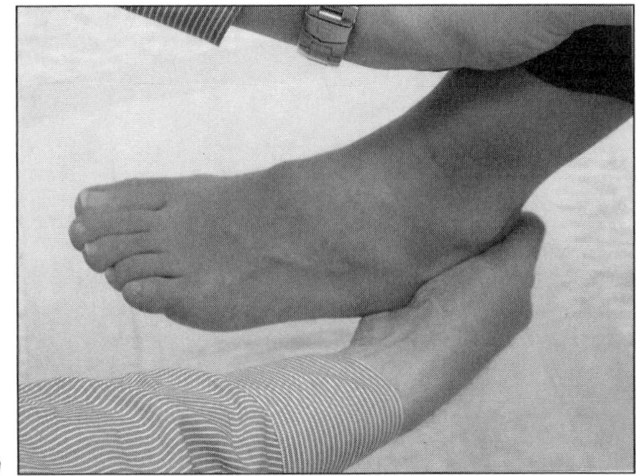

a

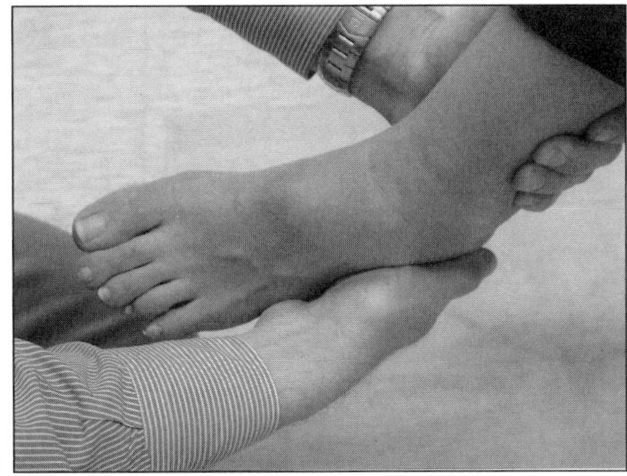

b

FIGURE 12.2 *(a)* Anterior drawer test demonstrates laxity in anterior talofibular ligament. *(b)* Inversion or talar tilt test demonstrates laxity of the calcaneo-fibular ligament.

athlete. However, stress images, with either fluoroscopy or plain X-ray, may demonstrate increased talar subluxation (anterior drawer test) or talar tilt (inversion test). Although absolute numbers have been suggested (15°), comparison to the contralateral (uninvolved) ankle may prove beneficial. Magnetic resonance imaging (MRI) may be useful in confirming the diagnosis; however, MRI is often too sensitive and will reveal ATFL signal change with a history of ankle sprain, even in the patient without chronic instability.

Treatment

Successful treatment of ankle sprains is almost exclusively nonoperative. The standard "RICE" protocol (Rest, Ice, Compression, Elevation) is followed by early mobilization in a lace-up brace and physical therapy. The goals of treatment are to (1) avoid reproducing the inversion ankle injury and (2) strengthen the peroneal tendons. The use of a brace is to protect the ankle from reinjury; it is not intended to substitute for poor peroneal tendon strength. Therefore, even when the acute injury has resolved, peroneal tendon strengthening should routinely continue, combined with generalized conditioning. Initially, the physical therapy can be supervised by a certified physical therapist, but eventually the exercises are performed independently by the athlete. Rehabilitation can be enhanced by physical therapy that includes proprioceptive exercises. Comorbidities such as diabetic neuropathy and other peripheral neuropathies are more common in adult recreational athletes, which compromises proprioception. The brace is worn during return to athletic activity, and then indefinitely during athletic competition to avoid reinjury.

It is essential to avoid prolonged immobilization in the adult recreational athlete. This can lead to muscle atrophy and stiffness, both of which are counterproductive. Whereas a cast or splint is often used to immobilize the ankle initially in a young athlete, a walking boot with a quick transition to taping or a stirrup brace is essential in the older athlete.

In a minority of ankle sprains, operative stabilization procedures may be required to allow for successful return to athletic competition. Rarely, if ever, are these procedures required in the immediate postinjury phase. Routinely, patients undergo the nonoperative protocol first, and only if this proves inadequate is surgical stabilization entertained. Referral to the orthopedic surgeon for surgical management of an acute sprain is rarely indicated in an adult recreational athlete but should be considered when complete ligamentous disruption occurs or an associated fracture or frank instability exists (Clanton 1999; Scioli 2000).

THE ANKLE SPRAIN THAT WON'T HEAL

In addition to persistent ankle instability despite proper nonoperative management, other factors need to be considered in ankle sprains that do not improve. Failure to respond to conventional methods of treating chronic ankle sprains may indicate misdiagnosis rather than improper treatment. This section concentrates on "the ankle sprain that won't heal" to bring an awareness to associated injuries that one may overlook when treating the patient with an ankle sprain.

In the older athlete, particularly one with previous ankle injuries, these associated injuries are probably more common than in younger patients with similar ankle injuries. Diagnoses other than ankle ligament instability include

- syndesmotic injuries ("high ankle sprain"),
- anterolateral ankle impingement,
- subtalar joint instability,
- peroneal tendon pathology,
- posterior ankle disorders,
- osteochondral lesions of the talus,
- fractures/nonunions, and
- neuralgias.

Syndesmotic Injury

The syndesmotic injury, or "high ankle sprain," can be a debilitating injury, particularly with a delay in diagnosis.

Mechanism of Injury

Although the mechanism of injury is described as that of a typical ankle sprain, it is actually slightly different. Whereas the typical ankle injury is one of inversion of the talus within the ankle mortise, a high ankle sprain usually occurs with supination and external rotation of the foot/talus relative to the tibia and fibula. The forces stress the deltoid ligament and the strong distal tibiofemoral ligaments (syndesmosis). The spectrum of this injury is wide: A mild sprain stretches the ligaments only slightly, whereas a severe sprain could completely disrupt the deltoid ligament and the majority of the distal tibiofemoral ligaments, exiting as a fracture through the proximal fibula. Often the injury is subtle; but a misdiagnosis and treatment by conventional methods for an ankle sprain is usually inadequate, because the injured area is not managed appropriately.

Evaluation

Evaluation of the syndesmotic injury may be nonspecific. The patient describes pain similar to that with any other patient who has an ankle sprain. Tenderness is medial (deltoid) and lateral (ATFL/CFL). However, this is where the similarities end. There is also tenderness over the anterolateral distal tibia and fibula, directly over the syndesmosis. Furthermore, a "squeeze test" (compression of the proximal tibia and fibula creates symptoms at the distal tibia/fibula syndesmosis) is often positive (figure 12.3). With severe syndesmotic injuries, the proximal fibula may also be tender (with an associated fibula fracture); this is termed a Maisonneuve fracture (Clanton 1999; Scioli 2000).

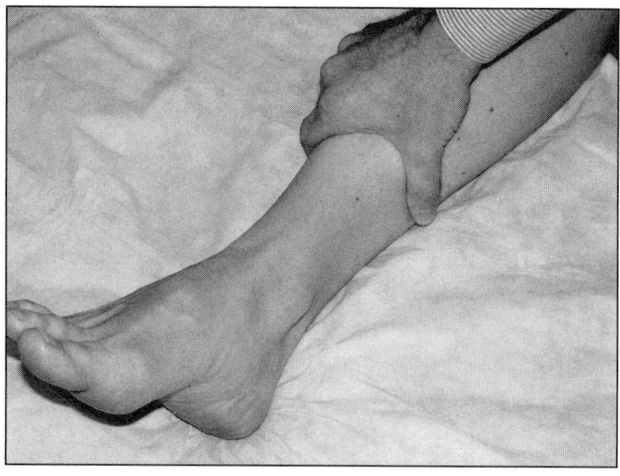

FIGURE 12.3 Squeeze test, diagnostic for syndesmotic injury.

Non-weight-bearing ankle radiographs do not typically demonstrate any abnormal findings; weight-bearing radiographs may demonstrate widening of the medial clear space (between the medial malleolus and the medial talar dome) and widening of the syndesmosis. Although radiographic findings defining normal anatomic ankle alignment have been delineated, usually it is easiest to compare the injured side to the uninjured contralateral ankle. Finally, with proximal fibular tenderness, an X-ray of the lower leg or knee may demonstrate a proximal fibular fracture. Stress views of the ankle can also be useful. In selected cases an MRI or computed tomography (CT) may be useful to delineate pathology prior to treatment.

Treatment

Required treatment is almost always longer than for a conventional ankle sprain. This is understandable considering that the strong deltoid and tibiofibular ligaments are disrupted. With more subtle sprains in which there is no demonstrable instability between the tibia and the fibula, initial non-weight bearing and immobilization followed by early transition to a stirrup brace or taping are recommended (figure 12.4). Recovery is usually twice as long as with an ankle sprain.

Treatment of a syndesmotic injury with instability as demonstrated by stress X-rays, but no frank diastasis, can be treated nonoperatively but should involve a non-weight-bearing short leg cast for at least four weeks followed by progressive weight bearing. This is in contrast to treatment of conventional ankle sprains, for which early weight bearing and mobilization are favored. With the conventional ankle sprain, the dynamic effect of the peroneal tendons can protect the healing ligaments and ankle joint; in the high

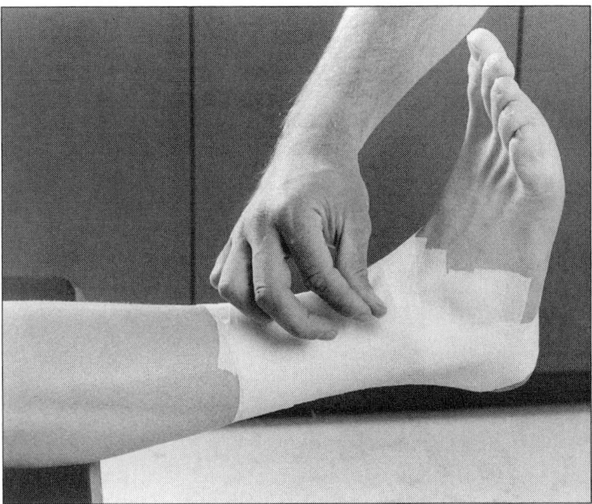

FIGURE 12.4 Taping for ankle sprains.

ankle sprain, there is no comparable dynamic stabilizer. Therefore physical therapy and proprioceptive exercises do not play a central role in the rehabilitation of a syndesmotic injury. The difficulty in this injury for active seniors is that immobilization tends to have far greater negative consequences on their mobility and risk for falling than in younger counterparts.

When instability between the tibia and fibula or medial malleolus and talus can be demonstrated, repeated stress radiographs of a nonoperatively treated syndesmotic injury are positive, or there is persistent clinical instability, a surgical stabilization procedure is required. These cases should be referred to the orthopedic surgeon for management.

Anterolateral Ankle Impingement ("Bassett's Ligament")

Patients may remain symptomatic despite regaining ankle stability following treatment for an ankle sprain. One relatively simple explanation is scarring (similar to a "plica" in the knee) that impinges on the anterolateral aspect of the talar dome. This can be more common in the adult recreational athlete who may have suffered multiple sprains over the years. The patient complains of lateral ankle pain, and tenderness is present on the anterolateral ankle. Radiographs are usually negative, but MRI may demonstrate fibrous bands or scar tissue on the anterolateral ankle.

Nonoperative management consists of reduction of inflammation with ice, nonsteroidal anti-inflammatory agents, and possibly a steroid injection, but does not eliminate the fibrous band. Therefore, orthopedic referral for arthroscopic debridement of this ankle impingement is frequently required and leads to excellent results, provided the diagnosis is limited to anterior ankle impingement (Ferkel 1999).

Subtalar Instability

Subtalar instability is frequently associated with lateral ankle ligament injury. Since the mechanism of injury and clinical presentation between ankle and subtalar lateral ligament injury are very similar, the latter usually comes to the attention of the orthopedist after failed conservative treatment of a typical ankle sprain.

Anatomy and Pathoanatomy

Inversion injuries to the lateral ankle may affect the subtalar joint. The subtalar joint lies between the talus and calcaneus. Whereas the tibiotalar, or ankle, joint is responsible for the majority of dorsiflexion and plantar flexion, the subtalar joint is primarily responsible for inversion and eversion of the hindfoot. Ligaments directly connecting the talus to the calcaneus, including the interosseous and cervical ligaments, provide subtalar stability; however, lateral stability is also conferred by the CFL, since it crosses both the ankle and subtalar joints. With a severe ankle sprain, the stability of the subtalar joint can be compromised in addition to the CFLs being disrupted, leading to increased stress across the ligaments of the subtalar joint.

Evaluation and Treatment

Evaluation of subtalar instability is not as well defined as for ankle instability. Increased inversion may be appreciated on clinical evaluation, but it is not until stress radiographs and dynamic fluoroscopy are performed with comparison to the contralateral subtalar joint that subtalar instability can be appreciated. With an inversion stress using stress radiographs or dynamic fluoroscopy, the ankle joint instability is only mild or is absent; however, the subtalar joint has considerable subluxation, particularly when compared to the contralateral extremity.

Treatment is similar to that of an ankle sprain. Some degree of subtalar instability is associated with any severe ankle sprain that involves the CFL. Early weight bearing with bracing and peroneal strengthening are typically adequate. However, subtalar instability is usually not appreciated until conventional treatment of a suspected ankle sprain fails. Orthopedic referral for surgical intervention is usually indicated at this point (Clanton 1999; Schon 2000; Scioli 2000).

Peroneal Tendinopathy

The peroneal tendons are important to the dynamic stability of the ankle as well as proper function of the foot and ankle during walking and running. Inflammation of the tendons or the peroneal tendon sheath can occur with repetitive stress and result in a painful mechanically weak tendon at or distal to the musculotendinous junction. Tendon tearing or complete rupture can occur as the final pathway. Presumably, the older athlete accumulates more tears and progressive tendinopathy through years of repetitive microtrauma and is at increased risk for peroneal tendon pathology.

Anatomy and Pathoanatomy

The peroneal tendons are plantar flexors and everters of the foot and ankle. The peroneus brevis lies on the posterior aspect of the fibula, the peroneus longus just posterior to it. The peroneus brevis attaches to the dorsal aspect of the fifth metatarsal base, while the peroneus longus courses around the cuboid, under the midfoot, to insert on the plantar base of the first metatarsal. While both peroneal tendons evert the foot and ankle, the peroneus longus also plantar flexes the first metatarsal. A varus heel alignment may predispose to peroneal pathology.

Evaluation

Patients complain of lateral lower leg, ankle, and foot discomfort or a combination of these. With increased strain and tendinopathy of the peroneal tendons, the lateral compartment muscles often ache; and with peroneal tendon tears, the lateral ankle and foot hurts directly over the tendons. Evaluation of the peroneal tendons should first include inspection of the hindfoot with the patient weight bearing to determine any varus malalignment. Peroneal strength testing and palpation should be performed with the foot plantar flexed and everted, to isolate peroneal tendon function. Comparison to the contralateral side may be diagnostic.

Imaging studies include radiographs that typically do not demonstrate any abnormality but may reveal a varus heel alignment. An MRI scan is most useful in analyzing the peroneal tendons, with the transverse and sagittal images showing most of the pathology (Armagan and Shereff 2000; Coughlin 1999b; Scioli 2000).

Peroneal Tendinitis and Tear Pathophysiology

Peroneal tendon problems typically arise from ligamentous ankle instability. With an initial ankle inversion injury, with subsequent sprains or ongoing inversion instability, the peroneal tendons may be injured. In functional instability, in which sprains may not occur with any frequency but in which the ankle tends to invert with each step because of loss of static restraint from the lateral ligaments, the peroneal tendons are constantly strained. This may lead to peroneal tendinitis (inflammation about the peroneal tendons within their sheaths). Acute injury to the peroneal tendons and persistent peroneal tendinitis may lead to chronic peroneal tendon tears. These tears are typically partial tears initially, but with constant strain may rarely become full tears. In patients with compromised lateral static restraints (lateral ankle ligaments) this is particularly problematic, because it is no longer possible to rely on dynamic lateral ankle stability conferred by the peroneal tendons. In the aging athlete, the combination of chronic lateral ankle instability and loss of functional peroneal tendons results in ankle arthritis.

Treating Peroneal Tendinitis

Treatment of peroneal tendinitis is no different than for any other tendinitis. RICE should be instituted. The tendons should be rested and inflammation should be controlled. Then supervised physical therapy is employed to progressively strengthen the tendon. To protect the tendons, a lateral heel wedge unloads the tendons; initially this can be added to a cam walker and then within a shoe with an ankle brace, eventually graduating to a heel wedge alone. Chronic tendinitis may be especially resistant to conservative treatment and can be referred to the orthopedist for surgical intervention.

Peroneal tendinitis will persist or recur, however, if the underlying problem is not addressed. Typically, this is lateral ankle instability. The peroneals are simply being overworked to correct the tendency for the heel and ankle to invert. Therefore, treatment may need to include repair/reconstruction of the lateral ankle ligaments or possibly even a lateral closing wedge osteotomy of the calcaneus if the tendency for heel varus is driven by hindfoot malalignment. If the problem is driven by a high arch and a relatively plantar flexed first ray, then a dorsiflexion osteotomy of the first metatarsal may be required. To distinguish between true hindfoot varus and hindfoot varus driven by the forefoot, one should perform a Coleman block test (Clanton 1999; Coughlin 1999b; Schon 2000).

Treating Peroneal Tendon Tears

Peroneal tendon tears typically do not heal adequately with nonoperative management. Although symptoms may diminish after the acute injury, persistent pain and the development of varus heel alignment is anticipated. Partial tears are usually longitudinal and may ultimately progress to complete tears. Surgical management varies between partial excision of degenerative tendon and more complicated reconstructions depending on the degree of tendon tearing.

Painful Os Peroneum Syndrome

A variant of a tendinitis/tear of the peroneus longus is the painful os peroneum syndrome ("POPS").

Many patients have an ossicle, similar to a patella, in the peroneus longus (PL) where it turns around the cuboid. This ossicle "articulates" with the cuboid. Occasionally, this ossicle can be injured. Tenderness is directly over the PL where it courses around the cuboid. Radiographically, the ossicle may be fragmented or separated (figure 12.5), and MRI may demonstrate signal change at this ossicle. Treatment is initially nonoperative as described for other peroneal injuries. Should nonoperative measures fail, surgery involves repair/reconstruction of the PL in this area of tendon/ossicle disruption (Armagan and Shereff 2000; Clanton 1999; Coughlin 1999b).

Peroneal Tendon Instability

Following ankle sprains, the peroneal tendons may become unstable and subluxate behind the fibula. A classification scheme has been proposed for the various types of peroneal instability. A considerable number of people have asymptomatic peroneal tendon subluxation/dislocation without prior injury.

Anatomy and Pathoanatomy

The primary restraint of the peroneal tendons is the superior peroneal retinaculum (SPR). The mechanism for peroneal tendon subluxation and disruption of the SPR is not typically with inversion, unless the peroneal tendons are eccentrically contracted simultaneously to resist the inversion; usually, a dorsiflexion/eversion stress of the peroneal tendons creates the disruption of the SPR and peroneal tendon subluxation or even dislocation.

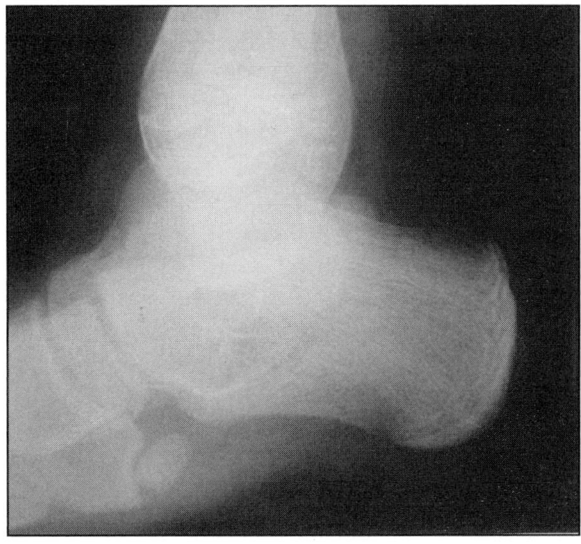

FIGURE 12.5 A lateral ankle X-ray demonstrates ossicle adjacent to the cuboid.

Evaluation

In the older athlete with a history of multiple inversion sprains or an eccentric contraction of the peroneal tendon, the peroneal tendons may sustain cumulative trauma developing into a symptomatic chronic subluxation/dislocation. The patient usually complains of pain posterior to the fibula. Tenderness is present directly over the peroneal tendons and the posterior fibula. Active dorsiflexion and eversion against resistance may demonstrate subluxation or even dislocation of the peroneal tendons around the posterior fibula. Imaging studies are important. The anteroposterior and mortise X-rays of the ankle may demonstrate a fibular "fleck" sign, indicating a bony avulsion of the posterior fibula suggestive of peroneal tendon dislocation. Magnetic resonance imaging scan shows some signal change in the posterior fibular region and possibly some displacement of the peroneal tendons. More importantly, however, it may show a signal change in the peroneus brevis suggestive of a tear. The peroneus brevis may tear as it repetitively subluxates around the posterior fibula.

Treatment

Nonoperative treatment may be successful with an acute subluxation, provided the SPR can adequately heal to the posterior fibula. Peroneal immobilization with a cast, cam walker, or at least a brace is combined with a pad placed directly over the distal fibula that compresses the retinacular tissues onto the fibula and maintains the reduction of the peroneal tendons. Nonoperative management is typically less successful in chronic cases.

Continued symptoms despite nonoperative management warrants orthopedic referral. The goal of surgery is to keep the peroneal tendons reduced behind the fibula; this can be accomplished with two different treatment concepts: (1) SPR reconstruction and (2) fibular groove deepening (Armagan and Shereff 2000; Clanton 1999; Coughlin 1999b; Schon 2000; Scioli 2000).

Osteochondral Lesions of the Talus

Occasionally, ankle sprains fail to heal because of articular damage to the talar dome, created by shear stresses or direct pressure incurred by the ankle injury. The natural history of osteochondral lesions of the talus (OLT) is not defined, but unlike younger patients, the older athlete may be predisposed to developing ankle arthritis.

Evaluation

Patients complain of ankle pain despite adequate ankle stability. However, mechanical symptoms from osteochondral lesion of the talus (OLT) such

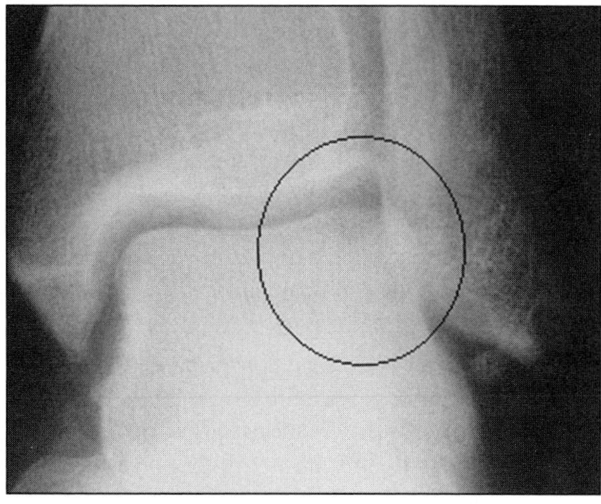

FIGURE 12.6 Anteroposterior ankle X-ray demonstrating large talar osteochondral lesion.

as locking, catching, and popping may lead to a sensation of ankle instability because of displacement of the loose articular fragment. Unfortunately, many of these lesions cannot be appreciated on plain radiographs alone (figure 12.6). Magnetic resonance imaging and CT have facilitated diagnosis of OLTs (Ferkel 1999; Toth and Easley 2000). Occasionally, purely articular OLTs (lesions that do not involve the subchondral bone) are not visible on any of the imaging studies and can be diagnosed only with direct visualization using arthroscopy.

Treatment

Nonoperative management is feasible for osteochondral lesions. It should be noted that OLTs are often incidental findings and asymptomatic for some patients. Rest, anti-inflammatory medications, and protective weight bearing may allow the lesion to gain some support in its defect; but unlike the situation in skeletally immature patients, healing of an OLT is unlikely in the older athlete. To control inflammation, a single steroid injection can help decrease symptoms. However, with persistent symptoms, typically related to unstable OLTs, nonoperative treatment is ineffective in symptom relief. Of note, there is no current evidence to suggest that the natural history of these focal OLTs is to eventually develop into diffuse ankle osteoarthritis.

Suspected or documented talar osteochondral lesions should be referred to the orthopedic surgeon if they are symptomatic. Several cartilage repair techniques have been developed to resurface OLTs, but the gold standard surgical management remains debridement to relieve the patient of mechanical symptoms. The drawback to the cartilage repair procedures is that the majority require harvesting cartilage from the knee joint and demand that the talar dome have the capacity to incorporate the transferred cartilage cells. While success has been reported for cartilage repair procedures applied to talar dome OLTs in small series, these studies include many younger patients and do not isolate results of cartilage repair procedures in athletic patients over the age of 50 (Ferkel 1999; Toth and Easley 2000).

Posterior Ankle Pain

Persistent ankle pain may also be secondary to posterior ankle pathology, including symptomatic lateral posterior talar process (os trigonum), symptomatic medial posterior talar process, posterior ankle impingement (scar tissue), and FHL tendinitis.

Evaluation

The patient typically complains of pain when walking down inclines or with ankle plantar flexion as occurs in sports such as soccer. Evaluation includes tenderness in the posterior ankle and pain with forced plantar flexion. FHL tendinitis can be elicited with hallux plantar flexion against resistance that produces pain in the posterior ankle, since the FHL courses over the posterior talus. Stenosing FHL tenosynovitis produces an audible crepitance with hallux range of motion.

Radiographs may suggest an os trigonum (figure 12.7) or separate posterior talar process; however, not every os trigonum is painful, and this may represent only an incidental finding. Occasionally, a diagnostic (and possibly therapeutic) anesthetic injection (with or without steroid) under fluoroscopic guidance in the posterior ankle at the posterior process may confirm the diagnosis. Magnetic resonance imaging or CT clearly defines the os trigonum or medial talar process and may suggest the detached fragment has acute changes. On MRI, change can be visualized on the posterior talar body and within the posterior process, and adjacent fluid can be seen; CT may demonstrate acute versus chronic changes at the separation between the fragment and the posterior talar body. Magnetic resonance imaging also may show signal change within the adjacent FHL tendon, suggestive of FHL tendinitis, and may demonstrate scar tissue in the posterior ankle.

Treatment

Rest, anti-inflammatory medications, physical therapy, and, as already noted, steroid injection into the posterior process area may diminish symptoms. Occasionally, in FHL tendinitis, a corticosteroid injection into the tendon sheath may be helpful; but care must be taken to avoid intratendinous injection. Should nonop-

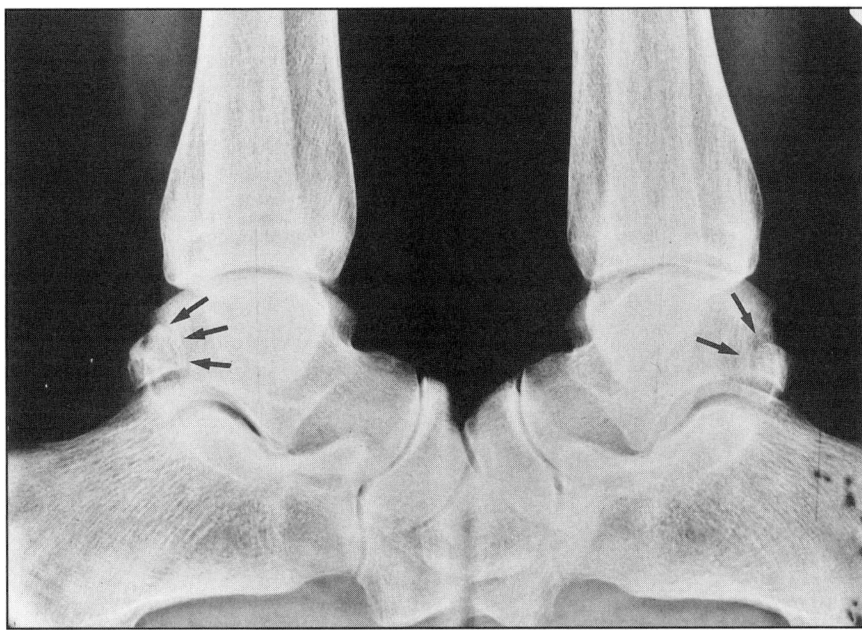

FIGURE 12.7 Lateral ankle X-ray demonstrating bilateral os trigonums.

erative measures fail, operative intervention typically relieves posterior ankle impingement symptoms. Open and arthroscopic procedures have been described to debride posterior ankle scar tissue and also to remove an os trigonum (Ferkel 1999; Hamilton and Hamilton 1999). Surgical treatment of FHL tendinitis is similar to that for tendinitis of any tendon. The affected areas are systematically debrided and impingement on the FHL relieved.

Fractures and Nonunions

Ankle sprains that fail to heal may be secondary to missed fractures about the hindfoot and ankle. Three common fractures that one should consider in chronic ankle injuries are (1) lateral talar process, (2) anterior calcaneal process, and (3) base of fifth metatarsal fracture. The last two are foot fractures, but may occur with inversion ankle injuries.

Lateral Talar Process

Lateral talar process fractures ("snowboarder's fracture") may be subtle. The patient continues to complain of lateral ankle pain, and tenderness is present in the lateral ankle and subfibular region. Pain is noted with ankle and subtalar range of motion. Routine ankle radiographs may not demonstrate the fracture, but it is typically observed on the mortise view. Foot X-rays may also fail to demonstrate the injury, but a Broden's view is often helpful as it directly focuses on the inferior articular surface of the talus. With any concern about this fracture, a CT scan will clearly define the fracture pattern and the involvement of the subtalar joint. Often, the fracture is not noted until an MRI is obtained as a screening tool for an occult injury; the CT is then typically still necessary to define the fracture pattern. Treatment involves open reduction internal fixation (ORIF) of the fracture (if the fragment is large enough) and excision if the fracture is comminuted or chronic with little chance for healing.

Anterior Calcaneal Process

The anterior process of the calcaneus can be avulsed with inversion ankle sprains and may lead to persistent symptoms if not recognized. A delayed union/nonunion continues to be symptomatic with stress from the bifurcate ligaments on the fragment; a malunion may impinge on the lateral aspect of the talar head. Pain is noted on the dorsolateral foot, and tenderness is present over the anterior process, directly deep the extensor digitorum brevis muscle. Radiographs, particularly the oblique X-ray of the foot, are helpful in diagnosing the injury; a CT scan typically fully defines the pathology. Nonoperative treatment is typically unsuccessful and, as with lateral talar process fractures, ORIF or excision is typically required.

Base of the Fifth Metatarsal Fractures

The base of the fifth metatarsal fracture is categorized into (1) avulsion, (2) Jones' fracture, and (3) stress fracture (figure 12.8). The avulsion fracture involves only the base of the fifth metatarsal and can typically be treated nonoperatively with immobilization in a cam walker or a cast. Acute care with RICE protocol and

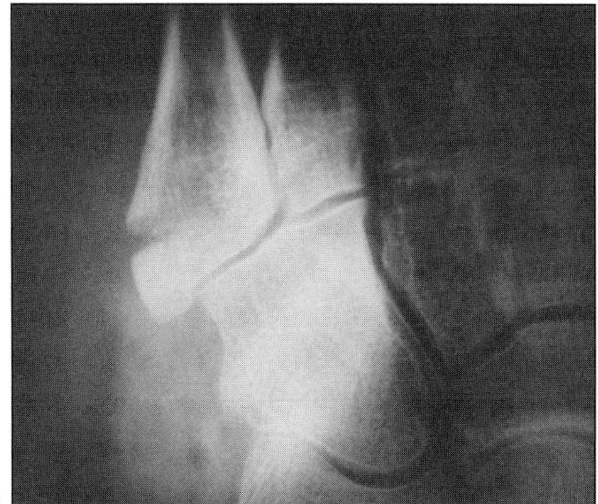
a

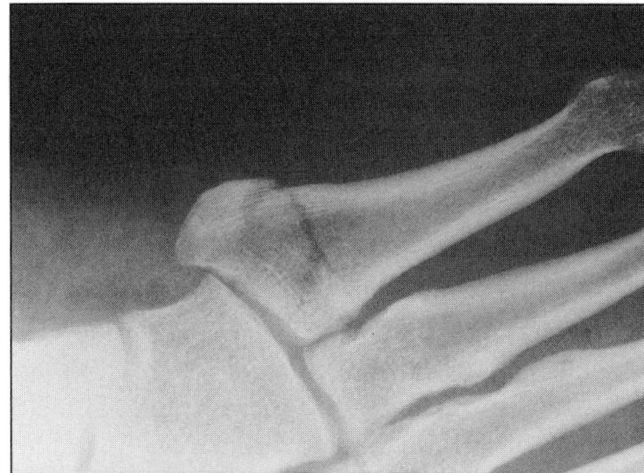
b

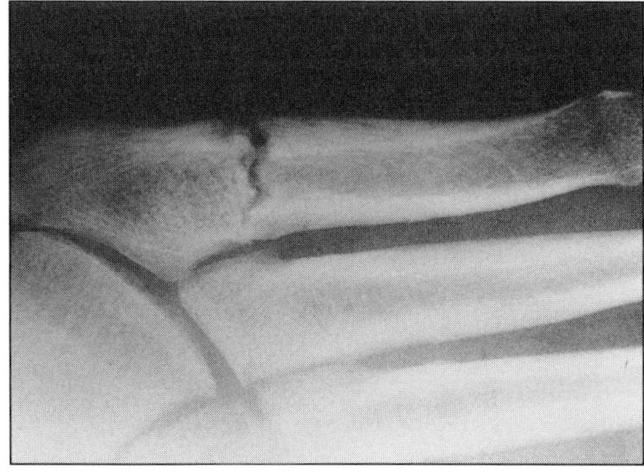
c

FIGURE 12.8 *(a)* Avulsion fracture of the tuberositas (also called "tennis fracture"), *(b)* acute Jones' fracture, and *(c)* diaphyseal stress fracture of the fifth metatarsal.

short-term immobilization should be followed by three to four weeks of rest with a gradual pain-guided return to sport. If necessary, the fragment can be excised if symptoms persist. Rarely is the fragment of adequate size to warrant ORIF. The peroneus brevis attachment must be preserved if excision is performed.

The Jones' fracture is notorious for poor healing, as it occurs in a watershed portion of the base of the fifth metatarsal (an area with poor vascular supply). The fracture is in the area where the base of the fifth metatarsal articulates with the base of the fourth metatarsal. Nondisplaced fractures may heal with cast immobilization and restricted weight bearing for six to eight weeks. Fractures that do not progress well toward union, or displaced fractures, should be managed operatively, typically with intramedullary screw fixation (with or without bone grafting).

Stress fractures occur slightly more distally than Jones' fractures, beyond the articulation of the bases of the fifth and fourth metatarsals. Treatment is similar to that for Jones' fractures.

Treatment for base of the fifth metatarsal fractures should include correction of any tendency for hindfoot varus. If hindfoot varus exists, there will be a continued tendency to overload the lateral aspect of the foot that will lead to continued stress on the base of the fifth metatarsal. Generally, orthotics are adequate, but one must entertain and correct other factors such as persistent ankle instability and peroneal tendon pathology (Sanders 1999). Operative management of hindfoot varus may be necessary.

Neuralgia

Finally, ankle inversion injuries may create excessive traction on the sural and superficial peroneal nerves. Despite improvement in the mechanical symptoms of an ankle inversion, hypersensitivity or numbness, or both, may persist in the sural and superficial peroneal nerve (SPN) distributions. The patient typically complains of lateral ankle pain not only with activity, but also at rest or with light touch on the skin of the lateral ankle and foot. Evaluation demonstrates the hypersensitivity of these two nerves not only with light touch but also with percussion of the nerves more proximally. A diagnostic injection of an anesthetic in either the location of the sural nerve or SPN confirms the diagnosis. Initial treatment consists of desensitization, antineuroleptics, and injection with steroid. Should this fail, it is necessary to consider referral to a pain management center.

ACHILLES TENDON PATHOLOGY

The middle-aged recreational athlete who has a rigorous passion for demanding sports such as basketball or tennis is a prime candidate for Achilles tendon pathology and rupture. The older recreational athlete has subjected the Achilles tendon to repeated microtrauma, which can result in a spectrum of tendonitis or manifest as rupture. There processes will be detailed below.

Achilles Tendon Ruptures

Rupture of the Achilles tendon usually occurs in the setting of tendon substance degeneration as a result of years of microtrauma and tendinitis. Tendon degeneration accompanied by rapid eccentric loading may result in a ruptured Achilles tendon.

Background, Anatomy, and Pathoanatomy

The Achilles tendon, formed by the confluence of the gastrocnemius-soleus aponeuroses, attaches on the posterior calcaneus. It is considered the strongest tendon in the human body and is enclosed in a paratenon or outer covering. With a tensile overload, Achilles tendon ruptures typically occur approximately 2 to 6 cm proximal to the insertion, in a watershed area of the tendon (area of poor vasculature). After age 30 the vasculature is less dense in this watershed area, and much of the nutrition for the tendon is derived from the paratenon. Tensile overload typically occurs with sudden ankle dorsiflexion with concurrent contraction of the gastrocnemius-soleus complex. There may be preexisting tendinopathy that promotes rupture in this watershed area. The typical patient with an Achilles rupture is the "weekend warrior" or poorly conditioned athlete between the ages of 30 to 50. This age is probably extended into the 60s with a more active older population. It is a concern that up to 25% of Achilles tendon ruptures are misdiagnosed initially because plantar flexion is still possible, using the other flexors of the foot and ankle.

Evaluation

The patient typically presents after an athletic injury, reporting that it felt as though someone had kicked him or her in the calf and the injury is often associated with an audible "pop." Examination reveals a palpable defect in the Achilles tendon in the hypovascular zone, 2 to 6 cm above the Achilles insertion. Plantar flexion is still possible but is notably weak, because flexion is occurring with the FHL, FDL, peroneals, and posterior tibial tendon. The pathomneumonic finding is a positive Thompson's test. With the patient prone, a calf squeeze fails to plantar flex the foot. This finding is in stark contrast to the plantar flexion observed with a calf squeeze on the contralateral extremity ("negative Thompson's test") (figure 12.9).

Imaging studies are rarely required. A lateral foot and ankle radiograph should be obtained to ensure that there is no bony avulsion of the Achilles tendon from its insertion. If a bony avulsion exists, then ORIF of the fragment is warranted. Magnetic resonance imaging will confirm the clinical diagnosis. Ultrasound can give some idea of how well the ruptured tendon ends can be opposed. If the tendon ends can be opposed with plantar flexion, then nonoperative treatment may be feasible. However, if the tendon ends cannot be opposed with plantar flexion alone, operative intervention should be entertained in the athletic patient.

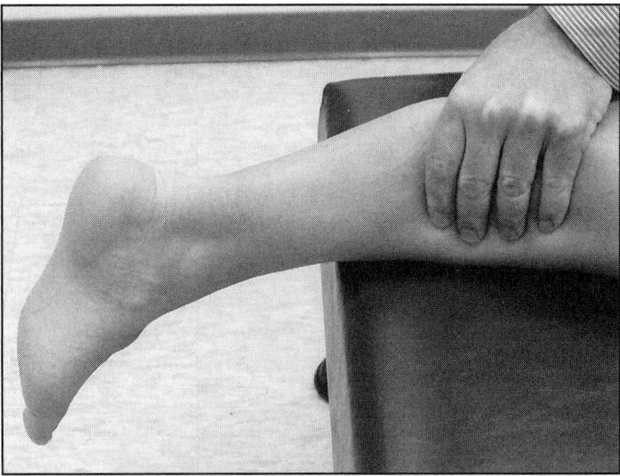

FIGURE 12.9 Thompson's test is best done with the patient prone and with comparison to the unaffected side. Plantar flexion signifies Achilles continuity.

Treatment

Controversy persists as to the ideal management of Achilles tendon ruptures. Favorable results have been reported with nonoperative management and surgical repair (including both open and percutaneous methods). Regardless of the treatment methods, the goals remain the same: (1) restore tendon integrity, (2) restore physiologic tendon function, (3) avoid complications. Traditionally, nonoperative treatment is favored in the older patient, but with the increasing number of athletically active individuals over the age of 50, operative management is being performed with greater frequency in older patients.

Regardless of whether one chooses surgical or nonsurgical treatment, a patient with an Achilles tendon rupture should be referred to an orthopedist. Nonoperative management requires that the ruptured tendon ends remain in contact. Typically, the ankle is immobilized in plantar flexion and gradually brought to a neutral position by 8 to 10 weeks. Although ultrasound may be useful to ensure that the tendon ends remain in contact. Between 10 to 12 weeks plantarflexion resistance exercises are initiated and a heel lift is worn. The patient is restricted from sports for at least six months.

Operative intervention allows for visualization of direct contact of the tendon ends. Intraoperatively, the desired resting tension of the Achilles tendon is equal to that of the unaffected side. With tendon contact maintained, earlier rehabilitation and range of motion are possible, which may lead to more effective reorganization of tendon fibers and an earlier return to athletics.

The advantages of each treatment method are obvious. Nonoperative management eliminates the risk of wound problems, infection, and nerve injury; operative management reduces the rerupture rate (operative 2% vs. nonoperative 10-18%). Percutaneous techniques are becoming increasingly popular as they may limit the risk of wound complications. A review of the recent literature suggests that the prevalence of surgical complications is relatively low, but the rerupture rate in nonoperative management is probably unacceptable for younger athletic patients. Again, with the aging population of athletes, this rerupture rate is probably also unacceptable for older athletically active patients (Coughlin 1999b; Myerson and Mendelbaum 2000).

Achilles Tendinopathy

Achilles tendinitis or tendinopathy represents a spectrum of disease from inflammation of the peritendinous structures and bursa to involvement of the tendon itself. The older recreational athlete is particularly prone to this disorder secondary to years of recurrent microtrauma as well as the greater tendency to be a weekend warrior. Risk factors for this disease process common to the weekend warrior include abruptly increasing or restarting a training program, as well as inadequate stretching. Achilles tendinopathy has been broadly classified as either insertional or non-insertional.

Non-Insertional Achilles Tendinopathy

Non-insertional Achilles tendinopathy is defined by its location and presentation. It is crucial to differentiate this entity from insertional Achilles tendinopathy in order to institute the correct treatment.

Background, Anatomy, and Pathoanatomy

Achilles tendinopathy proximal to the calcaneal insertion is a common lower extremity injury, with a 6.5% to 18% incidence among runners. This is not surprising given that six to eight times body weight is placed on the Achilles tendon during running. As with Achilles ruptures, non-insertional Achilles tendinopathy tends to occur in the hypovascular zone. As noted earlier, increasing age leads to decreasing elasticity, circulation, and collagen cross-linking/density in the Achilles tendon. Traditionally, this is a problem seen in young competitive athletes but may increase in frequency among the older competitive athletes of today. Non-insertional Achilles tendon pathology is classified into (1) peritendinitis, (2) peritendinitis-tendinosis, and (3) tendinosis. Generally, it is accepted that peritendinopathy ("peritendinitis") leads to pantendinopathy ("peritendinitis-tendinosis"), and eventually tendinopathy ("tendinitis"). Inflammation usually develops into a degenerative process, potentially leading to tendon incompetence.

Evaluation

The patient typically reports symptoms proximal to the Achilles tendon insertion. On examination, tenderness is noted within the Achilles tendon substance. A "painful arc sign" is useful in distinguishing between peritendinopathy and tendinopathy. With range of motion of the ankle, peritendinopathy symptoms remain localized in the same position over the mobile Achilles tendon, suggesting inflammation of the paratenon in that area, whereas migration of the symptomatic tendon is observed with range of motion in tendinopathy. Peritendinopathy does not have the same fusiform swelling of the tendon observed in tendinopathy. Magnetic resonance imaging may be useful in distinguishing tendinopathy from peritendinopathy. While axial views demonstrate the percentage of tendon involvement and define peritendinopathy (fluid around the tendon), sagittal images suggest the extent of tendon involvement.

Treatment

Acute pathology, whether peritendinitis or tendinopathy, typically responds well to nonoperative management, including activity modification, shoe modification, heel lift (figure 12.10), modalities to reduce inflammation, and nonsteroidal anti-inflammatory agents. Once symptoms improve, progressive gentle stretching (ankle dorsiflexion), shoe wear modifications (heel lift in all shoes), and improved training regimens that avoid uneven or slippery terrain, as well as abrupt changes in training regimens, often lead to 90% to 95% successful management.

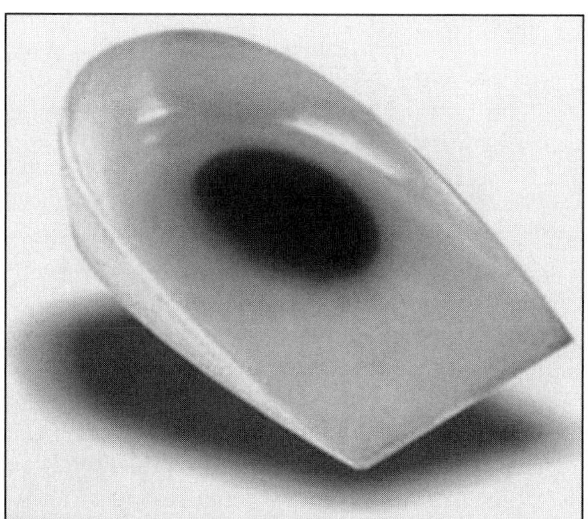

FIGURE 12.10 Heel lifts are essential for rehabilitation of Achilles tendinitis. Viscoelastic heel cups are available in most drugstores.

Aggressive Achilles stretching must be avoided as it will aggravate symptoms.

Once symptoms persist beyond three months, nonoperative measures tend to be less effective. Chronic peritendinopathy has been managed with a brisement procedure that allows for lysis of adhesion through injection of a minimal amount of local anesthetic in the peritendinous space, followed by immediate rehabilitation. Brisement has a reported success rate of 33%. Operative intervention for chronic peritendinopathy involves a limited medial incision to excise fibrotic tissue and lysis of adhesions. Progressive therapy is initiated once the wound has healed. Success with open management of chronic peritendinopathy is reported at 72% to 100% good-to-excellent results. Chronic pantendinopathy (disease with tendon involvement) has been managed with some success nonoperatively, but often requires surgical intervention for adequate functional recovery. A percutaneous longitudinal tenotomy technique has been described with 77% good to excellent results. The diseased portion of the Achilles tendon is subjected to five percutaneous stab incisions while the ankle is dorsiflexed and plantar flexed. Given minimal soft tissue disruption, early range of motion and return to activity are possible. Failures are generally attributed to associated peritendinitis that is not addressed with this procedure, and therefore this technique is recommended for pure tendinopathy. Open surgical management of chronic pantendinopathy addresses both the tendinopathy and the peritendinopathy. Through an open medial incision, the paratenon is debrided, lysis of adhesions is performed, and the diseased portion of the tendon is removed. Occasionally, an FHL transfer is required to augment the residual Achilles tendon when a substantial amount of Achilles tendon has to be debrided. Results of open debridement are varied, with 36% to 100% good to excellent results (Myerson and Mendelbaum 2000).

Insertional Achilles Tendinopathy

Insertional Achilles tendinopathy can be confused with other causes of heel pain. Its diagnosis rests on a comprehensive history and adequate radiographic examination.

Background, Anatomy, and Pathoanatomy

Posterior heel pain disorders include (1) insertional Achilles tendinopathy, (2) "pump bump" (prominent lateral calcaneal ridge), and (3) retrocalcaneal bursitis/Haglund's deformity. These diseases have some overlap and occur at the insertion of the Achilles tendon on the calcaneus. This problem is considered an overuse phenomenon but may be superimposed on a relatively minor injury to the Achilles tendon insertion. The repetitive trauma leads to degenerative changes in the Achilles tendon insertion. Symptoms are worsened by the bony impingement on the tendon by the Haglund's prominence, calcification within the tendon, associated retrocalcaneal bursitis, and shoe pressure. Traditionally, this is a common problem in the nonathletic, nonactive obese middle-aged patient (often with systemic disease). However, with the aging athletic population, older active patients are presenting with posterior heel disorders as well.

Evaluation

Patients complain of activity-related and post-activity-related posterior heel pain aggravated by increased mileage during running or running hills. An associated complaint is pain when wearing closed-heeled shoes that rub the painful prominent posterior calcaneus. The physical examination reveals fullness to the Achilles tendon insertion. With the disease process involving the tendon substance of the Achilles insertion, point tenderness is typically over the tendon insertion directly posteriorly in addition to the retrocalcaneal area. Without tendon involvement, tenderness is often limited to the retrocalcaneal area, particularly laterally over the prominent calcaneal tuberosity. Dorsiflexion of the ankle typically produces symptoms in the posterior heel. Because of pain, dorsiflexion is often limited; however, with tendon attenuation in chronic disease, hyperdorsiflexion may be observed. Lateral radiographs of the foot often demonstrate calcification in the Achilles insertion and a prominent posterior calcaneal process (Haglund's process). In calcific tendinopathy, calcification may also be seen extending more proximally within the Achilles tendon. Magnetic resonance imaging may be helpful for determining the extent of Achilles tendon involvement, but is usually not necessary in the management of insertional Achilles tendinopathy.

Treatment

Nonoperative management is typically successful (good-to-excellent in 95% of cases). Rest and alteration of the training routine, along with a heel lift, typically adequately relieve symptoms. However, immobilization in a cast or cam walker with a heel lift for four to six weeks is often necessary for adequate healing of the Achilles tendon insertion. As in noninsertional Achilles tendinopathy, aggressive stretching must be avoided. Gradual return to athletic activity is then permissible, and the patient wears a heel lift at all times while weight bearing. A full recovery may take six months to a year.

When nonoperative management fails, operative intervention may be considered. The goal of operative intervention is to (1) debride the degenerated portions of the diseased Achilles tendon and inflamed retrocalcaneal bursa, (2) remove the prominent Haglund's process, and (3) reattach the healthy tendon to a healthy cancellous calcaneal surface. Postoperative management includes two weeks of immobilization in a splint, then two to three weeks of weight bearing in a slightly plantar flexed short leg cast, followed by a cam walker with a heel lift and initiation of range of motion exercises. After three months, the patient wears a regular shoe with a heel lift and begins Achilles tendon strengthening exercises at 8 to 10 weeks. The best results are reported in surgical management of noncalcific tendinopathy (>90% satisfactory results) and are acceptable in calcific tendinopathy (approximately 80% satisfactory results) (Myerson and Mendelbaum 2000).

HINDFOOT

Hindfoot injuries in the older recreational athlete can be particularly resistant to treatment and can be debilitating.

Plantar Heel Pain

Plantar heel pain is one of the most common foot problems, and a precise diagnosis may be difficult given the complex heel anatomy and the close proximity of several structures that may generate symptoms. However, plantar heel pain can typically be categorized into (1) fat pad atrophy ("central heel pain syndrome"), (2) plantar fasciitis, (3) entrapment of the first branch of the lateral plantar nerve, and (4) calcaneal stress fractures. Regardless of diagnosis, plantar heel pain rarely requires surgical management.

Heel Fat Pad Atrophy

The central heel pain syndrome is generally a result of heel fat pad atrophy. Fat pad atrophy is rarely observed in younger patients; it typically occurs in older patients and therefore is particularly important in treating athletic patients over 50 years of age.

Evaluation

The patient complains of focal central heel pain with weight bearing; no radiating symptoms are noted. Clinical examination demonstrates focal tenderness directly over the prominent plantar calcaneal tuberosity, which reproduces the patient's symptoms.

Treatment

Treatment is aimed at substituting for the atrophic fat pad by increasing the padding on the plantar aspect of the heel with a viscoelastic heel or an orthotic. Alternatively, an orthotic or the athletic shoe can be relieved with a softer material directly under the most prominent area of the calcaneus to diminish pressure.

Plantar Fasciitis

Plantar fasciitis, or "proximal plantar fasciitis," typically creates symptoms at the origin of the plantar fascia on the medial plantar calcaneal tuberosity. With repetitive traction and stress on the plantar fascia, microscopic tears lead to a chronic proximal plantar fascial problem; an initial inflammatory response develops collagen degeneration and matrix calcification.

Evaluation

The patient usually notes medial plantar heel pain with weight bearing, particularly with the first steps after a period of rest ("start-up pain") and with prolonged standing or exercise. Evaluation localizes tenderness to the plantar medial calcaneal tuberosity, at the origin of the plantar fascia. Imaging studies are not typically helpful. If present, a plantar heel spur is at the origin of the flexor hallucis brevis and lies deep to the plantar fascia. The spur has no relation to plantar fasciitis; in fact, 15% of nonsymptomatic heels have a plantar heel spur on radiographs. The tendency is for patients and physicians to fixate on the accompanying spur. This is inappropriate.

Treatment

Treatment includes (1) activity modification, (2) cushioning with a heel pad or an orthotic, and, most importantly, (3) Achilles and plantar fascia stretching. Stretching is facilitated with the use of a night splint. Stretching is most effective if performed routinely and particularly after a period of rest (to stretch the plantar fascia and Achilles to limit excessive tension on the plantar fascia with the first steps after a period of non-weight bearing) (figure 12.11).

Should this combination of treatment methods fail to improve symptoms after three months, one may consider a steroid injection in the plantar fascia origin. Results of nonoperative treatment for plantar fasciitis are uniformly good, with a reported success rate of 90% to 95%. Surgical intervention is rarely indicated and can be performed endoscopically or with use of an open method; both are accepted methods. The goals of both techniques are to relieve tension in the plantar fascia by partially dividing it 33% to 50% medially. Complete division of the plantar fascia either by accidental transection of the entire plantar fascia or with rupture following multiple steroid injections can lead to further problems. Although the symptoms related to plantar fasciitis are typically relieved with transection, a lateral column syndrome (painful lateral foot) may develop due to loss of the plantar fascial support.

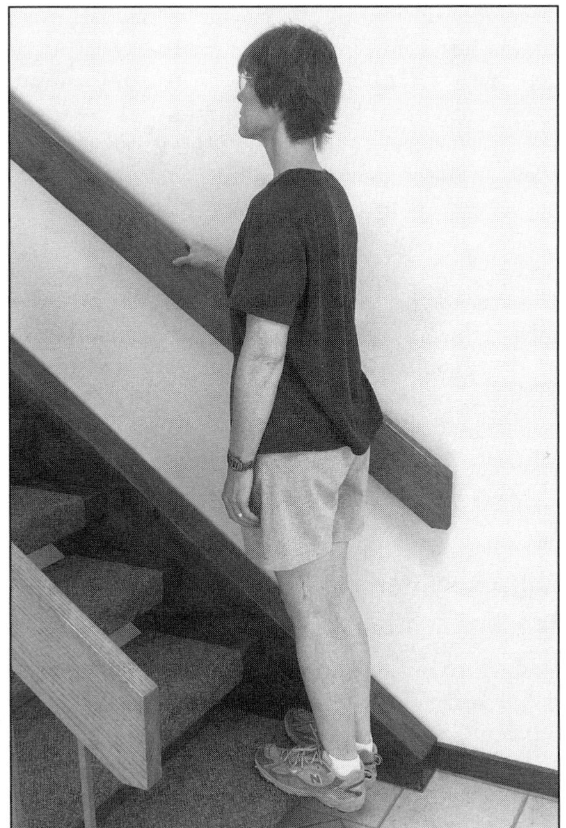

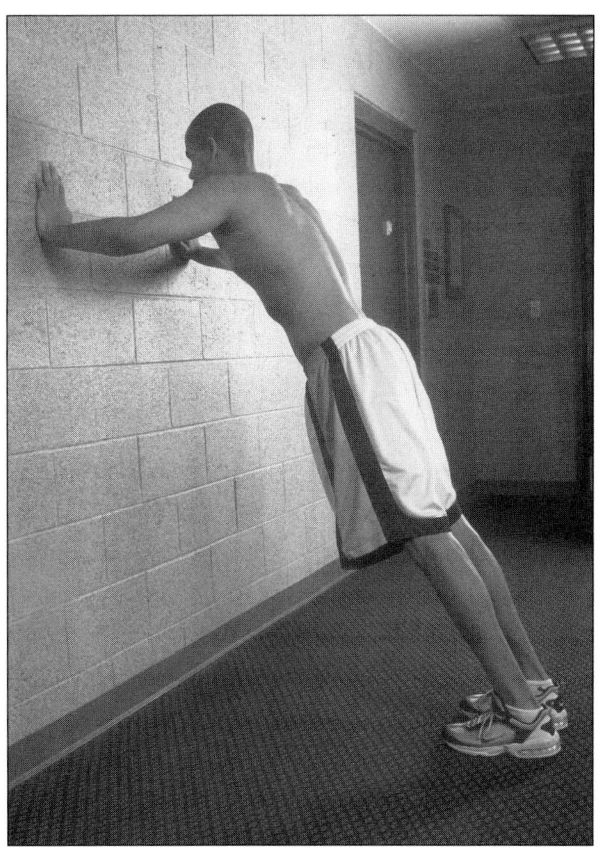

FIGURE 12.11 *(a)* Stair stretch and *(b)* wall stretch for Achilles and plantar fascia stretching.

Occasionally, acute ruptures of the plantar fascia occur in the athletic population, producing considerable heel and particularly arch pain. Without an adequate period of immobilization and subsequent arch support, the foot will have a tendency to assume a pes planus (flatfoot) alignment, creating the aforementioned lateral column syndrome. Immobilization after acute plantar fascia rupture should continue for several months, followed by a longitudinal arch support. Symptoms related to the lateral column syndrome may persist for 12 to 18 months (Pfeffer 2000).

Less frequently, plantar fasciitis may occur more distally than at the fascial origin on the calcaneus and is termed distal plantar fasciitis. Distal plantar fasciitis is an inflammation of the plantar fascia over the majority of its course. Tenderness is noted in the plantar fascia underlying the midfoot, and dorsiflexion of the toes exacerbates the symptoms (unlike what occurs with proximal plantar fasciitis). Treatment is similar to that for plantar fasciitis, with the addition of an arch support to avoid excessive tension across the plantar fascia (Pfeffer 2000).

Entrapment of the First Branch of the Lateral Plantar Nerve ("Baxter's Nerve")

Not all plantar heel pain is related to mechanical problems; in approximately 15% of patients with chronic plantar heel pain, one sees entrapment of the first branch of the lateral plantar nerve (FBLPN) between the deep fascia of the abductor hallucis muscle and the medial aspect of the quadratus plantae muscle. Even though the patient describes plantar heel pain similar to that of plantar fasciitis, examination demonstrates tenderness just slightly more medial than the origin of the plantar fascia, at the margin of the abductor hallucis where nerve entrapment occurs. Although this is a nerve compression disorder, electrodiagnostic studies are often inconclusive. Initial nonoperative treatment is similar to that of plantar fasciitis, particularly because hindfoot inflammation related to plantar fasciitis may contribute to nerve compression. With failure of conservative management over 6 to 12 months including stretching and observation, one should consider open surgical nerve decompression; typically less than 5% of patients require operative management. Decompression is performed through an open medial approach that simultaneously releases the abductor hallucis fascia and the medial aspect of the plantar fascia. The plantar fascia release is routinely included given the frequent coexistence of nerve compression and plantar fasciitis. With proper patient selection, good-to-excellent results are reported in >85% of patients (Pfeffer 2000).

Occasionally, runners develop medial hindfoot/midfoot pain with some radiation distally secondary to compression of the medial plantar nerve as it courses under the abductor hallucis fascia, similar to compression noted in "Baxter's nerve" problems. This is termed jogger's foot, and after failed nonoperative management for 6 to 12 months, nerve decompression may be considered (Baxter 1999).

Calcaneal Stress Fracture

Excessive training, particularly running on hard surfaces, rarely may lead to calcaneal stress fractures. Routine training, even in older athletes, typically does not result in a stress fracture. The patient usually reports heel pain with activity that is relieved by rest, similar to the situation with other plantar heel pain syndromes. However, uncharacteristic of these other entities is the physical finding of a positive calcaneal squeeze test that reproduces symptoms, both medially and laterally. If the stress fracture is chronic, plain radiographs may demonstrate a sclerotic line in the calcaneus; in more acute cases, a bone scan or MRI typically confirms the diagnosis (figure 12.12). Four to six weeks of non-weight bearing followed by gradual return to athletic activity is typically successful in treating calcaneal stress fractures. The patient should alter the training routine and use a shock-absorbing shoe or insert to prevent recurrence (Scranton 2000).

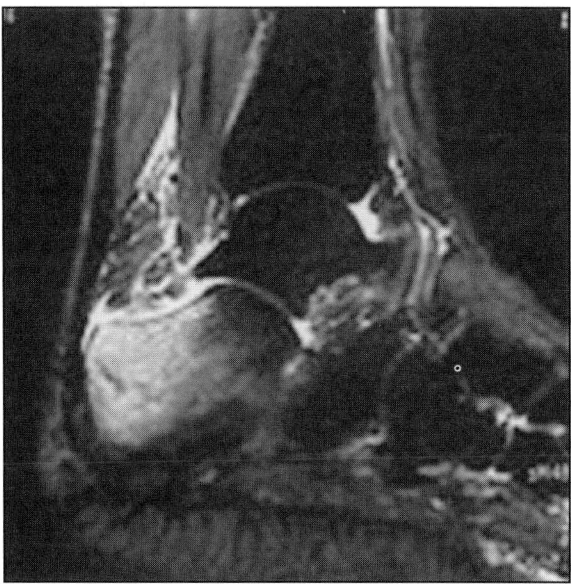

FIGURE 12.12 Magnetic resonance imaging demonstrating calcaneal stress fracture, often a subtle finding on X-rays. Sagittal transition zone (TZ) image displaying edema in the area of the stress fracture.

MIDFOOT

Injuries to the midfoot in older sport enthusiasts mirror those of the young and include posterior tibial tendon insufficiency, painful accessory navicular, and midfoot sprain. Treatment of the older recreational athlete may differ somewhat than that for the younger athlete as to the threshold for surgical intervention, but this demarcation is blurring as seniors continue to be competitive athletes at a later age.

Adult Acquired Flatfoot (Posterior Tibial Tendon Insufficiency)

Posterior tibial tendon (PTT) insufficiency can be debilitating. This tendon is largely responsible for efficient propulsion. Injury or associated pathology as seen in PTT insufficiency often translates into diminished athletic ability.

Background, Anatomy, and Pathoanatomy

Many athletes are flatfooted; pes planus in itself need not be symptomatic. During stance phase, a pes planus alignment is advantageous, as the foot is flexible and accommodates to most surfaces. However, for effective propulsion, the posterior tibial tendon must be functional. During push-off the posterior tibial tendon functions to invert the hindfoot, thereby locking the hindfoot and midfoot and reconstituting the arch to convert the foot into an effective lever arm against which the Achilles tendon can work. Without a functioning posterior tibial tendon, the hindfoot and midfoot are not locked, the foot is not converted into an effective lever arm, and the Achilles tendon works against a foot that is in an accommodative position. This situation stresses the static restraints of the hindfoot and midfoot and potentially worsens the patient's pes planus alignment. Posterior tibial tendon insufficiency is graded according its level of advancement.

Evaluation

The athletic patient usually complains of medial ankle and foot pain and occasionally lateral discomfort in the sinus tarsi. Participation in sport becomes increasingly difficult, and early fatigue in the affected extremity is reported. The patient may also note a loss of the longitudinal arch. Physical examination with the patient standing demonstrates heel valgus, loss of the longitudinal arch, and forefoot abduction ("too many toes sign"). A single-limb heel rise is difficult and may fail to reconstitute the longitudinal arch—a finding that is typically in stark contrast to that for the contralateral uninvolved foot, even if pes planus is noted bilaterally. Tenderness is along the posterior tibial tendon (PTT), with maximum tenderness occurring anywhere along its course, from behind the medial malleolus to the medial aspect of the navicular. With the foot held in plantar flexion to isolate the PTT, inversion strength is typically weaker than in the contralateral, uninvolved side. Radiographs may demonstrate loss of the longitudinal arch on the lateral view and talar head uncovering and forefoot abduction on the anteroposterior (AP) view. Although MRI or ultrasound may confirm the diagnosis, it is typically not necessary in the evaluation of PTT dysfunction. Associated with PTT insufficiency may be a spring ligament tear, which is attenuation of the calcaneonavicular ligaments that provide static medial ligamentous support to the foot (Anderson and Davis 2000; Mann 1999).

Treatment

Nonoperative treatment is often effective in less severe or chronic PTT tendinitis. Rest, immobilization in a cam walker for 4 to 12 weeks, and modalities to decrease inflammation typically control symptoms. Physical therapy to gradually strengthen the PTT, combined with a longitudinal arch support, typically allows for a return to athletic activity. With posterior tibial tendinosis as noted in more severe or acute disease, however, surgical management may be necessary to allow for successful return to athletic competition. Typically, both dynamic and static components need to be addressed to relieve symptoms. Reconstruction of the dynamic medial stabilizers includes

1. tendon debridement,
2. augmentation/substitution of the PTT with an adjacent tendon (FHL or FDL), and
3. possible spring ligament repair/tightening.

To protect this dynamic reconstruction, surgical management typically also includes repositioning of the static foot alignment with either (1) medial displacement calcaneal osteotomy or (2) lateral calcaneal lengthening osteotomy.

This combination of procedures does not violate joints and typically relieves symptoms while preserving hindfoot motion necessary for athletic competition. Results have been promising but typically focus on the nonathletic patient population, where the entity is more common. However, again with an increasing number of older athletes, this entity may become more common in this subset of athletes (Anderson and Davis 2000; Mann 1999).

Accessory Navicular

Occasionally, medial foot pain or an acquired flatfoot is secondary to an accessory navicular. Although an entity typically treated in the pediatric population, it may be observed in the adult population as well. Typically, it is a type II accessory navicular that affects the athletic population. The type II accessory navicular is associated with a synchondrosis or cartilaginous connection between the main body of the navicular and the accessory navicular. Typically, this is asymptomatic until a twisting injury to the foot produces persistent medial symptoms secondary to a disruption of the synchondrosis.

Evaluation

Evaluation may demonstrate some pes planus alignment, but this is usually not a major change from the patient's baseline foot alignment. Tenderness is noted directly over the medial navicular, and although a single-limb heel rise and PTT strength are intact with inversion against resistance, symptoms are exacerbated with these maneuvers. Routine AP and lateral radiographs may indicate that an accessory navicular is present, but an external oblique radiograph is most helpful in placing the navicular in profile to define the accessory navicular and the synchondrosis. Magnetic resonance imaging may demonstrate signal change about the accessory navicular and synchondrosis, suggesting acute or subacute injury. Furthermore, MRI can define if any associated injury to the PTT is present (Schon 2000).

Treatment

Nonoperative management includes rest, immobilization in a cast or cam walker, and four to six weeks of restricted weight bearing. With resolution of symptoms, an orthotic may prove to be beneficial but may create excessive pressure on the medial navicular. In the athletic population, surgery may be required to relieve symptoms. Traditionally, excision of the accessory navicular with attachment of the PTT to the remaining navicular has been successful, but it may lead to worsening of the pes planus alignment and renewed symptoms. Therefore, excision should probably be combined with a calcaneal osteotomy. More recently, attention has been given to debridement of the synchondrosis and reattachment of the accessory navicular to the main body of the navicular. This preserves the function of the PTT and allows for bone-to-bone healing (Schon 2000).

Midfoot Sprain ("Lisfranc Injury")

The Lisfranc injury can be a subtle finding; however, the results of an unrecognized Lisfranc fracture-dislocation dislocation can be devastating. There should be a high index of suspicion for this injury in any athlete who reports midfoot pain after the appropriate mechanism. This mechanism typically involves either direct blunt trauma or an axial load on the heel with the toes dorsiflexed on the ground.

Anatomy and Pathoanatomy

The Lisfranc joints are the tarsometatarsal joints between the cuneiforms/cuboid and the metatarsal bases. The second metatarsal base "keys" into the midfoot; the primary supporting ligaments course from the medial cuneiform to the second metatarsal base. High-energy injuries may produce easily recognizable fracture-dislocations across these articulations; however, in athletic competition, the findings may be subtle. It is imperative not to miss this injury. Without adequate stability across these articulations, the rigid lever arm of the foot is lost, and longitudinal arch collapse may be observed.

Evaluation

The patient typically complains of pain in the midfoot with weight bearing and with stress applied across the midfoot. Edema is noted throughout the midfoot, and ecchymosis is frequently observed on the plantar aspect of the foot. The midfoot is tender, and abduction or dorsiflexion/plantar flexion stress of the forefoot against the midfoot produces symptoms. Non-weight-bearing radiographs may be inconclusive; if possible, weight-bearing radiographs will typically demonstrate

- displacement of the second metatarsal base from its alignment with the middle cuneiform (AP view),
- displacement of the fourth metatarsal base from its alignment with the cuboid (oblique view), and
- dorsal displacement of the metatarsal bases (lateral view) (figure 12.13).

However, in subtle injuries these may not be demonstrated. Dynamic fluoroscopy, with comparison to the uninvolved foot, may demonstrate instability when an abduction force is placed across the tarsometatarsal joints. Magnetic resonance imaging, bone scan, and CT typically can define the subtle injuries.

Treatment

Treatment of this entity is rarely nonoperative. With no displacement evident, immobilization and non-weight-bearing for 10 to 12 weeks may be contemplated. It is the authors' preference to stabilize these fracture-dislocations in their anatomic position with ORIF using temporary screws or pins while adequate scar tissue forms to substitute for the preinjury ligamentous support. Typically non-weight bearing is instituted for 10 to 12 weeks, but screws are left in place for four to five months to ensure adequate ligamentous healing.

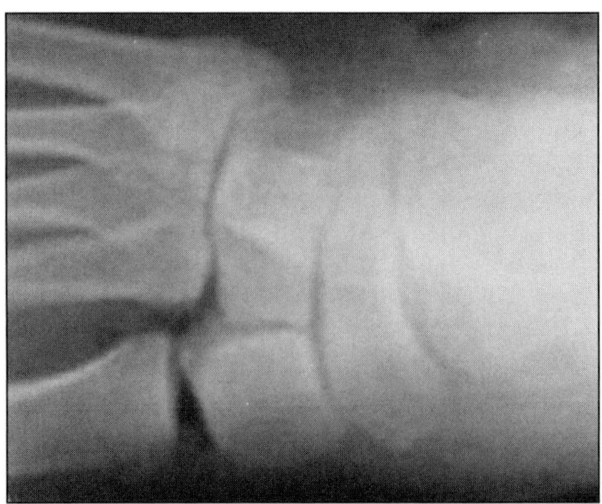

FIGURE 12.13 AP foot X-ray demonstrates malalignment of the proximal base of the second metatarsal and the medial margin of the middle cuneiform.

Occasionally, despite proper management, posttraumatic arthritis develops, necessitating arthrodesis (fusion). Since these articulations provide midfoot support and have virtually no motion physiologically, fusion does not restrict patients for athletic competition. However, it is imperative that only the first, second, and third tarsometatarsal (TMT) joints be fused and not the fourth and fifth, as motion at these lateral-most joints is essential for proper accommodation to various surfaces during gait (Clanton 1999).

FOREFOOT

Forefoot problems can be debilitating for the athlete at any age. Although it is convenient to view all forefoot problems as "metatarsalgia," the term is nondescript and probably should be reserved for tenderness under the metatarsal heads secondary to fat pad atrophy. Although fat pad atrophy is more prevalent in the older athlete, specific diagnoses are important for ensuring proper treatment. Forefoot diagnoses are typically separated into two main groups: disorders of the great toe and disorders of the lesser toes.

Hallux Valgus ("Bunion")

Although hallux valgus is not unique to the older athletic population, its treatment often differs in seniors compared to their younger counterparts. The bunion can present in many different forms, and the number of surgical and nonsurgical treatments is impressive.

Anatomy and Pathoanatomy

Hallux valgus ("bunion") results from an increased intermetatarsal angle (IMA) between the first and second metatarsals and an increased hallux valgus angle (HVA) between the first metatarsal and the proximal first phalanx (figure 12.14). Although a traumatic "bunion" may occur secondary to a valgus stress on the first MTP joint or injury to the first TMT joint, hallux valgus typically develops by atraumatic means. Some predisposition may exist, particularly with an increased distal metatarsal articular angle (DMAA), hypermobility of the first TMT joint, or pes planus and associated tight Achilles tendon. With malalignment of the first ray, transfer lesions (overload) may occur on the lesser metatarsal heads. This forefoot imbalance may impair push-off for the athlete.

Evaluation

The patient with a symptomatic hallux valgus typically describes forefoot discomfort, particularly with push-off when the forefoot is maximally loaded. The pain may be in the hallux MTP joint, on the lesser metatarsal heads, or both. Clinical evaluation includes (1) assessing the hindfoot alignment (rule out pes planus), (2) ruling out Achilles contracture, (3) evaluating for instability/hypermobility in the first TMT joint, (4) assessing pain in the first MTP joint, (5) determining the first ray alignment, and (6) eliciting secondary symptoms in the lesser metatarsals and MTP joints. Pes planus will promote hallux valgus and drive persistent symptoms at the first MTP joint. Hypermobility at the first ray tends to do the same and leads to lesser metatarsal overload. The easiest means of determining possible hypermobility is with a comparison to the contralateral foot. The first MTP joint may demonstrate some mechanical symptoms, such as crepitance or impingement. Assess range of motion to ensure that dorsiflexion is adequate for athletic participation. Finally, palpate the lesser metatarsals to rule out stress fractures (dorsal palpation) and under the metatarsal heads to assess transfer lesions (pure tenderness vs. callus formation).

Radiographic assessment includes a weight-bearing foot series (non-weight-bearing X-rays may not demonstrate the deformity adequately). Pes planus should be noted if present. The AP X-ray shows the increased IMA, HVA, DMAA, and any stress reactions to the lesser metatarsals from overload. The lateral X-ray may demonstrate instability at the first TMT joint.

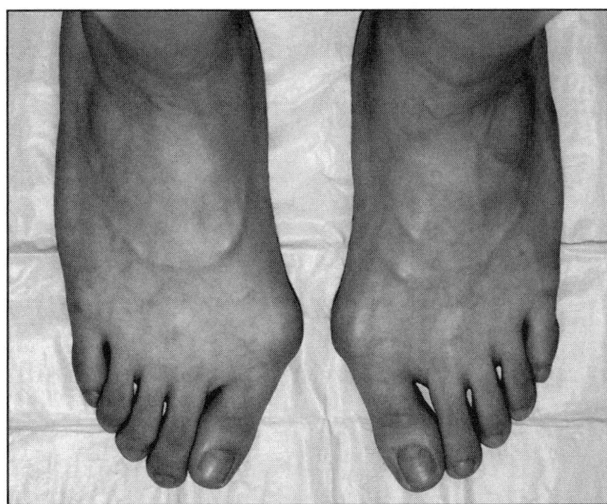

FIGURE 12.14 Hallux valgus demonstrating prominent medial eminence and partial overlap with the second toe.

Treatment

Management of hallux valgus in the athletic patient should be nonoperative if possible. With pes planus, orthotics with longitudinal arch and metatarsal support combined with accommodative athletic shoes should be effective, if prescribed in conjunction with Achilles stretching. If hallux valgus is not relieved with this treatment or if pes planus is not present, accommodative athletic shoes with a wider toe box are prescribed. With continued failure of nonoperative measures, it is appropriate to contemplate surgery, particularly if there is impingement of the first toe on the second (that may lead to second MTP joint instability/pain). The patient needs to understand that first MTP joint stiffness may result from hallux valgus correction and may restrict some athletic activity. The surgical algorithm is based on the IMA (Mann and Coughlin 1999; Myerson and Mendelbaum 2000). Failure of conservative treatment to alleviate symptoms necessitates orthopedic referral for the proper surgical intervention.

Hallux Rigidus

Hallux rigidus is first MTP joint osteoarthritis. It is far more common with advanced age and can be debilitating to senior fitness enthusiasts who speed walk, jog, or run.

Anatomy and Pathoanatomy

Physiologic first MTP joint range of motion is approximately 85° of dorsiflexion to 25° of plantar flexion. Generally, 60° of dorsiflexion is necessary for pain-free normal daily activities; hallux rigidus often prohibits this painless arc of motion. The cause of arthritis in the first MTP is controversial. Initially, the joint presents with synovitis followed by degeneration of the articular surface of the metatarsal head, predominantly the dorsal half. Osteophytes develop along the dorsal, medial, and lateral aspects of the metatarsal head, causing a mechanical impingement to dorsiflexion. This leads to a painful, stiff toe that prevents normal push-off.

Evaluation

Patients present with the complaint of first MTP joint pain, particularly during push-off. Range of motion is limited by dorsal impingement, noted with active and passive dorsiflexion. Often, the dorsal metatarsal head is tender to palpation. Certain athletic shoes may impinge on the dorsal osteophyte. Radiographs may demonstrate the hallmarks of degenerative arthritis including joint space narrowing, dorsal exostosis, and osteophytes. Hallux rigidus is typically graded based on radiographic findings (table 12.2).

Treatment

Nonoperative management is often successful in treating hallux rigidus. While a stiff-soled shoe is appropriate for work, a rocker sole insert across the MTP joint in a commercial sneaker is more appropriate for the athlete. Other custom orthotic inserts may be useful, but one must be careful to ensure that the toe box in the patient's shoe is wide enough to accommodate the enlarged MTP joint and insert.

Operative management is considered when pain becomes too disabling and conservative treatment has failed. For the athlete, surgical treatment should be restricted to joint-preserving procedures, if possible. Grade I and II hallux rigidus typically respond well to dorsal cheilectomy (removing overgrown bone—osteophyte). Removing the dorsal third of the metatarsal head (including the osteophyte) eliminates impingement and improves dorsiflexion. Cheilectomy should be considered for the initial operation since it is simple and does not preclude any further intervention. Arthrodesis of the first MTP joint is reserved for grade III hallux rigidus. This procedure may hinder some athletic activity, although with appropriate shoe wear and orthotic management, some patients may still be able to run provided the fusion is performed in the optimal position. Dorsal cheilectomy may prove beneficial even in advanced disease and should be considered in the athletic patient prior to arthrodesis (Coughlin 1999a; Horton 2000).

Sesamoid Disorders

It is difficult to believe that the sesamoids, relatively small bones seemingly arranged in space, have an important function in the mechanics of the foot. However, they do, and if they are traumatized or become pathologic they can cause significant pain and dysfunction.

Anatomy and Pathoanatomy

There may be three sesamoids located in the great toe. Two are almost always present at the level of the MTP joint, and one may be present at the level of the interphalangeal joint. The tibial sesamoid below the MTP joint is the most commonly injured due to its central location. The mechanism that most commonly results in sesamoid fracture or sprain of the capsuloligamentous complex is hyperextension and axial loading. However, overuse or repetitive stress in the athletic population can produce sesamoid symptoms. Occasionally, sesamoid fracture can occur, with either acute injury or repetitive stress. Not all sesamoid separation is a fracture; some patients may have a bipartite sesamoid. While a lateral bipartite sesamoid is unusual, a bipartite tibial sesamoid is present in 10% of the population and is bilateral in 25% of these individuals.

Other causes of hallucal sesamoid pain include sesamoiditis, osteochondritis, arthritis, and intractable plantar keratoses. Sesamoiditis usually occurs from repetitive trauma but typically occurs in the younger athlete. Osteochondritis frequently follows trauma with resultant osteonecrosis and subsequent regeneration and excessive calcification. Arthritis of the metatarsal sesamoid articulation can result from sesamoiditis, trauma, or chondromalacia. Plantar keratoses can be either localized or diffuse. A localized keratosis usually results from a sesamoid with a plantarly located osseous prominence or a first metatarsal with reduced dorsiflexion.

TABLE 12.2 Radiographic Classification of Hallux Rigidus

Grade	Radiographic findings
I	Minimal narrowing with dorsal osteophytes
II	More extensive narrowing with plantar joint preservation
III	Complete joint space narrowing and severe arthritis

Evaluation

Patients present with a uniform complaint of pain about the first MTP joint, predominantly on the plantar surface. The patient may demonstrate diffuse tenderness of the first MTP joint on examination, but more directed palpation of each sesamoid may localize the pain to these structures. Routine radiographs should include an AP and lateral X-rays. Axial sesamoid views may also be useful. Negative radiographs in a symptomatic patient should prompt a bone scan that is directed to the forefoot and sesamoids. Infiltration with a short-acting local anesthetic over the sesamoid may have diagnostic value.

Treatment

Treatment is generally nonoperative. Sesamoid disorders often respond to nonsteroidal anti-inflammatory agents, activity modification, temporary immobilization, and unloading of the first MTP joint, followed by orthotic use and shoe wear modifications. Rarely, excision of the sesamoid needs to be considered if conservative management proves inadequate. In select cases, nonunions of sesamoid fractures may benefit from bone grafting or partial excision.

Hallux Metatarsophalangeal Joint Sprain

Sprain of the hallux MTP, or "turf toe," is an injury to the capsule and ligaments that connect the foot to the great toe.

Etiology and Evaluation

Turf toe is typically caused by hyperextension of the first MTP joint. Usually it occurs in the older patient who still plays sports such as basketball, football, or soccer. Turf toe injuries are divided into three grades by severity. Severity increases from stretch of the joint capsule and ligaments to partial tear and complete tear of the joint capsule and ligaments. Trauma to the first MTP joint is a potentially devastating injury for the athlete, and one should maintain a high index of suspicion when a patient reports a hyperextension injury to the great toe. This history is usually accompanied by pain, tenderness, and swelling. Radiographs of both the affected and unaffected foot should be obtained to compare the position of the sesamoids. Magnetic resonance imaging may be useful in defining a soft tissue injury to the sesamoid complex.

Treatment

Treatment centers on rest in the acute stage of injury with light mobilization in the subacute stage. Since a turf toe is a sprain of the plantar first MTP joint, immobilization initially includes taping or splinting in slight plantarflexion. However, with a complete disruption of the sesamoid complex, surgical intervention should be delayed only as long as it takes the soft tissue swelling to resolve. If the sesamoid complex injury becomes chronic, successful reconstruction and return to sport may be limited. In milder-grade injuries, early range of motion is feasible. With more severe injuries, immobilization for several weeks is imperative, unless surgical reconstruction was performed, in which case gentle range of motion may begin once the incision has healed. Ultimately, stiff insoles, stiffer-soled shoes, or both, are worn for athletic competition to protect from reinjury (Clanton 1999).

Capsulitis

The diagnosis of capsulitis usually relies completely on physical exam. This condition can be debilitating, but almost never requires surgery.

Anatomy and Pathoanatomy

Capsulitis is an inflammation/degeneration of the plantar capsule or plantar plate complex. Patients typically describe focal discomfort under the "ball of the foot" and possibly even a specific metatarsal head or joint.

Evaluation

Symptoms are especially evident with walking barefooted on hard surfaces or with hard-soled shoes that lack padding; relief is noted with softer surfaces or insoles. Physical examination demonstrates tenderness under the involved MTP joint and metatarsal head. The Achilles tendon should be examined; even a slight equinus contracture may lead to forefoot overload in an athletic patient. Radiographs are typically unremarkable; however, X-rays may reveal that the involved metatarsal is relatively long compared to the adjacent metatarsals, leading to overload.

Treatment

Unloading the affected metatarsal head usually relieves symptoms. This can initially be accomplished by means of a temporary metatarsal pad and permanently by means of an orthotic designed with a metatarsal pad. If the heel cord shows tightness, then Achilles stretching should begin. Capsulitis is a nonsurgical problem, particularly in the athlete.

Synovitis

Synovitis, or inflammation of the MTP joint, is often due to direct trauma but more likely represents an overuse or overload phenomenon.

Anatomy and Pathoanatomy

Although the problem may arise in an athletic patient, several factors may predispose to increased stress at the MTP joint, including

- injury to the affected MTP joint,
- longer length of the involved metatarsal relative to the adjacent metatarsals, and
- transfer of stress from hallux valgus to the lesser MTP joints.

Without a period of activity modification and metatarsal unloading, the problem tends to persist, as the patient continues to stress the joint with weight bearing, particularly with athletic participation.

Evaluation

The patient notes dorsal and plantar pain at the involved MTP joint with associated swelling. Occasionally, the edema leads to inflammation of the adjacent interdigital nerve, and the entity can easily be confused with interdigital neuralgia. In advanced stages, the plantar capsular tissue, collateral ligaments, or both, become attenuated, leading to joint instability and resultant toe deformity. Instability can be demonstrated with a "drawer test."

Treatment

Management is nonoperative. Rest, anti-inflammatory agents, use of a hammertoe sling, and temporary use of a stiff-soled shoe typically relieve symptoms. Recalcitrant cases may benefit from a single steroid injection directly into the MTP joint (multiple injections should be avoided as they may exacerbate attenuation of the plantar plate and collateral ligaments). For maintenance, shoe wear should have stiffer soles or inserts with less flexion at the MTP joints.

Metatarsophalangeal Joint Instability

Chronic capsulitis or synovitis may eventually lead to capsular attrition with collateral insufficiency; therefore, it is important to properly treat inflammation of the lesser MTP joints.

Pathoanatomy

Left untreated, the MTP joint may subluxate/dislocate dorsally when the plantar plate degenerates or may subluxate medially or laterally, with loss of collateral capsular and ligamentous support. In severe cases, the MTP joint dislocates dorsally and deviates medially, particularly with associated hallux valgus. Pure plantar plate disease leads to dislocation into dorsiflexion; pure collateral disease typically leads to medial deviation. A more diffusely involved joint subluxates/dislocates dorsally and displaces medially. This entity becomes quite symptomatic because of the excess pressure on the involved metatarsal head. A grading scheme has been devised:

Grade I: synovitis/inflammation
Grade II: subluxation
Grade III: dislocatable
Grade IV: fixed dislocation

Evaluation

The patient complains of pain at the MTP joint and toe displacement, with worsening plantar pain at the metatarsal head and shoe wear difficulties dorsally. Tenderness is noted at the MTP joint, as with capsulitis and synovitis. In milder disease, a toe "drawer test" demonstrates MTP joint subluxation, dislocation, or both; in severe disease the toe is fixed in a dislocated position, either dorsally or dorsally and medially. Radiographs demonstrate subluxation/displacement/dislocation of the involved joint and may reveal a relatively long metatarsal of the involved joint.

Treatment

In milder disease, rest, anti-inflammatory agents, and a hammertoe sling or taping with a stiffer shoe can effectively limit symptoms. However, this fails to improve the attenuation of the capsular tissues. In moderate and severe disease, the treatment requires the realignment and soft tissue reconstruction to maintain MTP joint stability. Even with successful realignment, return to athletic activity may occassionally be limited by postsurgical stiffness and limitation of the toe dorsiflexion (Coughlin and Mann 1999).

Interdigital Neuralgia

While any of the interdigital nerves can be compressed, perhaps the most infamous is Morton's neuroma, which involves the nerve common to the third and fourth toes. This is actually not a true neuroma but rather a perineural fibrosis where the nerve passes under the metatarsal ligament.

Anatomy and Pathoanatomy

An interdigital nerve may become compressed under the transverse intermetatarsal ligament, particularly with repetitive athletic activity such as running. The third web space digital nerve is most commonly involved, probably for two reasons: (1) A thicker nerve is typically present in this location because it is formed by a confluence of the medial and lateral plantar nerves, and (2) the lateral two metatarsals have greater motion as compared to the relatively immobile medial three metatarsals. Although interdigital neuralgia may develop in the second web space, this is typically secondary to second MTP joint synovitis.

Evaluation

The patient typically complains of lateral foot pain and burning that radiates distally to the adjacent two toes.

Numbness may also be reported in the two toes. In addition, tighter shoe wear exacerbates the symptoms. Physical findings include

- web space/intermetatarsal tenderness,
- decreased web space sensation,
- a positive percussion test in the web space, and occasionally
- a positive Mulder's click with transverse forefoot compression.

Treatment

Nonoperative treatment includes wider toe box shoes with a stiffer forefoot to avoid hyperdorsiflexion that might compress the nerve. Although pads have been recommended, the concern is that padding may aggravate the symptoms. A web space injection of an anesthetic and corticosteroid may be both diagnostic and therapeutic. The transient effect of the anesthetic typically gives excellent relief of symptoms if the diagnosis is truly a Morton's neuroma; the steroid may provide longer relief. If the injection was successful in relieving symptoms but only temporarily, surgical release of the transverse intermetatarsal ligament and interdigital nerve excision usually is successful in permanently relieving symptoms. The nerve must be resected proximally, away from the weight-bearing surface of the forefoot, or the formation of a new neuroma may lead to recurrent or persistent symptoms.

Freiberg's Infraction

Avascular necrosis of a lesser metatarsal head ("Freiberg's infraction"), usually the second, is probably an overuse syndrome. With excessive stress, the metatarsal head loses its blood supply, particularly the dorsal one-half to one-third. With advanced disease, the arthritic changes develop in the MTP joint.

Evaluation

The patient complains of pain with push off in the affected MTP joint and pain with dorsiflexion. Tenderness is noted at the metatarsal head, as is painful range of motion, particularly dorsiflexion. Occasionally, a block to dorsiflexion is observed due to formation of a dorsal osteophyte. Radiographs may demonstrate a flattened metatarsal head, and MRI confirms the avascular changes.

Treatment

Nonoperative treatment may be successful in mild disease, with rest, anti-inflammatory agents, and a stiffer-soled shoe or insert. With moderate-to-severe disease, joint debridement and dorsal cheilectomy, similar to that recommended for hallux rigidus, may be successful. In order to further decompress the joint and possibly bring healthier articular cartilage from the plantar metatarsal head more dorsally, one may consider a capital dorsiflexion osteotomy of the metatarsal (Daniels 2000).

Metatarsal Stress Fracture

Stress fractures occur with excessive, repetitive overload of a metatarsal. Continued forefoot loading as in running may eventually create a fatigue failure of the metatarsal. In people with osteopenia, the same stress fracture may occur under physiologic conditions.

Evaluation

Patients complain of forefoot pain with weight bearing. Typically point tenderness is noted over the involved metatarsal; this is often associated with forefoot edema. Evaluation needs to include the Achilles tendon, as even a slight equinus contracture may lead to considerable forefoot overload. Radiographs may not reveal a fracture, but cortical hypertrophy may be present. The fracture is typically not evident radiographically for several weeks or even months after the onset of symptoms.

Treatment

Treatment is aimed at unloading the involved metatarsal. A postoperative shoe, cam walker, or cast is typically necessary for adequate pressure relief. The fracture may be considered healed when the involved metatarsal is no longer tender. Achilles stretching should be initiated if an equinus contracture is present. Once fracture healing has occurred, activity or shoe wear modifications are required to maintain pressure relief on the metatarsal. Occasionally, stress fractures are secondary to instability of the first ray, and a first TMT joint arthrodesis may be necessary (Sanders 1999; Scranton 2000).

Toenail Disorders

Toenail observation is of utmost importance in the aging athlete. Disorders of the toenail of special concern are traumatic onychodystrophy, onychomycosis, verrucae, and ingrown toenails. Some knowledge of other conditions such as melanoma, fibroma, and subungual/periungual epidermoid carcinoma is necessary to avoid misdiagnosis of a benign condition.

Traumatic Onychodystrophy

Trauma to a toenail may result in temporary or permanent onchodystrophy or discoloration of the nail. Often, the preceding trauma goes unnoticed by the patient, who presents with a brownish-blue to black discoloration of the subungual area, representing hematoma below the nail. This problem most often occurs in athletes who wear shoes with a tight toe box and participate in sudden-stopping sports such as tennis. When the foot slides forward creating toenail trauma, the problem may exist even in a shoe that is not too tight. It is important to rule out the possibility of subungual melanoma before proceeding with benign neglect or treatment. Two properties that favor the exclusion of melanoma are the existence of similar discoloration on a contralateral or adjacent toenail and greater size and length of the affected nail compared to its companions, which makes it more prone to injury. Biopsy is rarely necessary. Treatment is often benign neglect or paring of the nail plate overlying the area in question to allow blood extravasation if hematoma is present.

Onychomycosis

Infection with fungi is one of the most common abnormalities of toenails. The organism most commonly responsible for infection is *Trichophyton rubrum.* Changes to the nail plate and surrounding tissue include

- thickening of the nail plate;
- accumulation of keratin subungually;
- whitish, yellowish, or brownish discoloration of the nail; and
- of the periungual tissues (figure 12.15).

While the hallucal nail is most commonly involved, the second toenail is uncommonly involved. Patients often present for treatment because the thickened toe is painful when the shoe presses on it and socks catch on the rough dystrophic onychomycotic toenail. Many topical and oral agents help eradicate onychomycosis, but this can be a lengthy process and requires patience on the part of both the physician and patient. Seldom is surgical removal of an onychomycotic nail indicated. Local measures such as avoiding restrictive footwear, maintaining proper pedal hygiene, the restricted use of nylon socks or stockings, and use of absorbent powder can help prevent infection.

Verrucae

Verrucae, otherwise known as warts, may affect the periungual tissue of the toes. This can result in onchodystrophy and possibly a painful toe. Although these lesions are often easily diagnosed, they can frequently mimic a subungual fibroma or exostosis. Suspicious lesions should be biopsied. Treatment centers on desiccation and curettage if necessary. The nail plate may have to be lifted or trimmed to provide access to the wart.

Ingrown Toenails

An ingrown toenail often results from wearing constricting or foreshortened shoe wear. Often there is an associated subungual exostosis. Typically, the nail plate penetrates into the soft periungual tissues, usually the

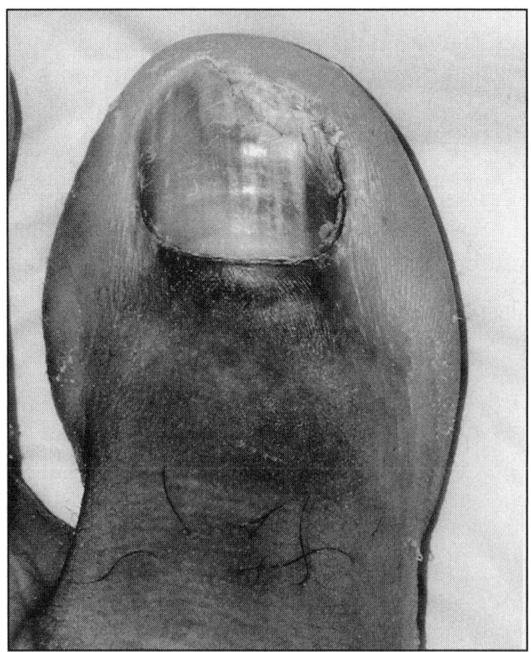

FIGURE 12.15 Onychomycotic changes of the great toe.

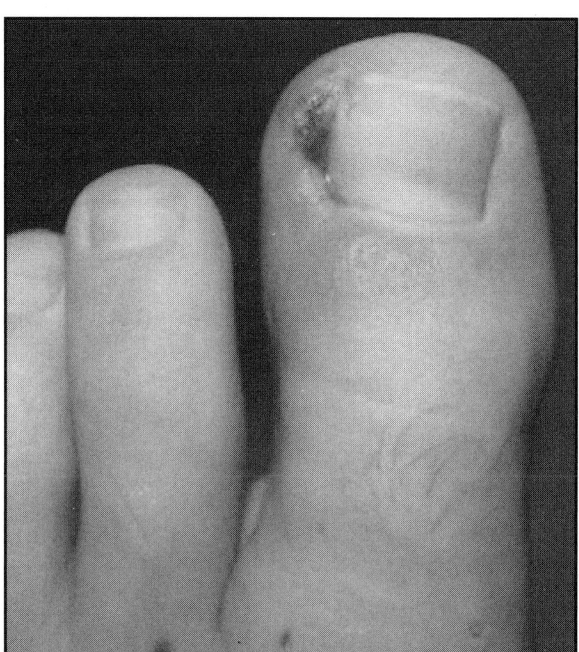

FIGURE 12.16 Characteristic changes of an ingrown toenail with superimposed infection.

lateral and distal nail folds. In chronic cases, granulation tissue may develop along the nail folds. Secondary bacterial infection can occur and necessitate antibiotic therapy (figure 12.16). Intervention entails removing the infiltrating portion of the nail plate with or without removal of the germinal matrix (from which nail growth emanates). Shoe wear modifications, including wider toe boxes, generally maintain adequate pressure relief on the toenails.

SUMMARY

A wide variety of foot and ankle disorders can affect the athlete. Active seniors are predisposed to many of these maladies due to repetitive microtrauma to soft tissues and bones over their many years of activity. In addition, many are "weekend warriors" secondary to their weekday responsibilities at work and at home. Predisposition to injury due to the decreased flexibility and muscle atrophy that occur with age, combined with sporadic training practices in these patients, dramatically increases these individuals' chance of injury. Many of these injuries are addressed with nonoperative means but occasionally demand an orthopedic referral for surgical intervention. When confronted with a foot or ankle injury or disease process in an active senior it is essential not only to diagnose the malady but also to assess the patient's biomechanics and foot and ankle alignment. Addressing any underlying abnormalities in gait or foot position with appropriate shoe wear and orthotics can be paramount to successful treatment. In addition, physical therapy for improved proprioception, strength, and range of motion is essential. It is imperative that the active senior athlete work closely with his or her primary care doctors, physical therapist, athletic trainer, and orthopedist to maximize performance and minimize most preventable injuries.

References

Chapter 1

Brown, J.E., Branch, T.P. 2000. Surgical alternatives for treatment of articular cartilage lesions. *J Am Acad Orthop Surg* 8: 180-189.

Buckwalter, J.A., Woo, S.L.-Y., Goldberg, V.M., Hadley, E.C., Booth, F., Oegema, T.R., Eyre, D.R. 1993. Soft tissue aging and musculoskeletal function. *J Bone Joint Surg Am* 75(10): 1533-1548.

Centers for Disease Control and Prevention. 1997. Impact of arthritis and other rheumatic conditions on the health care system: United States, 1997. *JAMA* 281: 2177-2178.

Clark, J.M., Harryman, D.T. II. 1992. Tendons, ligaments, and capsule of the rotator cuff: Gross and microscopic anatomy. *J Bone Joint Surg Am* 74(5): 713-725.

Cooper, D.E., Arnoczky, S.P., O'Brien, S.J., Warren, R.F., DiCarlo, E., Allen, A.A. 1992. Anatomy, histology, and vascularity of the glenoid labrum: An anatomical study. *J Bone Joint Surg Am* 74(1): 46-52.

Garrett, W.E. Jr., Best, T.M. 1994. Anatomy, physiology and mechanics of skeletal muscle. In *Orthopaedic basic science*. ed. S.R. Simon. Rosemont, IL: American Academy of Orthopaedic Surgeons, pp. 89-125.

Gohlke, F., Essigkrug, B., Schmitz, F. 1994. The pattern of collagen fiber bundles of the capsule of the gleno-humeral joint. *J Shoulder Elbow Surg* 3: 111-128.

Herndon, J.H., Robbins, P.D., Evans, C.H. 1999. Arthritis: Is the cure in your genes? *J Bone Joint Surg Am* 81(2): 152-157.

Lane, J.M., Russell, L., Khan, S.N. 2000. Osteoporosis. *Clin Orthop* 372: 139-150.

LaPrade, R.F., Swiontkowske, M.F. 1999. New horizons in the treatment of osteoarthritis of the knee. *JAMA* 281: 876-878.

Luff, A.R. 1998. Review: Age-associated changes in the innervations of muscle fibers an changes in the mechanical properties of motor units. *Ann NY Acad Sci* 854: 92-101.

Mont, M.A., Jones, L.C., Sotereanos, D.G., Amstutz, H.C., Hungerford, D.S. 2000. Understanding and treating orteonecrosis of the femoral head. *Instr Course Lect* 49: 169-185.

Mow, V.C., Ratcliffe, A., Chern, K.Y., Kelly, M.A. 1992. *Structure and function relationships of menisci of knee: Knee meniscus: Basic and clinical foundations.* New York: Raven Press, p. 40.

Spindler, K.P., Wright, R.W. 2002. Soft-tissue physiology and repair. *Orthopaedic Knowledge Update (OKU) 7: Home Study Syllabus*, pp. 3-18.

Terjung, R.L., Clarkson, P., Eichner, E.R., Greenhaff, P.L., Hespel, P.J., Israel, R.G., Kraemer, W.J., Meyer, R.A., Spriet, L.L., Tarnopolsky, M.A., Wagenmakers, A.J., Williams, M.H. 2000. American College of Sports Medicine roundtable: The physiological and health effects of oral creatine supplementation. *Med Sci Sports Exerc* 32(3): 706-717.

Chapter 2

Altchiler, L., Motta, R. 1994. Effects of aerobic and nonaerobic exercise on anxiety, absenteeism, and job satisfaction. *Journal of Clinical Psychology* 50: 829-840.

Åstrand, I. 1960. Aerobic work capacity in men and women with special reference to age. *Acta Physiol Scand* 49 (Suppl 169): 1-92.

Åstrand, P.O., Ryhming, I. 1954. A nomogram for calculation of aerobic capacity (physical fitness) from pulse rate during submaximal work. *J Appl Physiol* 7: 218-221.

Baker, K., McAlindon, T. 2000. Exercise for knee osteoarthritis. *Curr Opin Rheumatol* 12: 456-463.

Balady, G.J., Berra, K.A., Golding, L.A., Gordon, N.F., Mahler, D.A., Myers, J.N., Sheldahl, L.M. 2000. *ACSM's guidelines for exercise testing and prescription.* Baltimore: Lippincott Williams & Wilkins.

Balke, B., Ware, R.W. 1959. An experimental graded exercise test protocol. *U.S. Armed Forces Med J* 10: 675-688.

Beckham, S.G., Earnest, C.P. 2000. Metabolic cost of free weight circuit weight training. *J Sports Med Phys Fitness* 40: 118-125.

Bell, R.D., Hoshizaki, T.B. 1981. Relationships of age and sex with range of motion of seventeen joint actions in humans. *Can J Appl Sport Sci* 6: 202-206.

Bemben, D.A., Fetters, N.L., Bemben, M.B., Nabavi, N., Koh, E.T. 2000. Musculoskeletal responses to high- and low-intensity resistance training in early postmenopasal women. *Med Sci Sports Exerc* 32: 1949-1957.

Binder, E.F., Birge, S.J., Spina, R., Ehsani, A.A., Brown, M., Sinacore, D.R., Kohrt, W.M. 1999. Peak aerobic power is an important component of physical performance in older women. *J Gerontology A Biol Sci Med Sci* 54: M353-M356.

Blair, S.N., Kohl III, H.W., Paffenbarger, R.S. Jr., Clark, D.G., Cooper, K.H., Gibbons, L.W. 1989. Physical fitness and all-cause mortality: A prospective study of healthy men and women. *JAMA* 262: 2395-2401.

Booth, F.W., Weeden, S.H., Tseng, B.S. 1994. Effect of aging on human skeletal muscle and motor function. *Med Sci Sports Exerc* 26: 556-560.

Borg, G. 1970. Perceived exertion as an indicator of somatic stress. *Scand J Rehabil Med* 2: 92-98.

Borg, G. 1982. Ratings of perceived exertion and heart rates during short-term cycle exercise and their use in a new cycling strength test. *Int J Sports Med* 3: 153-158.

Borg, G., 1998. *Borg's perceived exertion and pain scales.* Champaign, IL: Human Kinetics.

Borst, S.E., De Hoyos, D.V., Garzarella, L., Vincent, K., Pollock, B.H., Lowenthal, D.T., Pollock, M.L. 2001. Effects of resistance training on insulin-like growth factor-I and IGF binding proteins. *Med Sci Sports Exerc* 33: 648-653.

Braith, R.W., Graves, J.E., Pollock, M.L., Leggett, S.L., Carpenter, D.M., Colvin, A.B. 1989. Comparison of 2 vs 3 days/week of variable resistance training during 10- and 18-week programs. *Int J Sports Med* 10: 450-454.

Brand, R.A., Pedersen, D.R., Friederich, J.A. 1986. The sensitivity of muscle force predictions to changes in physiologic cross-sectional area. *J Biomech* 19: 589-596.

Brill, P.A., Probst, J.C., Greenhouse, D.L., Schell, B., Macera, C.A. 1998. Clinical feasibility of a free-weight strength-training program for older adults. *Journal of the American Board of Family Practice* 11: 445-451.

Brischetto, M.J., Millman, R.P., Peterson, D.D., Silage, D.A., Pack, A.I. 1984. Effect of aging on ventilatory response to exercise and CO2. *J Appl Physiol* 56: 1143-1150.

Bruce, R.A., Kusumi, F., Hosmer, D. 1973. Maximal oxygen intake and nomographic assessment of functional aerobic impairment in cardiovascular disease. *Am Heart J* 85: 546-562.

Buchner, D.M., Cress, M.E., de Lateur, B.J., Esselman, P.C., Margherita, A.J., Price, R., Wagner, E.H. 1997. The effect of strength and endurance training on gait, balance, fall risk, and health services use in community-living older adults. *J Gerontology A Biol Sci Med Sci* 52: M218-M224.

Bunyard, L.B., Katzel, L.I., Busby-Whitehead, M.J., Wu, Z., Goldberg, A.P. 1998. Energy requirements of middle-aged men are modifiable by physical activity. *Am J Clin Nutr* 68: 1136-1142.

Burger, H., van Daele, P.L., Algra, D., van den Ouweland, F.A., Grobbee, D.E., Hofman, A., van Kuijk, C., Schutte, H.E., Birkenhager, J.C., Pols, H.A. 1994. The association between age and bone mineral density in men and women aged 55 years and over: The Rotterdam Study. *Bone and Mineral* 25: 1-13.

Campbell, W.W., Crim, M.C., Young, V.R., and Evans, W.J. 1994. Increased energy requirements and changes in body composition with resistance training in older adults. *Am J Clin Nutr* 60: 167-75.

Carpinelli, R.N., Otto, R.M. 1998. Strength training: Single versus multiple sets. *Sports Med* 26: 73-84.

Chien, M.Y., Wu, Y.T., Hsu, A.T., Yang, R.S., Lai, J.S. 2000. Efficacy of a 24-week aerobic exercise program for osteopenic postmenopausal women. *Calcif Tissue Int* 67: 443-448.

Convertino, V.A., Ludwig, D.A. 2000. Validity of VO(2 max) in predicting blood volume: implications for the effect of fitness on aging. *Am J Physiol Regul Integr Comp Physiol* 279: R1068-R1075.

Cooper, K.H. 1968. A means of assessing maximal oxygen intake. *JAMA* 3: 135-138.

Csuka, M., McCarty, D.J. 1985. Simple method for measurement of lower extremity muscle strength. *Am J Med* 78: 77-81.

Davy, K.P., Seals, D.R. 1994. Total blood volume in healthy young and older men. *J Appl Physiol* 76: 2059-2062.

DeLorme, T.L., Watkins, A.L. 1948. Techniques of progressive resistance exercise. *Arch Phys Med* 29: 263-273.

Dengel, D.R., Hagberg, J.M., Pratley, R.E., Rogus, E.M., Goldberg, A.P. 1998. Improvements in blood pressure, glucose metabolism, and lipoprotein lipids after aerobic exercise plus weight loss in obese, hypertensive middle-aged men. *Metabolism* 47: 1075-1082.

DiPietro, L., Seeman, T.E., Stachenfeld, N.S., Katz, L.D., Nadel, E.R. 1998. Moderate-intensity aerobic training improves glucose tolerance in aging independent of abdominal adiposity. *J Am Geriatr Soc* 46: 875-879.

Ebbeling, C.B., Ward, A., Puleo, E.M., Widrick, J., Rippe, J.M. 1991. Development of a single-stage submaximal treadmill walking test. *Med Sci Sports Exerc* 23: 966-973.

Eriksson, J., Taimela, S., Eriksson, K., Parviainen, S., Peltonen, J., Kujala, U. 1997. Resistance training in the treatment of non-insulin-dependent diabetes mellitus. *Int J Sports Med* 18: 242-246.

Etnier, J., Johnston, R., Dagenbach, D., Pollard, R.J., Rejeski, W.J., Berry, M. 1999. The relationships among pulmonary function, aerobic fitness, and cognitive functioning in older COPD patients. *Chest* 116: 953-960.

Ettinger, W.H. Jr., Afable, R.F. 1994. Physical disability from knee osteoarthritis: the role of exercise as an intervention. *Med Sci Sports Exerc* 26: 1435-1440.

Fiatarone, M.A., Marks, E.C., Ryan, N.D., Meredith, C.N., Lipsitz, L.A., Evans, W.J. 1990. High-intensity strength training in nonagenarians: Effects on skeletal muscle. *JAMA* 263: 3029-3034.

Foster, C., Jackson, A.S., Pollock, M.L., Taylor, M.M., Hare, J., Sennett, S.M., Rod, J.L., Sarwar, M., Schmidt, D.H. 1984. Generalized equations for predicting functional capacity from treadmill performance. *Am Heart J* 107: 1229-1234.

Frontera, W.R., Meredith, C.N., O'Reilly, K.P., Knuttgen, H.G., Evans, W.J. 1988. Strength conditioning in older men: Skeletal muscle hypertrophy and improved function. *J Appl Physiol* 64: 1038-1044.

Galloway, M.T., Jokl, P. 2000. Aging successfully: the importance of physical activity in maintaining health and function. *J Am Acad Orthop Surg* 8: 37-44.

Garfinkel, S., Cafarelli, E. 1992. Relative changes in maximal force, EMG, and muscle cross-sectional area after isometric training. *Med Sci Sports Exerc* 24: 1220-1227.

Garhammer, J. 1993. A review of power output studies of olympic and power lifting: methodology, performance prediction, and evaluation tests. *J Strength Cond Res* 7: 76-89.

Garhammer, J., McLaughlin, T. 1980. Power output as a function of load variation in olympic and power lifting. *J Biomech* 3: 198.

Gregg, E.W., Pereira, M.A., Caspersen, C.J. 2000. Physical activity, falls, and fractures among older adults: A review of the epidemiologic evidence. *J Am Geriatr Soc* 48: 883-893.

Haff, G.G. 2000. Roundtable discussion: machines versus free weights. *Strength and Conditioning Journal* 22: 18-30.

Hakkinen, K., Alen, M., Kallinen, M., Newton, R.U., Kraemer, W.J. 2000. Neuromuscular adaptation during prolonged strength training, detraining and re-strength-training in middle-aged and elderly people. *Eur J Appl Physiol* 83: 51-62.

Halbert, J.A., Silagy, C.A., Finucane, P., Withers, R.T., Hamdorf, P.A., Andrews, G.R. 1997. The effectiveness of exercise training in lowering blood pressure: a meta-analysis of randomised controlled trials of 4 weeks or longer. *J Human Hyperten* 11: 641-649.

Hepple, R.T., Mackinnon, S.L., Goodman, J.M., Thomasm, S.G., Plyley, M.J. 1997. Resistance and aerobic training in older men: Effects on VO2peak and the capillary supply to skeletal muscle. *J Appl Physiol* 82: 1305-1310.

Hettinger, R., Muller, E. 1953. Muskelleistung und Muskeltraining. *Arbeits Physiologie* 15: 111-126.

Hoeger, W.W.K., Hopkins, D.R., Barette, S.L., Hale, D.F. 1990. Relationship between repetitions and selected percentages of one repetition maximum: A comparison between untrained and trained males and females. *J Appl Sport Sci Res* 4: 47-54.

Honkola, A., Forsen, T., Eriksson, J. 1997. Resistance training improves the metabolic profile in individuals with type 2 diabetes. *Acta diabetologica* 34: 245-248.

Johnson, J.H., Colodny, S., Jackson, D. 1990. Human torque capability versus machine resistive torque for four Eagle resistive machines. *J Appl Sport Sci Res* 4: 83-87.

Judge, J.O., Underwood, M., Gennosa, T. 1993. Exercise to improve gait velocity in older persons. *Arch Phys Med Rehabil* 74: 400-406.

Kannus, P., Jozsa, L., Natri, A., Jarvinen, M. 1997. Effects of training, immobilization and remobilization on tendons. *Scan J Med Sci Sports* 7: 67-71.

Karvonen, M., Kentala, E., Mustala, O. 1957. The effects of training on heart rate. *Ann Med Exp Biol Fenn* 35: 307-315.

Kelley, G.A., Sharpe Kelley, K. 2001. Aerobic exercise and resting blood pressure in older adults: $a meta-analytic review of randomized controlled trials. *J Gerontology A Biol Sci Med Sci* 56: M298-M303.

Kline, G.M., Porcari, J.P., Hintermeister, R., Freedson, P.S., Ward, A., McCarron, R.F., Ross, J., Rippe, J.M. 1987. Estimation of VO2max from a one-mile track walk, gender, age, and body weight. *Med Sci Sports Exerc* 19: 253-259.

Kohrt, W.M., Malley, M.T., Coggan, A.R., Spina, R.J., Ogawa, T., Ehsani, A.A., Bourey, R.E., Martin, 3rd, W.H., Holloszy, J.O. 1991. Effects of gender, age, and fitness level on response of VO2max to training in 60-71 yr olds. *J Appl Physiol* 71: 2004-2011.

Komi, P.V., Viitasalo, J.T., Rauramaa, R., Vihko, V. 1978. Effect of isometric strength training of mechanical, electrical, and metabolic aspects of muscle function. *Eur J Appl Physiol and Occupational Physiology* 40: 45-55.

Kraemer, W.J., Hakkinen, K., Newton, R.U., Nindl, B.C., Volek, J.S., McCormick, M., r Gotshalk, L.A., Gordon, S.E., Fleck, S.J., Campbell, W.W., Putukian, M., Evans, W.J. 1999. Effects of heavy-resistance training on hormonal response patterns in younger vs. older men. *J Appl Physiol* 87: 982-992.

Kraemer, W.J., Ratamess, N., Fry, A.C., Triplett-McBride, T., Koziris, L.P., Bauer, J.A., Lynch, J.M., Fleck, S.J. 2000. Influence of resistance training volume and periodization on physiological and performance adaptations in collegiate women tennis players. *Am J Sports Med* 28: 626-633.

Kraemer, W.J., Stone, M.H., O'Bryant, H.S., Conley, M.S., Johnson, R.L., Nieman, D.C., Honeycutt, D.R., Hoke, T.P. 1997. Effects of single vs. multiple sets of weight training: Impact of volume, intensity, and variation. *J Strength Cond Res* 11: 143-147.

Kuhlman, K.A. 1993. Cervical range of motion in the elderly. *Arch Phys Med Rehabil* 74: 1071-1079.

Kyle, U.G., Genton, L., Hans, D., Karsegard, L., Slosman, D.O., Pichard, C. 2001. Age-related differences in fat-free mass, skeletal muscle, body cell mass and fat mass between 18 and 94 years. *Eur J Clin Nutr* 55: 663-672.

Layne, J.E., Nelson, M.E. 1999. The effects of progressive resistance training on bone density: A review. *Med Sci Sports Exerc* 31: 25-30.

Lee, I.M., Hsieh, C.C., Paffenbarger, R.S. Jr. 1995. Exercise intensity and longevity in men. The Harvard Alumni Health Study. *JAMA* 273: 1179-1184.

Lemmer, J.T., Ivey, F.M., Ryan, A.S., Martel, G.F., Hurlbut, D.E., Metter, J.E., Fozard, J.L., Fleg, J.L., Hurley, B.F. 2001. Effect of strength training on resting metabolic rate and physical activity: Age and gender comparisons. *Med Sci Sports Exerc* 33: 532-541.

Lemon, P.W. 1998. Effects of exercise on dietary protein requirements. *Int J Sport Nutr* 8: 426-447.

Mannion, A.F., Jakeman, P.M., Willan, P.L. 1992. Effects of isokinetic training of the knee extensors on isometric strength and peak power output during cycling. *Eur J Appl Physiol and Occupational Physiology* 65: 370-375.

Marley, W.P., Linnerud, A.C. 1976. A three-year study of the Astrand-Ryhming step test. *Res Q* 47(2): 211-217.

Martel, G.F., Hurlbut, D.E., Lott, M.E., Lemmer, J.T., Ivey, F.M., Roth, S.M., Rogers, M.A., Fleg, J.L., Hurley, B.F. 1999. Strength training normalizes resting blood pressure in 65- to 73-year-old men and women with high normal blood pressure. *J Am Geriatr Soc* 47: 1215-1221.

Mayhew, J.L., Ware, J.R., Prinster, J.L. 1993. Using lift repetitions to predict muscular strength in adolescent males. *National Strength and Conditioning Association Journal* 15: 35-38.

Mazzeo, R.S., Cavanagh, P., Evans, W.J., Fiatarone, M.A., Hagberg, J.M., McAuley, E., Startzell, J. 1998. American College of Sports Medicine position stand. Exercise and physical activity for older adults. *Med Sci Sports Exerc* 30: 992-1008.

McLester, J.R., Bishop, P., Guilliams, M.E. 2000. Comparison of 1 day and 3 days per week of equal-volume resistance training in experienced subjects. *J Strength Cond Res* 14: 273-281.

Messier, S.P., Royer, T.D., Craven, T.E., O'Toole, M.L., Burns, R., Ettinger Jr., W.H. 2000. Long-term exercise and its effect on balance in older, osteoarthritic adults: Results from the Fitness, Arthritis, and Seniors Trial (FAST). *J Am Geriatr Soc* 48: 131-138.

Miller, T.R., Grossman, S.J., Schectman, K.B., Biello, D.R., Ludbrook, P.A., Ehsani, A.A. 1986. Left ventricular diastolic filling and its association with age. *Am J Cardiol* 58: 531-535.

Miller, W.C., Wallace, J.P., Eggert, K.E. 1993. Predicting max HR and the HR-VO2 relationship for exercise prescription in obesity. *Med Sci Sports Exerc* 25: 1077-1081.

Moore, K.A., Blumenthal, J.A. 1998. Exercise training as an alternative treatment for depression among older adults. *Altern Ther Health Med* 4: 48-56.

Morrissey, M.C., Harman, E.A., Johnson, M.J. 1995. Resistance training modes: specificity and effectiveness. *Med Sci Sports Exerc* 27: 648-660.

Motoyama, M., Sunami, Y., Kinoshita, F., Irie, T., Sasaki, J., Arakawa, K., Kiyonaga, A., Tanaka, H., Shindo, M. 1995. The effects of long-term low intensity aerobic training and detraining on serum lipid and lipoprotein concentrations in elderly men and women. *European J Appl Physiol* 70: 126-131.

Nelson, M.E., Fiatarone, M.A., Morganti, C.M., Trice, I., Greenberg, R.A., Evans, W.J. 1994. Effects of high-intensity strength training on multiple risk factors for osteoporotic fractures. A randomized controlled trial. *JAMA* 272: 1909-1914.

Nieman, D.C. 1999. *Exercise testing and prescription: A health-related approach*. Mountain View, CA: Mayfield Publishing.

Paffenbarger, R.S. Jr., Hyde, R.T., Wing, A.L., Hsieh, C.C. 1986. Physical activity, all-cause mortality, and longevity of college alumni. *N Engl J Med* 314: 605-613.

Panton, L.B., Graves, J.E., Pollock, M.L., Garzarella, L., Carroll, J.F., Leggett, S.H., Lowenthal, D.T., Guillen, G.J. 1996. Relative heart rate, heart rate reserve, and VO2 during submaximal exercise in the elderly. *J Gerontology A Biol Sci Med Sci* 51: M165-M171.

Poehlman, E.T., McAuliffe, T.L., Van Houten, D.R., Danforth, E. Jr. 1990. Influence of age and endurance training on metabolic rate and hormones in healthy men. *Am J Physiol* 259: E66-E72.

Pollock, M.L., Bohannon, R.L., Cooper, K.H., Ayres, J.J., Ward, A., White, S.R., Linnerud, A.C. 1976. A comparative analysis of four protocols for maximal treadmill stress testing. *Am Heart J* 92: 39-46.

Pollock, M.L., Foster, C., Schmidt, D., Hellman, C., Linnerud, A.C., Ward, A. 1982. Comparative analysis of physiologic responses to three different maximal graded exercise test protocols in healthy women. *Am Heart J* 103: 363-373.

Pollock, M.L., Gaesser, G.A., Butcher, J.D., Despres, J.P., Dishman, R.K., Franklin, B.A., Garber, C.E. 1998. American College of Sports Medicine position stand: The recommended quantity and quality of exercise for developing and maintaining cardiorespiratory and muscular fitness, and flexibility in healthy adults. *Med Sci Sports Exerc* 30: 975-991.

Pyka, G., Lindenberger, E., Charette, S., Marcus, R. 1994. Muscle strength and fiber adaptations to a year-long resistance training program in elderly men and women. *J Gerontol* 49: M22-M27.

Quinn, T.J., Vroman, N.B., Kertzer, R. 1994. Postexercise oxygen consumption in trained females: Effect of exercise duration. *Med Sci Sports Exere* 26: 908-913.

Schilke, J.M. 1991. Slowing the aging process with physical activity. *J Gerontol Nurs* 17: 4-8.

Schlicht, J., Camaione, D.N., Owen, S.V. 2001. Effect of intense strength training on standing balance, walking speed, and sit-to-stand performance in older adults. *J Gerontology A Biol Sci Med Sci* 56: M281-M286.

Schuit, A.J., Schouten, E.G., Miles, T.P., Evans, W.J., Saris, W.H., Kok, F.J. 1998. The effect of six months training on weight, body fatness and serum lipids in apparently healthy elderly Dutch men and women. *Int J Obes Rel Metab Disord* 22: 847-853.

Seals, D.R., Hagberg, J.M., Spina, R.J., Rogers, M.A., Schechtman, K.B., Ehsani, A.A. 1994. Enhanced left ventricular performance in endurance trained older men. *Circulation* 89: 198-205.

Shimokata, H., Kuzuya, F. 1993. Aging, basal metabolic rate, and nutrition. *Nippon Ronen Igakkai Zasshi* 30: 572-576.

Shimokata, H., Muller, D.C., Fleg, J.L., Sorkin, J., Ziemba, A.W., Andres, R. 1991. Age as independent determinant of glucose tolerance. *Diabetes* 40: 44-51.

Silver, K.H., Macko, R.F., Forrester, L.W., Goldberg, A.P., Smith, G.V. 2000. Effects of aerobic treadmill training on gait velocity, cadence, and gait symmetry in chronic hemiparetic stroke: A preliminary report. *Neurorehabil Neural Repair* 14: 65-71.

Siscovick, D.S., Weiss, N.S., Fletcher, R.H., Lasky, T. 1984. The incidence of primary cardiac arrest during vigorous exercise. *N Engl J Med* 311: 874-877.

Stone, M.H. 1990. Muscle conditioning and muscle injuries. *Med Sci Sports Exerc* 22: 457-462.

Stone, M.H., O'Bryant, H., Garhammer, J. 1981. A hypothetical model for strength training. *J Sports Med Phys Fitness* 21: 342-351.

Storer, T.W., Davis, J.A., Caiozzo, V.J. 1990. Accurate prediction of VO2max in cycle ergometry. *Med Sci Sports Exerc* 22: 704-712.

Stratton, J.R., Levy, W.C., Cerqueira, M.D., Schwartz, R.S., Abrass, I.B. 1994. Cardiovascular responses to exercise. Effects of aging and exercise training in healthy men. *Circulation* 89: 1648-1655.

Sunami, Y., Motoyama, M., Kinoshita, F., Mizooka, Y., Sueta, K., Matsunaga, A., Sasaki, J., Tanaka, H., Shindo, M. 1999. Effects of low-intensity aerobic training on the high-density lipoprotein cholesterol concentration in healthy elderly subjects. *Metabolism* 48: 984-988.

Taaffe, D.R., Duret, C., Wheeler, S., Marcus, R. 1999. Once-weekly resistance exercise improves muscle strength and neuromuscular performance in older adults. *J Am Geriatr Soc* 47: 1208-1214.

Taaffe, D.R., Pruitt, L., Pyka, G., Guido, D., Marcus, R. 1996. Comparative effects of high- and low-intensity resistance training on thigh muscle strength, fiber area, and tissue composition in elderly women. *Clin Physiol* 16: 381-392.

Tanasescu, M., Leitzmann, M.F., Rimm, E.B., Willett, W.C., Stampfer, M.J., Hu, F.B. 2002. Exercise type and intensity in relation to coronary heart disease in men. *JAMA* 288(16): 1994-2000.

Toth, M.J., Beckett, T., Poehlman, E.T. 1999. Physical activity and the progressive change in body composition with aging: Current evidence and research issues. *Med Sci Sports Exerc* 31: S590-S596.

Tsutsumi, T., Don, B.M., Zaichkowsky, L.D., Takenaka, K., Oka, K., Ohno, T. 1998. Comparison of high and moderate intensity of strength training on mood and anxiety in older adults. *Percept Mot Skills* 87: 1003-1011.

Tucci, J.T., Carpenter, D.M., Pollock, M.L., Graves, J.E., Leggett, S.H. 1992. Effect of reduced frequency of training and detraining on lumbar extension strength. *Spine* 17: 1497-1501.

US Department of Commerce. 2000. Bureau of the Census. *Statistical abstract of the united states: the national data book*. Washington DC: US Government Printing Office.

US Department of Health and Human Services, Centers for Disease Control and Prevention, National Center for Chronic Disease Prevention and Health Promotion, and the President's Council on Physical Fitness and Sports. 1996. *Physical activity and health: a report of the surgeon general*. McLean: International Medical Publishing.

Welle, S., Totterman, S., Thornton, C. 1996. Effect of age on muscle hypertrophy induced by resistance training. *J Gerontology A Biol Sci Med Sci* 51: M270-M275.

Whaley, M.H., Kaminsky, L.A., Dwyer, G.B., Getchell, L.H., Norton, J.A. 1992. Predictors of over- and underachievement of age-predicted maximal heart rate. *Med Sci Sports Exerc* 24: 1173-1179.

Wilmore, J.H., Parr, R.B., Girandola, R.N., Ward, P., Vodak, P.A., Barstow, T.J., Pipes, T.V., Romero, G.T., Leslie, P. 1978. Physiological alterations consequent to circuit weight training. *Med Sci Sports* 10: 79-84.

Withers, R.T., Smith, D.A., Tucker, R.C., Brinkman, M., Clark, D.G. 1998. Energy metabolism in sedentary and active 49- to 70-yr-old women. *J Appl Physiol* 84: 1333-1340.

Woods, J.A., Ceddia, M.A., Wolters, B.W., Evans, J.K., Lu, Q., McAuley, E. 1999. Effects of 6 months of moderate aerobic exercise training on immune function in the elderly. *Mech Ageing Dev* 109: 1-19.

Woolf-May, K., Kearney, E.M., Jones, D.W., Davison, R.C., Coleman, D., Bird, S.R. 1998. The effect of two different 18-week walking programmes on aerobic fitness, selected blood lipids and factor XIIa. *J Sports Sci* 16: 701-710.

Zinovieff, A. 1951. Heavy resistance exercise: The Oxford technique. *Brit J Phys Med* 14: 129-132.

Chapter 3

Bobbert, M.V. and A.J. van Soest. 2000. Why do people jump the way they do. *Exerc Sport Sci Rev* 2: 95-103.

Bosco, C. and P.V. Komi. 1980. Influence of aging on the mechanical behavior of leg extensor muscles. *Eur J Appl Physiol* 45: 209-219.

Burkhart, S.S., C.D. Morgan, and W.B. Kibler. 2000. Shoulder injuries in throwing athletes: The dead arm revisited. *Clin Sports Med* 19: 125-158.

Cordo, P.J. and L.M. Nashner. 1982. Properties of postural adjustment with rapid arm movements. *J Neurophysiol* 47: 287-303.

Elliott, B.C., R.N. Marshall, and G. Noffal. 1995. Contributions of upper limb segment rotations during the power serve in tennis. *J Biomech* 11: 433-442.

Glousman, R., F.W. Jobe, J. Tibone, D. Moynes, D. Antonelli, and J. Perry. 1988. Dynamic electromyographic analysis of the throwing shoulder with glenohumeral instability. *J Bone Joint Surgery Am* 70(2): 220-226.

Hirashima, M., H. Kadota, S. Sakurai, K. Kudo, and T. Ohtsuki. 2002. Sequential muscle activity and its functional role in the upper extremity and trunk during overarm throwing. *J Sports Sci* 20(4): 301-310.

Kibler, W.B. 1995. Biomechanical analysis of the shoulder during tennis activities. *Clin J Sports Med* 14: 79-86.

Kibler, W.B., T.J. Chandler, and B.K. Pace. 1992. Principles of rehabilitation after chronic tendon injuries. *Clin J Sports Med* 11: 661-673.

Kibler, W.B., C. Goldberg, and T.J. Chandler. 1991. Functional biomechanical deficits in running athletes with plantar fasciitis. *Am J Sports Med* 19: 66-71.

Kibler, W.B., S.A. Herring, and J.M. Press. 1998. *Functional rehabilitation of sports and musculoskeletal injuries*. Frederick, MD: Aspen.

Kibler, W.B., and B.P. Livingston. 2001. Closed chain rehabilitation for the upper and lower extremity. *J Am Acad Orthop Surg* 9: 412-421.

Kibler, W.B., and J. McMullen. 2003. Scapular dyskinesis and its relation to shoulder pain. *J Am Acad Orthop Surg* 11:142-152.

Kibler, W.B., J. McMullen, and T.L. Uhl. 2001. Shoulder rehabilitation strategies, guidelines, and practice. *Orthop Clin North Am* 32: 527-538.

Knapik, J.J., C.L. Bauman, B.H. Jones, J.M. Harris, L. Vaughan. 1991. Preseason strength and flexibility imbalances associated with athletic injuries in female collegiate athletes. *Am J Sports Med* 19(1): 76-81.

Larsson, L. 1978. Morphological and functional characteristics of aging skeletal muscle in man. *Acta Physiol Scand* 457: 1-36.

MacIntyre, J.G., D.R. Lloyd-Smith. 1993. Overuse running injuries. In *Sports injuries, principles of prevention and care*. London: Blackwell Scientific.

Marshall, R.N., B.C. Elliott. 2000. Long axis rotation: The missing link in proximal to distal segmental sequencing. *J Sports Sci* 18: 247-254.

McQuade, K.J., J. Dawson, G.L. Smidt. 1998. Scapulothoracic muscle fatigue associated with alteration in scapulohumeral rhythm kinematics during maximum resistive shoulder elevation. *J Orthop Sports Phys Ther* 5: 71-87.

Nichols, J.F., D. Medina, E. Dean. 2001. Effects of strength, balance, and trunk stabilization training on measures of functional fitness in older adults. *Am J Sports Med* 3: 279-285.

Nichols, T.R. 1994. A biomechanical perspective on spinal mechanisms of coordinated muscle activation. *Acta Anatomica* 15: 1-13.

Nieminen, H., J. Niemi, E.P. Takala, E. Viikari-Juntura. 1995. Load sharing patterns in the shoulder during isometric flexion tasks. *J Biomech* 28(5): 555-566.

Putnam, C.A. 1993. Sequential motions of body segments in striking and throwing skills. *J Biomech* 26: 125-135.

Toyoshima, S., T. Hoshikawa, M. Miyashita. 1974. Contribution of body parts to throwing performance. In *Biomechanics IV*. Baltimore: University Park Press.

Van Ingen Schenau, G.J., M.F. Bobbert, R.H. Rozendahl. 1987. The unique action of bi-articular muscles in complex movements. *J Anat* 155: 1-5.

Warner, J.J.P., L. Micheli. 1992. Scapulothoracic motion in normal shoulders and shoulders with impingement and instability. *Clin Orthop Rel Res* 285: 199-215.

Wilmore, J.H. 1991. The aging of bone and muscle. *Clin Sports Med* 10: 231-243.

Young, J.L., S.A. Herring, J.M. Press. 1996. The influence of the spine on the shoulder in throwing athletes. *J Back Musculoskeletal Rehabil* 7: 5-17.

Zattara, M., S. Bouisset. 1988. Posturo-kinetic organization during the early phase of voluntary limb movement. *J Neurol Neurosurg Psychiatry* 51: 956-965.

Zhang, S.N., B.T. Bates, J.S. Dufek. 2000. Contributions of lower extremity joints to energy dissipation during landings. *Med Sci Sports Exerc* 32: 812-819.

Chapter 4

Bandy, W.D., Irion, J.M. 1994. The effect of time on static stretch on the flexibility of the hamstring muscles. *Phys Ther* 77(9): 845-850.

Bell, G.W. 1999. Aquatic sports massage therapy. *Clin Sports Med* 18(2): 427-435.

Buckwalter, J.A., Woo, S.L., Goldbert, V.M., Hadley, E.C., Booth, F., Oegema, T.R., Eyer, D.R. 1993. Current concepts review: Soft-tissue aging and musculoskeletal function. *J Bone Joint Surg Am* 75(10): 1533-1548.

Cafarelli, E., Flint F. 1992. The role of massage in preparation for and recovery from exercise. *Sports Med* 14(1): 1-9.

Cyriax, J.H., Cyriax, P.J. 1983. *Illustrated manual of orthopedic medicine*. 2nd ed. Boston: Butterworth & Heinemann.

Crosman, L.J., Chateauvert, S.R., Weisburg, J. 1984. The effect of massage to the hamstring muscle group on range of motion. *J Orthop Sports Phys Ther* 6: 168-172.

Feland, J.B., Myrer, J.B., Schulthies, S.S., Fellingham, G.W., Measom, G.W. 2001. The effect of duration of stretching of the hamstring muscle group for increasing range of motion in people aged 65 years or older. *Phys Ther* 81(5): 1110-1117.

Ferrell-Torry, A.T., Glick, O.J. 1993. The use of therapeutic massage as a nursing intervention to modify anxiety and the perception of cancer pain. *Cancer Nurs* 16(2): 93-101.

Field, T., Grizzle, N., Scafidi, F., Schanberg, S. 1996. Massage and relaxation therapies' effect on depressed adolescent mothers. *Adolescence* 31(124): 903-911.

Goats, G.C. 1994. Massage: The scientific basis of an ancient art: Part 2. Physiological and therapeutic effects. *Brit J Sports Med* 28(3): 153-156.

Hernandez-Reif, M., Field, T., Krasnegor, J., Theakston, H. 2001. Lower back pain is reduced and range of motion increased after massage therapy. *Int J Neurosci* 106(3-4): 131-145.

Hovind, H., Nielsen, S.L. 1974. Effects of massage on blood flow in skeletal muscle. *Scan J Rehabil Med* 6(2): 74-77.

Kamenetz, H.L. 1976. *History of massage*. New York: Robert E. Krieger.

Kisner, C., Colby, L.A. 1996. *Therapeutic exercise: Foundations and techniques*. 3rd ed. Philadelphia: F.A. Davis.

Kleen, E.A. 1921. *Massage and medical gymnastics*. New York: William Wood.

Martin, N.A., Zoeller, R.F., Robertson, R.J., Lephart, S.M. 1998. The comparative effects of sports massage, active recovery, and rest in promoting blood lactate clearance after supramaximal leg exercise. *J Athl Train* 33(1): 30-35.

Mazzeo, R.S., Cavanagh, P., Evans, W.J., Fiatrone, M., Hagberg, J., McAuly, E., Startzell, J. 1998. ACSM Position Stand on Exercises and Physical Activity for Older Adults. *Med Sci Sports Exerc* 30(6): 992-1008.

Menard, D., Stanish, W.D. 1989. The aging athlete. *Am J Sports Med* 17(2): 187-196.

Preyde, M. 2000. Effectiveness of massage therapy for subacute low-back pain: A randomized controlled trial. *CMAJ* 162(13): 1815-1820.

Seto, J.L. and Brewster, C.E. 1991. Musculoskeletal conditioning of the older athlete. *Clin Sports Med* 10(2): 401-429.

Smith, L.L., Keating, M.N., Holbert, D., Spratt, D.J., McCammon, M.R., Smith, S.S., Israel, R.G. 1994. The effects of athletic massage on delayed onset muscle soreness, creatine kinase, and neutrophil count: A preliminary report. *J Orthop Sports Phys Ther* 19(2): 93-99.

Tappan, F.M., Benjamin, P.J. 1998. *Tappan's handbook of healing massage techniques*. 3rd ed. Stamford, CT: Appleton & Lang.

Taylor, D.C., Dalton, J.D., Seaber, A.V., Garrett, W.E. 1990. Viscoelastic properties of muscle-tendon units: The biomechanical effects of stretching. *Am J Sports Med* 18: 300-309.

Tiidus, P.M., Shoemaker, J.K. 1995. Effleurage, massage, muscle blood flow and long-term post-exercise strength recovery. *Int J Sports Med* 16(7): 478-483.

Travell, J.G., Simons, D.G. 1983. *Myofascial pain and dysfunction: The trigger point manual*. Vol. 1. Baltimore: Williams & Wilkins.

Travell, J.G., Simons D.G. 1992. *Myofascial pain and dysfunction, The trigger point manual: The lower extremities*. Vol. 2. Baltimore: Williams & Wilkins.

Weber, M.D., Servedio F.J., Woodall, W.R. 1994. The effects of three modalities on delayed onset muscle soreness. *J Orthop Sports Phys Ther* 20(5): 236-242.

Chapter 5

American College of Sports Medicine, American Dietetic Association, Dietitians of Canada. Joint Position Statement. 2000. Nutrition and athletic performance. *Med Sci Sports Exerc* 32(12): 2130-2145.

Antonio, J., Stout, J. 2001. Glucosamine and chondroitin sulfate. In *Sports supplments*, 250-253. New York: Lippincott Williams & Wilkins.

Ayus, J.C., Arieff, A.I. 1996. Abnormalities of water metabolism in elderly. *Sem Nephrol* 16(4): 277-288.

Bermon, S., Veneembre, P., Sachet, C., Valour, S., Dolisi, C. 1998. Effects of creatine monohydrate ingestion in sedentary and weight-trained older adults. *Acta Physiol Scand* 164(2): 147-155.

Bingham, III, C.O. 2002. Development and clinical application of COX-2-selective inhibitors for the treatment of osteoarthritis and rheumatoid arthritis. *Cleve Clin J Med* 69(Suppl 1): SI5-S12.

Bonnefoy, M., Constans, T., Ferry, M. 2000. Influence of nutrition and physical activity on muscle in the very elderly. Review. *Presse Medicale* 29(39): 2177-2182.

Carr, H.R. 2002. A randomized, double-blind, placebo-controlled trial of glucosamine sulphate as an analgesic in osteoarthritis of the knee. *Rheumatol* 41(3): 279-284.

Catella-Lawson, F., Reilly, M., Kapoor, S.C., et al. 2001. Cyclooxygenase inhibitors and the antiplatelet effects of aspirin. *N Engl J Med* 345: 1809-1817.

ConsumerLab.com. August 2000. Product review: Glucosamine and chondroitin. Internet.

Crofford, L.J. 2002. Specific cyclooxygenase-2 inhibitors: What have we learned since they came into widespread clinical use? *Curr Opin Rheumatol* 14(3): 225-230.

De los Reyes, G.C., Koda, R.T., Lien, E.J. 2000. Glucosamine and chondroitin sulfates in the treatment of osteoarthritis: a survey. Review. *Prog Drug Res* 55: 81-103.

Eikelenboom, P., Rozemuller, A.J.M., Hoozemans, J.J.M., Veerhuis, R., van Gool, W.A. 2000. Neuroinflammation and Alzheimer disease: Clinical and therapeutic implications. *Alzheimer Dis Assoc Disord* 14: S54-S61.

Evans, W.J., and Cyr-Campbell, D. 1997. Nutrition, exercise, and healthy aging. *J Am Dietetic Assoc* 97: 632-638.

Farquhar, B., Kenney, W.L. 1997. Anti-inflammatory drugs, kidney function, and exercise. Sports Science Exchange. *Gatorade Sports Science Institute* 11(4).

Fitzgerald, G.A. 2004. Coxibs and cardiovascular disease. *N Engl J Med* 351(17): 1709-1711.

Fogelholm, M. 2000. Vitamins: metabolic functions. In *Nutrition in sport.* ed. R. Maughan. Oxford: Blackwell Science.

Food Insight. 1998a. Antioxidants: Working toward a definition. International Food Information Council.

Food Insight. 1998b. Better eating for better aging. International Food Information Council.

Frederickson, R.C.A., Brunden, K.R. 1994. New opportuntities in AD research: Roles of immunoinflammatory responses and glia. *Alzheimer Dis Assoc Disord* 8: 159-165.

Gerrior, S.A. 2001a. Assessing body composition and dietary intakes of older men who meet ACSM guidelines for exercise intensity and frequency. Yet unpublished. Poster Session at Sports, Cardiovascular and Wellness Nutritionists Annual meeting in Washington, DC.

Gerrior, S.A. 2001b. Information not yet published, poster presentation. Examining total fat and saturated fat intakes (as a % of kilocalories) and anthropometric status of physically active older women.

Greaves, K.A., Thomson, K. April 2001. Soy protein comes to the aid of women. In *Today's dietitian.* Great Valley Publishing Company, PA.

Holtzman, M.J., Turk, J., Sharnick, L.P. 1992. Identification of a pharmacologically distinct prostaglandin H in synthetase in cultured epithelial cells. *J Biol Chem* 267: 21438-21445.

Incledon, T. May/June 2001. Bone health. In *Dietitian's edge,* 30-35. Ramsey, NJ.

Ivy, J.L. 1999. Role of carbohydrate in physical activity. Review. *Clin Sports Med* 18(3): 469-484, v.

Kawamori, T., Rao, C.V., Seibert, K., Reddy, B.S. 1998. Chemopreventative activity of celecoxib, a specific cyclooxygenase-2 inhibitor, against colon carcinogenesis. *Cancer Res* 58: 409-412.

Kendrick, Z.V., Nelson-Steen, S., Scafidi, K. 1994. Exercise, aging and nutrition. *South Med J* 87(5): S50-S60.

Konstam, M.A., Weir, M.R. 2002. Current perspective on the cardiovascular effects of coxibs. *Cleve Clin J Med* 69(Suppl 1): S147-S152.

Lamb, D.R., Helmy Shehata, A. 1999. Benefits and limitations to prehydration. *Gatorade Sports Science Exchange* 12(2).

Lawrence, R.C., Helmick, C.G., Arnett, F.C., et al. 1998. Estimates of the prevalence of arthritis and selected musculoskeletal disorders in the United States. *Arthritis Rheum* 41: 778-799.

Maughan, R.J., Nadel, E.R. 2000. Temperature regulation and fluid and electrolyte balance. In *Nutrition in sport.* ed. R. Maughan. Oxford: Blackwell Science.

McArdle, W., Katch, F., Katch, V. 2001. *Exercise physiology,* 5th ed. New York: Lippincott Williams & Wilkins.

McMurray, R.W., Hardy, K.J. 2002. Cox-2 inhibitors: Today and tomorrow. *Am J Med Sci* 323(4): 181-189.

National Academy of Sciences. September 2002. *Report on new eating and physical activity targets to reduce chronic disease risk.* The National Academies News. www4.national acdademies.org.

National Research Council. 1989. Minerals. In *Diet and health: Implications for reducing chronic disease risk,* 347-366. Washington, DC: National Academy Press.

Nieman, D.C. 2000. Exercise immunology: Future directions for research related to athletes, nutrition and the elderly. *Int J Sports Med* 21(Suppl 1): S61-S68.

Oshima, M., Murai (Hata), N., Kargman, S., et al. 2001. Chemoprevention of intestinal polyposis in the $Apc^{\Delta 716}$ mouse by rofecoxib, a specific cyclooxygenase-2 inhibitor. *Cancer Res* 61: 1733-1740.

Raisz, L.G. 2001. Potential impact of selective cyclooxygenase-2 inhibitors on bone metabolism in health and disease. *Am J Med* 110(3A): 43S-45S.

Reaven, G. 2000. *Syndrome X.* New York: Simon and Schuster.

Reents, S. 2000. *Sport and exercise pharmacology,* 244-249. Champaign, IL: Human Kinetics.

Rosenbloom, C. 2000. In *Sports nutrition,* 55. Chicago: The American Dietetic Association.

Russell, R.M., Mason, J.B. 2000. Future health needs: Nutrition and aging. Cyberrounds.com.

Saltzman, J.R., Russell, R.M. 1998. The aging gut: Nutritional issues. *Gastroenterol Clin North Am* 27(2): 309-324.

Schwartz, J.I., Malice, M.P., Lasseter, K.C., Holmes, G.B., Gottesdiener, K.M., Brune, K. 2001. Effects of rofecoxib, celecoxib, and naproxen on urinary sodium excretion in elderly volunteers. Presented at The Congress of the European League Against Rheumatism (EULAR), Prague, Czech Republic, June 13-16.

Silverstein, F.E., Faich, G., Goldstein, J.L., et al. 2000. Gastrointestinal toxicity with celecoxib vs nonsteroidal anti-inflammatory drugs for osteoarthritis and rheumatoid arthritis. The CLASS study: A randomized controlled trial. *JAMA* 284(10): 1247-1255.

Stading, J.A., Skrabal, M.Z., Faulkner, M.A. 2001. Seven cases of interaction between warfarin and cyclooxygenase-2 inhibitors. *Am J Health-Syst Pharm* 58: 2076-2080.

Stout, N.R., Kenny, R.A., Baylis, P.H. 1999. A review of water balance in aging in health and disease. *Gerontol* 45(2): 61-66.

Subbaramaiah, K., Norton, L., Gerald, W., Dannenberg, A.J. 2002. Cyclooxygenase-2 is overexpressed in HER-2/neu-positive breast cancer: Evidence for involvement of AP-1 and PEA3. *J Biol Chem* 277(21): 18649-18657.

Subudhi, A.W., Davis, S.L., Kipp, R.W., Askew, E.W. 2001. Antioxidant status and oxidative stress in elite alpine ski racers. *Int J Sport Nutr Exerc Metab* 11(1): 32-41.

Swan, S.K., Rudy, D.W., Lasseter, K.C., et al. 2000. Effect of cyclooxygenase-2 inhibition on renal function in elderly persons receiving a low-salt diet: A randomized, controlled trial. *Ann Intern Med* 133(1): 1-9.

Wardlaw, G.M. 2003. *Contemporary nutrition: Issues and insights.* 5th ed. Boston: McGraw-Hill. P. 534.

Webb, D. 2002. Glycemic index: Gateway to good health or grand waste of time? *Environmental Nutrition* 25(November): 11.

Webb, D., Ward, E.M. 1999. *Super nutrition after 50,* 110-112. Lincolnwood, IL: Publications International.

Williams, M.H. 1998. Ginseng. In *The ergogenics edge,* 204-208. Champaign, IL: Human Kinetics.

Zawadzki, K.M., Yaspelkis, III., B.B., Ivy, J.L. 1992. Carbohydrate-protein complex increases the rate of muscle glycogen storage after exercise. *J Appl Physiol* 72(5): 1854-1859.

Chapter 6

Allen, G.M., Wilson, D.J. 2001. Ultrasound of the shoulder. *Eur J Ultrasound* 14(1): 3-9.

Barnes, C.J., Van Steyn, S.J., Fischer, R.A. 2001. The effects of age, sex, and shoulder dominance on range of motion of the shoulder. *J Shoulder Elbow Surg* 10(3): 242-246.

Bateman, J.E. 1978. *The shoulder and neck.* 2nd ed. Philadelphia: WB Saunders.

Beaufils, P., Prevot, N., Boyer, T., Allard, M., Dorfmann, H., Frank, A., Kelberine, F., Kempf, J.F., Mole, D., Walch, G. 1999. Arthroscopic release of the glenohumeral joint in shoulder stiffness: A review of 26 cases. French Society for Arthroscopy. *Arthroscopy* 15(1): 49-55.

Bennett, W.F. 2001. Subscapularis, medial, and lateral head coracohumeral ligament insertion anatomy. Arthroscopic appearance and incidence of "hidden" rotator interval lesions. *Arthroscopy* 17(2): 173-180.

Bigliani, L.U., Kimmel, J., McCann, P.D., Wolfe, I. 1992. Repair of rotator cuff tears in tennis players. *Am J Sports Med* 20(2): 112-117.

Bigliani, L.U., Morrison, D.S., April, E.W. 1986. The morphology of the acromion and rotator cuff impingement. *Orthop Trans* 10: 288.

Bonsell, S., Pearsall, A.W., IV., Heitman, R.J., Helms, C.A., Major, N.M., Speer, K.P. 2000. The relationship of age, gender, and degenerative changes observed on radiographs of the shoulder in asymptomatic individuals. *JBone Joint Surg Br* 82(8): 1135-1139.

Brandt, T.D., Cardone, B.W., Grant, T.H., Post, M., Weiss, C.A. 1989. Rotator cuff sonography: A reassessment. *Radiology* 173(2): 323-327.

Brenneke, S.L., Morgan, C.J. 1992. Evaluation of ultrasonography as a diagnostic technique in the assessment of rotator cuff tendon tears. *Am J Sports Med* 20(3): 287-289.

Brewer, B.J. 1979. Aging of the rotator cuff. *Am J Sports Med* 7(2): 102-110.

Bunker, T.D., Anthony, P.P. 1995. The pathology of frozen shoulder. A Dupuytren-like disease. *J Bone Joint Surg Br* 77(5): 677-683.

Burkhead, W.Z. Jr., Hutton, K.S. 1995. Biologic resurfacing of the glenoid with hemiarthroplasty of the shoulder. *J Shoulder Elbow Surg* 4(4): 263-270.

Calvert, P., Wallace, W.A., Kelly, I.G., et al. 2001. The clinical outcome from a randomized controlled study of rotator cuff repairs reviewed at 6 and 12 months. European Shoulder and Elbow Society in Sept 2001.

Chambler, A.F., Carr, A.J. 2003. The role of surgery in frozen shoulder. *J Bone Joint Surg Br* 85(6): 789-795.

Chronopoulos, E., Kim, T.K., Park, H.B., Ashenbrenner, D., McFarland, E.G. 2004. Diagnostic value of physical tests for isolated chronic acromioclavicular lesions. *Am J Sports Med* 32(3): 655-661.

Cofield, R.H., Parvizi, J., Hoffmeyer, P.J., Lanzer, W.L., Ilstrup, D.M., Rowland, C.M. 2001. Surgical repair of chronic rotator cuff tears: A prospective long-term study. *J Bone Joint Surg Am* 83: 71-77.

Davidson, P.A., ElAttrache, N.S., Jobe, C.M., Jobe, F.W. 1995. Rotator cuff and posterior-superior glenoid labrum injury associated with increased glenohumeral motion: A new site of impingement. *J Shoulder Elbow Surg* 4(5): 384-390.

de Laat, E.A., Visser, C.P., Coene, L.N., Pahlplatz, P.V., Tavy, D.L. 1994. Nerve lesions in primary shoulder dislocations and humeral neck fractures. A prospective clinical and EMG study. *J Bone Joint Surg Br* 76(3): 381-383.

Demicis, T.A., Wilkins, D.A., McFarland, E.G. 2000. "AC Spot Views." *Phys Sportsmed* 28(3): 40-52.

DePalma, A.F. 1983. *Surgery of the shoulder.* 3rd ed. Philadelphia: JB Lippincott.

Dines, D.M., Warren, R.F., Inglis, A.E., Pavlov, H. 1990. The coracoid impingement syndrome. *J Bone Joint Surg Br* 72(2): 314-316.

Drakeford, M.K., Quinn, M.J., Simpson, S.L., Pettine, K.A. 1990. A comparative study of ultrasonography and arthrography in evaluation of the rotator cuff. *Clin Orthop Rel Res* 253: 118-122.

Fink, B., Sallen, V., Guderian, H., Tillmann, K., Ruther, W. 2001. Resection interposition arthroplasty of the shoulder affected by inflammatory arthritis. *J Shoulder Elbow Surg* 10(4): 365-371.

Flatow, E.L., Raimondo, R.A., Kelkar, R., Wang, V.M., Pollock, R.G., Pawluk, R.J., Mow, V.C., Bigliani, L.U. 1997. Active and passive restraints against superior humeral translation: The contribution of the rotator cuff, the biceps tendon, and the coracoacromial arch (abstract). 12th Open Meeting, American Shoulder Elbow Surgeon, Atlanta, GA; 1996. *J Shoulder Elbow Surg* 6: 172.

Furtschegger, A., Resch, H. 1988. Value of ultrasonography in preoperative diagnosis of rotator cuff tears and postoperative follow-up. *Eur J Radiol* 8: 69-75.

Galatz, L.M., Ball, C.M., Teefey, S.A., Middleton, W.D., Tamaguchi, K. 2004. The outcome and repair integrity of completely arthroscopically repaired large and massive rotator cuff tears. *J Bone Joint Surg Am* 86(2): 219-224.

Gerber, C., Galantay, R.V., Hersche, O. 1998. The pattern of pain produced by irritation of the acromioclavicular joint and the subacromial space. *J Shoulder Elbow Surg* 7(4): 352-355.

Gerber, C., Sebesta, A. 2000. Impingement of the deep surface of the subscapularis tendon and the reflection pulley on the anterosuperior glenoid rim: A preliminary report. *J Shoulder Elbow Surg* 9(6): 483-490.

Gerber, C., Terrier, F., Ganz, R. 1985. The role of the coracoid process in the chronic impingement syndrome. *J Bone Joint Surg Br* 67(5):703-708.

Gill, T.J., McIrvin, E., Mair, S.D., Hawkins, R.J. 2001. Results of biceps tenotomy for treatment of pathology of the long head of the biceps brachii. *J Shoulder Elbow Surg* 10(3): 247-249.

Hawkins, R.J., Mohtadi, N.G. 1991. Clinical evaluation of shoulder instability. *Clin J Sports Med* 159-164.

Healy, W.L., Iorio, R., Lemos, M.J. 2001. Athletic activity after joint replacement. *Am J Sports Med* 29(3): 377-388.

Jacob, A.K., Sallay, P.I. 1997. Therapeutic efficacy of corticosteroid injections in the acromioclavicular joint. *Biomedical Sciences Instrumentation* 34: 380-385.

Jando, D.H., Hawkins, R.J. 1993. Shoulder manipulation in patients with adhesive capsulitis and diabetes mellitus: A clinical note. *J Shoulder Elbow Surg* 2: 36-38.

Jones, L. 1942. The Shoulder joint: Observations on an anatomy and physiology with an analysis of a reconstructive operation following extensive surgery. *Surgery, Gynecology & Obstetrics* 75: 433-444.

Keyes, E.L. 1935. Anatomical observations on senile changes in the shoulder. *J Bone Joint Surg* 17: 953-960.

Kibler, W.B., Chandler, T.J., Livingston, B.P., Roetert, E.P. 1996. Shoulder range of motion in elite tennis players: Affect of age and years of tournament play. *Am J Sports Med* 24(3): 279-285.

Lee, T.Q., Black, A.D., Tibone, J.E., McMahon, P.J. 2001. Release of the coracoacromial ligament can lead to glenohumeral laxity: A biomechanical study. *J Shoulder Elbow Surg* 10(1): 68-72.

Lindblom, K. 1939. Arthrography and roentgenography in ruptures of the tendon of the shoulder joint. *Acta Radiologica* 20: 548.

Liu, S.H., Boynton, E. 1993. Posterior superior impingement of the rotator cuff on the glenoid rim as a cause of shoulder pain in the overhead athlete. *Arthroscopy* 9(6): 697-699.

Mack, L.A., Matsen, F.A., III, Kilcoyne, R.F., Davies, P.K., Sickler, M.E. 1985. US evaluation of the rotator cuff. *Radiology* 157(1): 205-209.

Mallon, W.J., Liebelt, R.A., Mason, J.B. 1996. Total joint replacement and golf. *Clin Sports Med* 15(1): 179-190.

Martin-Hervas, C., Romero, J., Navas-Acien, A., Reboiras, J.J., Munuera, L. 2001. Ultrasonographic and magnetic Resonance images of rotator cuff lesions compared with arthroscopy or open surgery findings. *J Shoulder Elbow Surg* 10(5): 410-415.

McFarland, E.G., Hsu, C.Y, Neira, C., O'Neil, O. 1999. Internal impingement of the shoulder: A clinical and arthroscopic analysis. *J Shoulder Elbow Surg* 8(5): 458-460.

McLaughlin, H.L. 1952. Posterior dislocation of the shoulder. *J Bone Joint Surg Am* 34: 584-590.

Milgrom, C., Schaffler, M., Gilbert, S., van Holsbeeck, M. 1995. Rotator-cuff changes in asymptomatic adults: The affect of age, hand dominance and gender. *J Bone Joint Surg Br* 77(2): 296-298.

Neer, C.S., II. 1970. Displaced proximal humeral fractures. I. Classification and evaluation. *J Bone Joint Surg Am* 52(6): 1077-1089.

Neer, C.S., II. 1972. Anterior acromioplasty for the chronic impingement syndrome in the shoulder: A preliminary report. *J Bone Joint Surg Am* 54(1): 41-50.

Neer, C.S., II. 1983. Impingement lesions. *Clin Orthop Rel Res* 173: 70-77.

Neviaser, R.J. 1987. Radiologic assessment of the shoulder: Plain and arthrographic. *Orthop Clin North Am* 18(3): 343-349.

Nixon, J.E., DiStefano, V. 1975. Ruptures of the rotator cuff. *Orthop Clin North Am* 6(2): 423-447.

Nobuhara, K., Sugiyama, D., Ikeda, H., Makiura, M. 1990. Contracture of the shoulder. *Clin Orthop Rel Res* 254: 105-110.

Ogilvie-Harris, D.J., Myerthall, S. 1997. The diabetic frozen shoulder: Arthroscopic release. *Arthroscopy* 13(1): 1-8.

Olive, R.J. Jr., Marsh, H.O. 1992. Ultrsonography of rotator cuff tears. *Clin Orthop Rel Res* 282: 110-113.

Paavolainen, P., Ahovuo, J. 1994. Ultrasonography and arthrography in the diagnosis of tears of the rotator cuff. *J Bone Joint Surg Am* 76(3): 335-340.

Paley, K.J., Jobe, F.W., Pink, M.M., Kvitne, R.S., ElAttrache, N.S. 2000. Arthroscopic findings in the overhand throwing athlete: Evidence for posterior internal impingement of the rotator cuff. *Arthroscopy* 16(1): 35-40.

Pattee, G.A., Snyder, S.J. 1998. Sonographic evaluation of the rotator cuff: Correlation with arthroscopy. *Arthroscopy* 4(1): 15-20.

Penny, J.N., Welsh, R.P. 1981. Shoulder impingement syndromes in athletes and their surgical management. *Am J Sports Med* 9(1): 11-15.

Petersson, C.J. 1983. Degeneration of the acromioclavicular joint: A morphological study. *Acta Orthopaedica Scandinavica* 54(3): 434-438.

Petersson, C.J., Redlund-Johnell, I. 1983. Radiographic joint space in normal acromioclavicular joints. *Acta Orthop Scand* 54(3): 431-433.

Post, M. 1978. Diagnosis. In *The shoulder*, 8-34. ed. M. Post. Philadelphia: Lea & Febiger.

Post, M., Cohen, J. 1986. Impingement syndrome: A review of late stage II and early stage III lesions. *Clin Orthop Rel Res* 207: 126-132.

Roberts, C.S., Beck, D.J. Jr., Heinsen, J., Seligson, D. 2002. Review article: Diagnostic ultrasonography: Applications in orthopaedic surgery. *Clin Orthop Rel Res* 401: 248-264.

Rothman, R.H., Parke, W.W. 1965. The vascular anatomy of the rotator cuff. *Clin Orthop Rel Res* 41: 176-186.

Rowe, C.R. 1988. *The shoulder.* New York: Churchill Livingstone.

Sano, H., Ishii, H., Trudel, G., Uhthoff, H.K. 1999. Histologic evidence of degeneration at the insertion of 3 rotator cuff tendons: A comparative study with human cadaveric shoulders. *J Shoulder Elbow Surg* 8(6): 574-579.

Sano, H., Ishii, H., Yeadon, A., Backman, D.S., Brunet, J.A., Uhthoff, H.K. 1997. Degeneration at the insertion weakens the tensile strength of the supraspinatus tendon: A comparative mechanical and histologic study of the bone-tendon complex. *J Orthop Res* 115(5): 719-726.

Sarkar, K., Uhthoff, H.K. 1996. Pathophysiology of rotator cuff degeneration, calcification, and repair. In *Rotator cuff disorders*, 36-44. ed. W.Z. Burkhead, Jr. Baltimore: Lippincott Williams & Wilkins.

Sher, J.S., Uribe, J.W., Posada, A., Murphy, B.J., Zlatkin, M.B. 1995. Abnormal findings on magnetic resonance images of asymptomatic shoulders. *J Bone Joint Surg Am* 77(1): 10-15.

Slatis, P., Aalto, K. 1979. Medial dislocation of the tendon of the long head of the biceps brachii. *Acta Orthopaedica Scandinavica* 50(1): 73-77.

Sonnery-Cottet, B., Edwards, T.B., Noel, E., Walch, G. 2002. Rotator cuff tears in middle-aged tennis players: Results of surgical treatment. *Am J Sports Med* 30(4): 558-564.

Spencer, R., Skirving, A.P. 1986. Silastic interposition arthroplasty of the shoulder. *J Bone Joint Surg Br* 68(3): 375-377.

Stein, B.E., Wiater, J.M., Pfaff, H.C., Bigliani, L.U., Levine, W.N. 2001. Detection of acromioclavicular joint pathology in asymptomatic shoulders with magnetic resonance imaging. *J Shoulder Elbow Surg* 10(3):204-208.

Swen, W.A., Jacobs, J.W., Algra, P.R., M. 1999. Sonography and magnetic resonance imaging equivalent for the assessment of full-thickness rotator cuff tears. *Arthritis Rheumatism* 42(10): 2231-2238.

Teefey, S.A., Hasan, S.A., Middleton, W.D., Patel, M., Wright, R.W., Yamaguchi, K. 2000. Ultrasonography of the rotator cuff: A comparison of ultrasonographic and arthroscopic findings in one hundred consecutive cases. *J Bone Joint Surg Am* 82(4): 498-504.

Teefey, S.A., Middleton, W.D., Yamaguchi, K. 1999. Shoulder sonography: State of the art. *Radiol Clin N Am* 37(4):767-785.

ten Have, H.A., Eulderink, F. 1981. Mobility and degenerative changes of the ageing cervical spine: A macroscopic and statistical study. *Gerontol* 27(1-2): 42-50.

Tibone, J.E., Jobe, F.W., Kerlan, R.K., Carter, V.S., Shields, C.L., Lombardo, S.J., Yocum, L.A. 1985. Shoulder impingement syndrome in athletes treated by an anterior acromioplasty. *Clin Orthop Rel Res* 198: 134-140.

Ticker, J.B., Beim, G.M., Warner, J.J. 2000. Recognition and treatment of refractory posterior capsular contracture of the shoulder. *Arthroscopy* 16(1): 27-34.

Tillmann, K., Braatz, D. 1989. Resection-interposition arthroplasty of the shoulder in rheumatoid arthritis. In *Rheumatoid arthritis: Surgery of the shoulder*, 126-133. eds. A.W.F. Lettin, C. Petersson. Basel: S. Karger.

Toivonen, D.A., Tuite, M.J., Orwin, J.F. 1995. Acromial structure and tears of the rotator cuff. *J Shoulder Elbow Surg* 4(5): 376-383.

Tuite, M.J., Toivonen, D.A., Orwin, J.F., Wright, D.H. 1995. Acromial angle on radiographs of the shoulder: Correlation with the impingement syndrome and rotator cuff tears. *AJR. Am J Roentgenol* 165(3): 609-613.

Uhthoff, H.K., Sano, H. 1997. Pathology of failure of the rotator cuff tendon. *Orthop Clin North Am* 28(1): 31-41.

Uhthoff, H.K., Sarkar, K. 1993. The affect of aging on the soft tissues of the shoulder. In *The shoulder: A Balance of mobility and stability*, 269-278. eds. F.A. Matsen, III, F.H. Fu, R.J. Hawkins. Rosemont. IL: American Academy of Orthopaedic Surgeons.

Vecchio, P.C., Hazleman, B.L., King, R.H. 1993. A double-blind trial comparing subacromial methylprednisolon and lidocaine in acute rotator cuff tendinitis. *Br J Rheumatol* 32(8): 743-745.

Vick, C.W., Bell, S.A. 1990. Rotator cuff tears: diagnosis with sonography. *AJR. Am J Roentgenol* 154(1):121-123.

Walch, G., Boileau, P., Noel, E., Donell, S.T. 1992. Impingement of the deep surface of the supraspinatus tendon on the posterosuperior glenoid rim: An arthroscopic study. *J Shoulder Elbow Surg* 1: 238-245.

Walch, G., Maconia, G., Pozzi, I., et al. 1997. Arthroscopic tenotomy of the long head of the biceps in rotator cuff ruptures. In *The cuff*, 350-355: eds. D.F. Gazielly, P. Gleyze, T. Thomas. Paris: Elsevier.

Walch, G., Nove-Josserand, L., Boileau, P., Levigne, C. 1998. Subluxations and dislocations of the tendon of the long head of the biceps. *J Shoulder Elbow Surg* 7(2): 100-108.

Wallny, T., Wagner, U.A., Prange, S., Schmitt, O., Reich, H. 1999. Evaluation of chronic tears of the rotator cuff by ultrasound. *J Bone Joint Surg Br* 81(4): 675-678.

Warner, J.J. 1997. Frozen shoulder: Diagnosis and management. *The J Am Acad Orthop Surg* 5(3): 130-140.

Weinstein, D.M., Bucchieri, J.S., Pollock, R.G., Flatow, E.L., Bigliani, L.U. 2000. Arthroscopic debridement of the shoulder for osteoarthritis. *Arthroscopy* 16(5): 471-476.

Wiley, A.M. 1991. Arthroscopic appearance of frozen shoulder. *Arthroscopy* 7(2): 138-143.

Yamaguchi, K., Tetro, A.M., Blam, O., Evanoff, B.A., Teefey, A. 2001. Natural history of asymptomatic rotator cuff tears: A longitudinal analysis of asymptomatic tears detected sonographically. *J Shoulder Elbow Surg* 10(3): 199-203.

Yamakata, K., Fukuda, H. 1991. Ageing process of the supraspinatus tendon with reference to rotator cuff tears. In *Surgical disorders of the shoulder*, 247-258. ed. M.S. Watson. London: Churchill Livingstone.

Yocum, L.A., Conway, J.E. 1996. Rotator cuff tear: Clinical assessment and treatment. In *Operative techniques in upper extremity sports injuries*, 223-245. ed. F.W. Jobe. St. Louis: Mosby-Year Book.

Zanca, P. 1971. Shoulder pain: Involvement of the acromioclavicular joint. (Analysis of 1,000 cases). *Am J Roentgenol Radium Ther Nucl Med* 112(3): 493-506.

Chapter 7

Adelsberg, S. 1986. An EMG analysis of selected muscles with rackets of increasing grip size. *Am J Sports Med* 14: 139-142.

Andrews, J.R., Heggland, E.J.H., Fleisig, G.S., Zheng, N. 2001. Relationship of ulnar collateral ligament strain to amount of medial olecranon osteotomy. *Am J Sports Med* 29(6): 716-721.

Andrews, J.R., Soffer, SR. 1994. *Elbow arthroscopy*. St. Louis: Mosby Year Book.

Andrews, J.R., Timmerman, L.A. 1995. Outcome of elbow surgery in professional baseball players. *Am J Sports Med* 23: 407-4134.

Andrews, J.R., Wilk, K.E., Satterwhite, Y.E., Tedder, J.L. 1993. Physical Examination of the thrower's elbow. *J Orthop Sports Phys Ther* 6: 296-304.

Ballantyne, B.T., O'Hare, S.J., Paschall, J.L., Pavia-Smith, M.M., Pitz, A.M., Gillon, J.F., Soderberg, G.L. 1993. Electromyographic activity of selected shoulder muscles in commonly used therapeutic exercises. *Physical Therapy* 73(10): 668-682.

Basford, J.R., Sheffield, C.G., Cieslak, K.R. 2000. Laser therapy: A randomized, controlled trial of the effects of low intensity Nd: YAG laser irradiation on lateral epicondylitis. *Arch Phys Med and Rehabilitation* 81:1504-1510.

Bennett, G.E. 1959. Elbow and shoulder lesions of baseball players. *Am J Surg* 98: 484-492.

Bernhang, A.M., Dehner, W., Fogarty, C. 1974. Tennis elbow: A biomechanical approach. *Am J Sports Med* 2: 235-260.

Blackburn, T.A., McLeod, W.D., White, B., et al. 1990. EMG analysis of posterior rotator cuff exercises. *Athl Train* 25: 40-45.

Bowling, R.W., Rockar, P.A. 1985. The elbow complex. In G.J. Davies and J.A. Gould (Eds.) *Orthopaedic and sports physical therapy*, 476-496. St. Louis: Mosby.

Boyer, M.I. Hastings, H. 1999. Lateral tennis elbow: Is there any science out there? *J Shoulder Elbow Surgery* 8: 481-491.

Brattberg, G. 1983. Acupuncture therapy for tennis elbow. *Pain* 16: 285-288.

Carroll, R. 1981. Tennis elbow: Incidence in local league players. *Br J Sports Med* 15: 250-255.

Chinn, C.J., Priest J.D., Kent B.E. 1974. Upper extremity range of motion, grip strength, and girth in highly skilled tennis players. *Phys Ther* 54: 474-482.

Cyriax, J.H, Cyriax, P.J. 1983. *Illustrated manual of orthopaedic medicine*. London: Butterworths.

Dijs, H., Mortier, G., Driessens, M., DeRidder, A., Willems, J., Devroey, T. 1990. A retrospective study of the conservative treatment of tennis elbow. *Medica Physica* 13: 73-77.

Ellenbecker, T.S. 1991. A total arm strength isokinetic profile of highly skilled tennis players. *Isokinetics and Exercise Science* 1: 9-21.

Ellenbecker, T.S. 1995. Rehabilitation of shoulder and elbow injuries in tennis players. *Clin Sports Med* 14: 87-110.

Ellenbecker, T.S., Davies, G.J. 2001. *Closed kinetic chain exercise*. Champaign, IL: Human Kinetics.

Ellenbecker, T.S., Mattalino, A.J. 1997. *The elbow in sport*. Champaign, IL: Human Kinetics.

Ellenbecker, T.S., Mattalino, A.J., Elam, E.A., Caplinger, R.A. 1998. Medial elbow laxity in professional baseball pitchers: A bilateral comparison using stress radiography. *Am J Sports Med* 26(3): 420-424.

Ellenbecker, T.S., Roetert, E.P. 1994. Unpublished data from the USTA on Range of Motion of the Elbow and Wrist in Senior Tennis Players 1994.

Ellenbecker, T.S., Roetert, E.P. 2003a. Isokinetic profile of elbow flexion and extension strength in elite junior tennis players. *J Orthop Sports Phys Ther* 33(2): 79-84.

Ellenbecker, T.S., Roetert, E.P. 2003b. Isokinetic profile of wrist and forearm strength in female elite junior tennis players. Platform presentation presented at the APTA Annual Conference and Exposition, Washington DC, June 2003.

Ellenbecker, T.S., Roetert, E.P., Bailie, D.S., Davies, G.J., Brown, S.W. 2002. Glenohumeral joint total rotation range of motion in elite tennis players and baseball pitchers. *Med Sci Sports Exerc* 34(12): 2052-2056.

Fleck, S.J, Kraemer, W.J. 1987. *Designing resistance training programs*. Champaign, IL: Human Kinetics.

Gam, A.N., Warming, S., Larsen, L.H., Jensen, B., Hoydalsmo, O., Allon, I., Andersen, B., Gotzsche, N.E., Petersen, M., Mathiesen, B. 1998. Treatment of myofascial trigger-points with ultrasound combined with massage and exercise: A randomized controlled trial. *Pain* 77(1): 73-79.

Glousman, R.E, Barron, J., Jobe, F.W., Perry, J., Pink, M. 1992. An electromyographic analysis of the elbow in normal and injured pitchers with medial collateral ligament insufficiency. *Am J Sports Med* 20(3): 311-317.

Goldie, I. 1964. Epicondylitis lateralis humeri. *Acta Chir Scand Suppl* 339: 1-114.

Gould, J.A., Davies, G.J. 1985. Orthopaedic and sports rehabilitation concepts. In G.J. Davies and J.A. Gould (Eds,) *Orthopaedic and sports physical therapy*, 181-198. C.V. Mosby.

Greenbaum, B., Itamura J., Vangsness, C.T., Tibone, J., Atkinson, R. 1999. Extensor carpi radialis brevis. *J Bone Joint Surg Br* 81(5): 926-929.

Groppel, J.L., Nirschl, R.P. 1986. A mechanical and electromyographical analysis of the effects of counterforce braces on the tennis player. *Am J Sports Med* 14(3): 195-200.

Haake, M., Konig, I.R., Decker, T., Riedel, C., Buch, M., Muller, H.H., Vogel, M., Auersperg, V., Maier-Boerries, O., Betthauser, A., Fischer, J., Loew, M., Muller, I., Rehak, H.C., Gerdesmeyer, L., Maier, M., Kanovsky, W. 2002. Extracorporeal shock wave therapy in the treatment of lateral epicondylitis: A randomized multicenter trial. *J Bone Joint Surg* 84-A(11):1982-1991.

Hang, Y.S, Peng, S.M. 1984. An epidemiological study of upper extremity injury in tennis players with particular reference to tennis elbow. *J Formos Med Assoc* 83: 307-316.

Hawkins, R.J., Kennedy, J.C. 1980. Impingement syndrome in athletes. *Am J Sports Med* 8: 151-158.

Indelicato, P.A, Jobe, F.W, Kerlan, R.K, Carter, V.S, Shields, C.L, Lombardo, S.J. 1979. Correctable elbow lesions in professional baseball players: a review of 25 cases. *Am J Sports Med* 7: 72-75.

Ingham, B. 1981. Transverse cross friction massage. *Phys Sportsmed* 9(10): 116.

Inman, V.T., Saunders, J.B., de CM, Abbot L.C. 1944. Observations on the function of the shoulder joint. *J Bone Joint Surg Am* 26: 1-30.

Jensen, B.R., Sjogaard, G., Bornmyr, S., Arborelius, M., Jorgensen, K. 1995. Intramuscular laser-Doppler flowmetry in the supraspinatus muscle during isometric contractions. *Eur J Appl Physiol Occup Physiol* 71(4): 373-378.

Jobe, F.W., Kvitne, R.S. 1989. Shoulder pain in the overhand or throwing athlete: The relationship of anterior instability and rotator cuff impingement. *Orthop Rev* 18(9): 963-975.

Joyce, M.E., Jelsma, R.D., Andrews, J.R. 1995. Throwing injuries to the elbow. *Sports Med Arthroscopy Rev* 3: 224-236.

Kamien, M. 1990. A rational management of tennis elbow. *Sports Med* 9: 173-191.

Kibler, W.B. 1991. Role of the scapula in the overhead throwing motion. *Contemp Orthop* 22(5): 525-532.

Kibler, W.B. 1998. The role of the scapula in athletic shoulder function. *Am J Sports Med* 26(2): 325-337.

Kibler, W.B., Chandler, T.J., Livingston, B.P., Roetert, E.P. 1996. Shoulder range of motion in elite tennis players. *Am J Sports Med* 24(3): 279-285.

Kibler, W.B., Uhl, T.L., Maddux, J.W.Q., Brooks, P.V., Zeller, B., McMullen, J. 2002. Qualitative clinical evaluation of scapular dysfunction: A reliability study. *J Shoulder Elbow Surg* 11: 550-556.

King, J.W., Brelsford, H.J, Tullos, H.S. 1969. Analysis of the pitching arm of the professional baseball pitcher. *Clin Orthop* 67: 116-123.

Kitai, E., Itay, S., Ruder, A., Engel, J., Modan, M. 1986. An epidemiological study of lateral epicondylitis (tennis elbow) in amateur male players. *Ann Chir Main* 5(2): 113-121.

Kraushaar, B.S., Nirschl, R.P. 1999. Tendinosis of the elbow (tennis elbow). Clinical features and findings of histopathological, immunohistochemical and electron microscopy studies. *J Bone Joint Surg* 81-A(2): 259-278.

Kulund, D.N, Rockwell, D.A, Brubaker, C.E. 1979. The long term effects of playing tennis. *Phys Sportsmed* 7: 87-92.

Labelle, H., Guibert, R., Joncas, J., Newman, N., Fallaha, M., Rivard, C.H. 1992. Lack of scientific evidence for the treatment of lateral epicondylitis of the elbow. *J Bone Joint Surg Br* 74: 646-651.

Leadbetter, W.B. 1992. Cell matrix response in tendon injury. *Clin Sports Med* 11: 533-579.

McFarland, E.G., Torpey, B.M., Carl, L.A. 1996. Evaluation of shoulder laxity. *Sports Medicine* 22: 264-272.

Morrey, B.F. 1993. *The elbow and its disorders.* 2nd ed. Philadelphia: Saunders.

Morrey, B.F, An, K.N. 1983. Articular and ligamentous contributions to the stability of the elbow joint. *Am J Sports Med* 11: 315.

Neer, C.S. 1973. Impingment lesions. *Clin Orthop* 173: 70-77.

Nirschl, R.P. 1992. Elbow tendinosis/tennis elbow. *Clin Sports Med* 11: 851-870.

Nirschl, R.P. 1993. Rehabilitation of the athlete's elbow. In B.F. Morrey, ed., *The elbow and its disorders.* 2nd ed., 537-552. Philadelphia: Saunders.

Nirschl, R.P., Rodin, D.M., Ochiai, D.H., Maartmann-Moe, C. 2003. Iontophoretic administration of Dexamethasone Sodium Phosphate for acute epicondylitis: A randomized, double blind, placebo controlled study. *Am J Sports Med* 31(2): 189-195.

Nirschl, R., Sobel, J. 1981. Conservative treatment of tennis elbow. *Phys Sportsmed* 9: 43-54.

O'Driscoll, S.W, Morrey, B.F. 1992. Arthroscopy of the elbow: Diagnostic and therapeutic benefits and hazards. *J Bone Joint Surg* 74-A(1): 84-94.

Ogilvie-Harris, D.J., Gordon, R., MacKay, M. 1995. Arthroscopic treatment for posterior impingement in degenerative arthritis of the elbow. *Arthroscopy* 11(4): 437-443.

Percy, E.C, Carson, J.D. 1981. The use of DMSO in tennis elbow and rotator cuff tendinitis. A double blind study. *Med Sci Sports Exerc* 13: 215-219.

Priest, J.D., Jones, H.H., Nagel, D.A. 1974. Elbow injuries in highly skilled tennis players. *Journal of Sports Medicine* 2(3): 137-149.

Priest, J.D., Jones, H.H., Tichenor, C.J., Nigel, D.A. 1977. Arm and elbow changes in expert tennis players. *Minn Med* 60(5): 399-404.

Reddy, A.S., Kvitne, R.S., Yocum, L.A., Elattrache, N.S., Glousman, R.E., Jobe, F.W. 2000. Arthroscopy of the elbow: A long term clinical review. *Arthroscopy* 16(6): 588-594.

Rijke, A.M., Goitz, H.T., McCue, F.C. 1994. Stress radiography of the medial elbow ligaments. *Radiology* 191: 213-216.

Roetert, E.P., Ellenbecker, T.S. 1998. *Complete conditioning for tennis.* Champaign, IL: Human Kinetics.

Roetert, E.P., Ellenbecker, T.S., Brown, S.W. 2000. Shoulder internal and external rotation range of motion in nationally ranked junior tennis players: A longitudinal analysis. *J Strength Cond Res* 14(2): 140-143.

Rosenthal, M. 1984. The efficacy of flurbiprofen versus piroxicam in the treatment of acute soft tissue rheumatism. *Curr Med Res Opin* 9: 304-309.

Runge, F. 1873. Zur genese unt behand lung bes schreibekramp fes Berl Kun Woschenschr 10: 245.

Ryu, R.K, McCormick, J., Jobe, F.W, Moynes, D.R., Antonelli, D.J. 1988. An electromyographic analysis of shoulder function in tennis players. *Am J Sports Med* 16(5): 481-485.

Slocum, D.B. 1978. Classification of the elbow injuries from baseball pitching. *Am J Sports Med* 6: 62.

Sullivan, P.E., Markos, P.D, Minor, M.D. 1982. *An integrated approach to therapeutic exercise: Theory and clinical application.* Reston, VA: Reston Publishing.

Svernlov, A.B., Adolfsson, L. 2001. Non-operative treatment regime including eccentric training for lateral humeral epicondylalgia. *Scand J Med Sci Sports* 11(6): 328-334.

Townsend, H., Jobe, F.W, Pink, M. 1991. Electromyographic analysis of the glenohumeral muscles during a baseball rehabilitation program. *Am J Sports Med* 19(3): 264-272.

Verhaar, J.A.N., Walenkamp, G.H.I.M., Kester, A.D.M., Linden, A.J.V.D. 1995. Local corticosteroid injection versus Cyriax-type physiotherapy for tennis elbow. *J Bone Joint Surg Br* 77: 128-132.

Waslewski, G.L., Lund, P., Chilvers, M., Taljanovic, M., Krupinski, E. 2002. MRI Evaluation of the Ulnar Collateral Ligament of the Elbow in Asymptomatic, Professional Baseball Players. Presented at the AOSSM Meeting 2002.

Wilk, K.E., Arrigo, C.A., Andrews, J.R. 1993. Rehabilitation of the elbow in the throwing athlete. *J Orthop Sports Phys Ther* 17: 305-317.

Wilson, F.D., Andrews, J.R., Blackburn, T.A., McCluskey, G. 1983. Valgus extension overload in the pitching elbow. *Am J Sports Med* 11(2): 83-88.

Winge, S., Jorgensen, U., Nielsen, A.L. 1989. Epidemiology of injuries in Danish championship tennis. *Int J Sports Med* 10: 368-371.

Wolf, B.R., Altchek, D.W. 2003. Elbow problems in elite tennis players. *Techniques in Shoulder and Elbow Surgery* 4(2): 55-68.

Chapter 8

Ashmead, D. IV, Watson, H., Damon, C., Herber, S., Paly, W. 1994. Scapholunate advanced collapse wrist salvage. *J Hand Surg Am* 19: 741-750.

Ayres, J., Goldstrohm, G., Miller, G., Dell, P. 1988. Proximal interphalangeal joint arthrodesis with the Herbert screw. *J Hand Surg Am* 13: 600-603.

Bamberger, H., Stern, P., Kiefhaber, T., McDonaough, J., Cantor, R. 1992. Trapeziometacarpal joint arthrodesis: A functional evaluation. *J Hand Surg Am* 17: 605-611.

Bande, S., De Smet, L., Fabry, G. 1994. The results of carpal tunnel release: open versus endoscopic technique. *J Hand Surg Br* 19: 14-17.

Berger, R. 1998. Partial denervation of the wrist: A new approach. *Techniques in Hand and Upper Extremity Surgery* 2(1): 25-35.

Blevens, A., Light, T., Jablonsky, W., Smith, D., Patwardhan, A., Guay, M., Woo, T. 1989. Radiocarpal articular contact characteristics with scaphoid instability. *J Hand Surg Am* 14: 781-790.

Brown, R., Gelberman, R., Seiler, J., Abrahamsson, S., Weiland, A., Urbaniak, J., et al. 1993. Carpal tunnel release: A prospective, randomized assessment of open and endoscopic methods. *J Bone Joint Surg Am* 75: 1265-1275.

Brown, R., E. Zook, R. Russell, J. Kucan, E. Smoot. 1991. Fingernail deformities secondary to ganglions of the distal interphalangeal joint (mucous cysts). *J Plas Reconstr Surg* 87: 718-725.

Burgess, R. 1987. The effect of rotatory subluxation of the scaphoid on radio-scaphoid contact. *J Hand Surg Am* 12: 771-774.

Burton, R. 1973. Basal joint arthrosis of the thumb. *Orthop Clin North Am* 4: 331-348.

Burton, R., Pellegrini, V. Jr. 1986. Surgical management of basal joint arthritis of the thumb. Part II: Ligament reconstruction with tendon interposition arthroplasty. *J Hand Surg Am* 11: 324-332.

Caspi, D., G. Flusser, I. Farber, J. Ribak, A. Leibovitz, B. Habot, M. Yaron, and R. Segal. 2001. Clinical, radiologic, demographic, and occupational aspects of hand osteoarthritis in the elderly. *Seminars in Arthritis and Rheumatism* 30(5): 321-331.

Chow, J. 1990. Endoscopic release of the carpal ligament for carpal tunnel syndrome: 22-month clinical result. *Arthroscopy* 6: 288-296.

Cohen, M., Kozin, S. 2001. Degenerative arthritis of the wrist: Proximal row carpectomy versus scaphoid excision and four-corner arthrodesis. *J Hand Surg Am* 26: 94-104.

Cooney, W., Chao, E. 1977. Biomechanical analysis of static forces in the thumb during hand function. *J Bone Joint Surg Am* 59: 27-36.

Cooney, W., Linscheid, R., Askew, L. 1987. Total arthroplasty of the thumb trapeziometacarpal joint. *Clin Orthop Rel Res* 220: 35-45.

Douglas, D., Peimer, C., Koniuch, M. 1987. Motion of the wrist after simulated limited intercarpal arthrodeses: An experimental study. *J Bone Joint Surg Am* 69: 1413-1418.

Durkan, J. 1991. A new diagnostic test for carpal tunnel syndrome. *J Bone Joint Surg Am* 73: 535-538.

Eaton, R., Dobranski, A., Littler, J. 1973. Marginal osteophyte excision in treatment of mucous cysts. *J Bone Joint Surg Am* 55: 570-574.

Eaton, R., Glickel, S., Littler, J. 1985. Tendon interposition arthroplasty for degenerative arthritis of the trapeziometacarpal joint of the thumb. *J Hand Surg Am* 10: 645-654.

Eaton, R., Littler, J. 1969. A study of the basal joint of the thumb (treatment of its disabilities by fusion). *J Bone Joint Surg Am* 51: 661-668.

Eaton, R., Malerich, M. 1980. Volar plate arthroplasty of the proximal interphalangeal joint: A review of ten years' experience. *J Hand Surg Am* 5: 260-268.

Froimson, A. 1970. Tendon arthroplasty of the trapeziometacarpal joint. *Clin Orthop Rel Res* 70: 191-199.

Frykman, E., Af Ekenstam, F., Wadin, K. 1988. Triscaphoid arthrodesis and its complications. *J Hand Surg Am* 13: 844-849.

Fulton, D., Stern, P. 2001. Trapeziometacarpal arthrodesis in primary osteoarthritis: A minimum two-year follow up study. *J Hand Surg Am* 26: 109-114.

Gelberman, R., Cooney, III, W., Szabo, R. 2001. Carpal instability. In *AAOS Instructional Course Lectures*, ed. F.H. Sim. Rosemont, IL: American Academy of Orthopaedic Surgeons.

Gelberman, R., Aronson, D., Weisman, M. 1980. Carpal tunnel syndrome: Results of a prospective trial of steroid injection and splinting. *J Bone Joint Surg Am* 62: 1181-1184.

Gellman, H., Gelberman, R., Tan, A., Botte, M. 1986. Carpal tunnel syndrome: An evaluation of the provacative diagnostic tests. *J Bone Joint Surg Am* 68: 735-737.

Gellman, H., D. Kauffman, M. Lenihan, M. Botte, and A. Sarmiento. 1988. An in vitro analysis of wrist motion: the effect of limited intercarpal arthrodesis and the contributions of the radiocarpal and midcarpal joints. *J Hand Surg Am* 13: 378-383.

Gervis, W. 1949. Excision of the trapezium for osteoarthritis of the trapeziometacarpal joint. *J Bone Joint Surg Br* 31: 537-539.

Gilula, L. 1979. Carpal injuries: analytic approach and case exercises. *American Journal of Roentgenology* 133(3): 503-517.

Glickel, S., Millender, L. 1984. Ligamentous reconstruction for chronic intercarpal instablity. *J Hand Surg Am* 9: 514-527.

Green, D. 1984. Diagnostic and therapeutic value of carpal tunnel injection. *J Hand Surg Am* 9: 850.

Hage, J., Yoe, E., Zevering, J., de Groot, P. 1999. Proximal interphalangeal joint silicone arthroplasty for posttraumatic arthritis. *J Hand Surg Am* 24: 73-77.

Hastings, H. II, Weiss, A., Strickland, J. 1993. Wrist fusion: Indication, technique, functional consequences for the hand and wrist. *Orthopade* 22: 86-91.

Herndon, J. 1987. Trapeziometacarpal arthroplasty: A clinical review. *Clin Orthop Rel Res* 220: 99-105.

Howell, D. 1985. Etiopathogenesis of osteoarthritis. In *Arthritis and allied conditions*, 10th ed., ed. D. McCarty. Philadelphia: Lea & Febiger.

Ishida, O., Tsai, T. 1993. Complications and results of scapho-trapezio-trapezoid arthrodesis. *Clin Orthop Rel Res* 287: 125-130.

Jacobsen, M., Rahme, H. 1996. A prospective, randomized study with an independent observer comparing open carpal tunnel release with endoscopic carpal tunnel release. *J Hand Surg Am* 21: 202-204.

Kasdan, M., Stallings, S., Leis, V., Wolens, D. 1994. Outcome of surgically treated mucous cysts of the hand. *J Hand Surg Am* 19: 504-507.

Kauer, J.M.G. 1974. The interdependence of carpal articulation chains. *Acta Anatomica* 88: 481-501.

Kleinert, W., Kutz, J., Fishman, J., McCraw, L. 1972. Etiology and treatment of the so-called mucous cyst of the finger. *J Bone Joint Surg Am* 54: 1455-1458.

Kleinman, W. 2001. Dynamics of carpal instability. In *The wrist*, edited by H. Watson and J. Weinzweig. Philadelphia: Lippincott Williams & Wilkins.

Knirk, J., Jupiter, J. 1986. Intra-articular fractures of the distal end of the radius in young adults. *J Bone Joint Surg Am* 68: 647-659.

Krakauer, J., Bishop, A., Cooney, W. 1994. Surgical treatment of scapholunate advanced collapse. *J Hand Surg Am* 19: 751-759.

Kvarnes, L., Reikeras, O. 1985. Osteoarthritis of the carpometacarpal joint of the thumb: An analysis of operative procedures. *J Hand Surg Br* 16: 117-120.

Lanzetta, M., Foucher, G. 1995. A comparison of different surgical techniques in treating degenerative arthrosis of the carpometacarpal joint of the thumb: A retrospective study of 98 cases. *J Hand Surg Br* 20: 105-110.

Lavernia, C., Cohen, M., Taleisnik, J. 1992. Treatment of scapholunate dissociation by ligamentous repair and capsulodesis. *J Hand Surg Am* 17: 354-359.

Leibovic, S., Strickland, J. 1994. Arthrodesis of the proximal interphalangeal joint of the finger: Comparison of the use of the Herbert screw with other fixation methods. *J Hand Surg Am* 19: 181-188.

Levin, S., Pearsell, G., Ruderman, R. 1978. Von Frey's method of measuring pressure sensibility in the hand: An engineering analysis of the Weinstein-Semmes pressure aethesiometer. *J Hand Surg Am* 3: 211-216.

Lins, R., Gelberman, R., McKeown, L., Katz, J., Kadiyala, R. 1996. Basal joint arthritis: Trapeziectomy with ligament reconstruction and tendon interposition arthroplasty. *J Hand Surg Am* 21: 202-209.

Linscheid, R. 2000. Implant arthroplasty of the hand: Retrospective and prospective considerations. *J Hand Surg Am* 25: 796-816.

Linscheid, R., Dobyns, J., Beabout, J., Bryan, R. 1972. Traumatic instability of the wrist. *J Bone Joint Surg Am* 54: 1612-1632.

Linscheid, R., Murray, P., Vidal,M., Beckenbaugh, R. 1997. Development of a surface replacement arthroplasty for proximal interphalangeal joints. *J Hand Surg Am* 22: 286-298.

Mankin, H. 1976. Biochemical changes in articular cartilage in osteoarthritis. *Symposium on osteoarthritis*. St. Louis, MS: C.V. Mosby.

Mankin, H., Johnson, M., Lippiello, L. 1981. Biochemical and metabolic abnormalities in articular cartilage from osteoarthritic human hips. *J Bone Joint Surg Am* 63: 131-139.

Mathoulin, C., Gilbert, A. 1999. Arthroplasty of the proximal interphalangeal joint using the Sutter implant for traumatic joint destruction. *J Hand Surg Br* 24: 565-569.

McAuliffe, J., Dell, P., Jaffe, R. 1993. Complications of intercarpal arthrodesis. *J Hand Surg Am* 18: 1121-1128.

Mih, A. 1997. Limited wrist fusion. *Hand Clin* 13: 615-625.

Minami, A., Kato, H., Iwaski, N., Minami, M. 1999. Limited wrist fusions: Comparison of results 22 and 89 months after surgery. *J Hand Surg Am* 24: 133-137.

Napier, J. 1955. The form and function of the carpo-metacarpal joint of the thumb. *J Anat* 89: 362-369.

Nath, R., Mackinnon, S., Weeks, P. 1993. Ulnar nerve transection as a complication of two-portal endoscopic carpal tunnel release: A case report. *J Hand Surg Am* 18: 896-898.

Nylen, S., Johnson, A., Rosenquist, A. 1993. Trapeziectomy and ligament reconstruction for osteoarthrosis of the base of the thumb: A prospective study of 100 operations. *J Hand Surg Br* 18: 616-619.

Peimer, C. 1987. Long-term complications of trapeziometacarpal silicone arthroplasty. *Clin Orthop Rel Res* 220: 86-97.

Pelligrini, V. 1991. Osteoarthritis of the trapeziometacarpal joint: The pathophysiology of articular cartilage degeneration. I. Anatomy and pathology of the aging joint. *J Hand Surg Am* 16: 967-974.

Pellegrini, V., Burton, R. 1990. Osteoarthritis of the proximal interphalangeal joint of the hand: Arthroplasty or fusion? *J Hand Surg Am* 15: 194-209.

Pellegrini, V., Olcott, C., Hollenberg, G. 1993. Contact patterns in the trapeziometacarpal joint: The role of the palmer oblique ligament. *J Hand Surg Am* 18: 238-244.

Phalen, G.S. 1966. The carpal tunnel syndrome: 17 years' experience in diagnosis and treatment of 654 hands. *J Bone Joint Surg Am* 48: 211-228.

Phalen, G.S. 1972. The carpal tunnel syndrome: Clinical evaluation of 598 hands. *Clin Orthop Rel Res* 83: 29-40.

Phalen, G.S., Kendrick, J. 1957. Compression neuropathy of the median nerve in the carpal tunnel. *JAMA* 164: 524-530.

Pribyl, C., Omer, G., McGinty, L. 1996. Effectiveness of the chevron arthrodesis in small joints of the hand. *J Hand Surg Am* 21: 1052-1058.

Sebald, S., Dobyns, J., Linscheid, R. 1974. The natural history of collapse deformities of the wrist. *Clin Orthop Rel Res* 104: 104-108.

Sonnex, T. 1986. Digital myxoid cysts: A review. *Cutis* 37: 89-94.

Stern, P., Gates, N., Jones, T. 1993. Tension band arthrodesis of small joints in the hand. *J Hand Surg Am* 18: 194-197.

Stern, P., Ho, S. 1987. Osteoarthritis of the proximal interphalangeal joint. *Hand Clin* 3(3): 405-412.

Swanson, A., de Groot, G. 1985. Osteoarthritis in the hand. *Clin Rheumatic Dis* 11(2): 393-420.

Swanson, A., Maupin, B., Gajjar, N., de Groot, G. 1985. Flexible implant arthroplasty in the proximal interphalangeal joint of the hand. *J Hand Surg Am* 10: 796-805.

Szabo, R. 1991. Carpal tunnel syndrome-general. *Operative Nerve Repair and Reconstruction*, ed. R. Gelberman. Philadelphia: Lippincott.

Szabo, R. 1993. Entrapment and compression neuropathies. In *Green's operative hand surgery*, 4th ed., ed. D. Green, R. Hotchkiss, and W. Pederson. New York: Churchill Livingstone.

Tinel, J. 1915. Le signe du "fourmillement" dans les lesions des nerfs peripheriques. *Presse Medicale* 23: 385.

Tomaino, M., Delsignore, J., Burton, R. 1994. Long-term results following proximal row carpectomy. *J Hand Surg Am* 19: 694-703.

Tomaino, M., Miller, R., Cole, I., Burton, R. 1994. Scapholunate advanced collapse wrist: proximal row carpectomy or limited wrist arthrodesis with scaphoid excision? *J Hand Surg Am* 19: 134-142.

Tomaino, M., Pellegrini, V., Burton, R. 1995. Arthroplasty of the basal joint of the thumb: Long-term follow-up after ligament reconstruction with tendon interposition. *J Bone Joint Surg Am* 77: 346-354.

Trumble, T., Culp, R., Hanel, D., et al. 1998. Intra-articular fractures of the distal aspect of the radius. *J Bone Joint Surg Am* 80: 582-600.

Van Heest, A., Waters, P., Simmons, B., Schwartz, J. 1995. A cadaveric study of the single-portal endoscopic carpal tunnel release. *J Hand Surg Am* 20: 363.

Watson, H.K., Ashmead, D., Makhlouf, M. 1988. Examination of the scaphoid. *J Hand Surg Am* 13: 657-660.

Watson, H.K., Ballet, F. 1984. The SLAC wrist: scapholunate advanced collapse pattern of degenerative arthritis. *J Hand Surg Am* 9: 358-365.

Watson, H.K., Hempton, R. 1980. Limited wrist arthrodesis: The triscaphoid joint. *J Hand Surg Am* 5: 320-327.

Watson, H.K., Weinzweig, J. 1997. Physical examination of the wrist. *Hand Clin* 13: 17-34.

Watson, H.K., Weinzweig, J. 2001. Dorsal wrist syndrome: Predynamic carpal instability. In *The wrist*, edited by H.K. Watson and J. Weinzweig. Philadelphia: Lippincott Williams & Wilkins.

Weber, E. 1984. Concepts governing the rotational shift of the intercalated segment of the carpus. *Orthop Clin North Am* 15: 193-207.

Weiss, A.P., Hastings II, H. 1995. Wrist arthrodesis for post-traumatic conditions: A study of plate and local bone graft application. *J Hand Surg Am* 20: 50-56.

Weiss, A.P., Sachar, K., Gendreau, M. 1994. Conservative management of carpal tunnel syndrome: A reexamination of steroid injection and splinting. *J Hand Surg Am* 19: 410-415.

Weiss, A.P., Wiedeman, G.Jr., Quenzer, D., Hanington, H., Hastings II, H., Strickland, J. 1995. Upper extremity function after wrist arthrodesis. *J Hand Surg Am* 20: 813-817.

Wilgis, E.F. 1997.Distal interphalangeal joint silicone interpositional arthroplasty of the hand. *Clin Orthop Rel Res* 342: 38-41.

Wilhelm, A. 1966. Die Gelenkdenervation und ihre anatomische Grundlagen. *Hefte Unfallheilkd* 86: 1-109.

Wintman, B., Gelberman, R., Katz, J. 1995. Dynamic scapholunate instability: Results of operative treatment with dorsal capsulodesis. *J Hand Surg Am* 20: 971-979.

Wyrick, J., Stern, P., Kiefhaber, T. 1995. Motion-preserving procedures in the treatment of scapholunate advanced collapse wrist: Proximal row carpectomy versus four-corner arthrodesis. *J Hand Surg Am* 20: 965-970.

Wyrick, J., Youse, B., Kiefhaber, T. 1998. Scapholunate ligament repair and capsulodesis for the treatment of static scapholunate dissociation. *J Hand Surg Br* 23: 776-780.

Wyrsch, B., Dawson, J., Aufranc, S., Weikert, D., Milek, M. 1996. Distal interphalangeal joint arthrodesis comparing tension-band wire and Herbert screw: A biomechanical and dimensional analysis. *J Hand Surg Am* 21: 438-443.

Yamaguchi, D., Lipscomb, P., Soule, E. 1965. Carpal tunnel syndrome. *Minn Med* 48: 22-33.

Chapter 9

Airaksinen, O., Herno, A., et al. 1997. Surgical outcome of 438 patients treated surgically for lumbar spinal stenosis. *Spine* 22(19): 2278-2282.

Akuthota, V., Willick, S., et al. 2001. The Adult spine: A practical approach to low back pain. In *Low back pain: A symptom-based approach to diagnosis and treatment*, 15-42. eds. K. Rucker, A. Cole and S. Weinstein. Woburn, MA: Butterworth-Heinemann.

Amundsen, T., Weber, H., et al. 2000. Lumbar spinal stenosis: Conservative or surgical management? A prospective 10-year study. *Spine* 25(11): 1424-1436.

Amundsen, T., Weber, H., et al. 1995. Lumbar spinal stenosis: Clinical and radiologic features. *Spine* 20(10): 1178-1186.

Atlas, S.J., Deyo, R.A., et al. 1996a. The Main Lumbar Spine Study, Part II. 1-year outcomes of surgical and nonsurgical management of sciatica. *Spine* 21(15): 1777-1786.

Atlas, S.J., Deyo, R.A., et al. 1996b. The Maine Lumbar Spine Study, Part III. 1-year outcomes of surgical and nonsurgical management of lumbar spinal stenosis. *Spine* 21(15): 1787-1794; discussion 1794-1795.

Barr, J.D., Barr, M.S., et al. 2000. Percutaneous vertebroplasty for pain relief and spinal stabilization. *Spine* 25(8): 923-928.

Bergquist-Ullman, M., Larsson, U. 1977. Acute low back pain in industry: A controlled prospective study with special reference to therapy and confounding factors. *Acta Orthop Scand* (170): 1-117.

Bergmark, A. 1989. Stability of the lumbar spine: A study in mechanical engineering. *Acta Orthop Scand Suppl* 230: 1-54.

Bernard, T.N., Cassidy, D. 1997. The sacroiliac joint syndrome: Pathophysiology, diagnosis, and management. *The adult spine: Principles and practice*, 2343-2366. ed. J.W. Frymoyer. Philadelphia: Lippincott-Raven.

Bernick, S., Cailliet, R. 1982. Vertebral end-plate changes with aging of human vertebrae. *Spine* 7: 97-102.

Bigos, S. et al. 1994. *Acute low back problems in adults: Clinical practice guideline*. Rockville, MD: U.S. Department of Health and Human Services.

Boden, S.D., Davis, D.O., et al. 1990. Abnormal magnetic-resonance scans of the lumbar spine in asymptomatic subjects: A prospective investigation. *J Bone Joint Surg Am* 72(3): 403-408.

Bogduk, N. 1997. *Clinical anatomy of the lumbar spine and sacrum.* New York: Churchill Livingstone.

Bortz, W.M. II. 1982. Disuse and aging. *JAMA* 248(10): 1203-1208.

Botwin, K.P., Gruber, R.D., et al. 2000. Complications of fluoroscopically guided transforaminal lumbar epidural injections. *Arch Phys Med Rehabil* 81(8): 1045-1050.

Botwin, K.P., Gruber, R.D., et al. 2001. Complications of fluoroscopically guided caudal epidural injections. *Am J Phys Med Rehabil* 80(6): 416-424.

Butler, D. 1991. *Mobilisation of the nervous system.* Melbourne: Churchill Livingstone.

Butler, D. 2000. *The sensitive nervous system.* Adelaide, Australia: Noigroup Publications.

Cassinelli, E., Hall, R., et al. 2001. Biochemistry of Intervertebral Disc Degeneration and the Potential for Gene Therapy Applications. *SpineLine* II: 5-10.

Cholewicki, J., Juluru, K., McGill, S.M. 1999. Intra-abdominal pressure mechanism for stabilizing the lumbar spine. *J Biomech* 32(1): 13-17.

Ciric, I., Mikhael, M., et al. 1980. The lateral recess syndrome: A variant of spinal stenosis. *J Neurosurg* 53: 433-443.

Cypress, B.K. 1983. Characteristics of physician visits for back symptoms: A national perspective. *Am J Public Health* 73(4): 389-395.

Deyo, R.A. 1986. Early diagnostic evaluation of low back pain. *J Gen Intern Med* 1(5): 328-338.

Dreyfuss, P., Dryer, S., et al. 1994. Positive sacroiliac screening tests in asymptomatic adults. *Spine* 19(10): 1138-1143.

Dreyfuss, P., Halbrook, B., et al. 2000. Efficacy and validity of radiofrequency neurotomy for chronic lumbar zygapophysial joint pain. *Spine* 25(10): 1270-1277.

Dreyfuss, P., Michaelsen, M., et al. 1996. The value of medical history and physical examination in diagnosing sacroiliac joint pain [see comments]. *Spine* 21(22): 2594-2602.

Dyck, P., Doyle, J.B. Jr. 1977. Bicycle test of van Gelderen in diagnosis of intermittent cauda equina compression syndrome: Case report. *Journal of Neurosurgery* 46(5): 667-670.

Ekin, J.A., Sinaki, M. 1993. Vertebral compression fractures sustained during golfing: report of three cases. *Mayo Clinic Proceedings* 68(6): 566-570.

Eskola, A., Pohjolainen, T., et al. 1992. Calcitonin treatment in lumbar spinal stenosis: A randomized, placebo-controlled, double-blind, cross-over study with one-year follow-up. *Calcified Tissue Intl* 50(5): 400-403.

Fairbank, J.C., Couper, J., et al. 1980. The Oswestry low back pain disability questionnaire. *Physiotherapy* 66(8): 271-273.

Fairbank, J.C., Pynsent, P.B. 2000. The Oswestry Disability Index. *Spine* 25(22): 2940-2952; discussion 2952.

Fardon, D. 1997. Differential diagnosis of low back disorders. In *The adult spine: Principles and practice*, 1745-1768. ed. J. Frymoyer. Philadelphia: Lippincott-Raven.

Fast, A., Robin, G. 1985. Surgical treatment of lumbar spinal stenosis in the elderly. *Arch Phys Med Rehab* 66: 149-151.

Favus, M., ed. 1999. *Primer on the metabolic bone diseases and disorders of mineral metabolism*. Philadelphia: Lippincott Williams & Wilkins.

Fischer, B., Watkins, R. 1996. Golf. In *The spine in sports*, 505-514. ed. R. Watkins. St. Louis: Mosby.

Foundation, N.O. 1998. *Physician's guide to prevention and treatment of osteoporosis*. Belle Mead, NJ: Excerpta Medica.

Fritz, J.M., Delitto, A., et al. 1998. Lumbar spinal stenosis: A review of current concepts in evaluation, management, and outcome measurements. *Arch Phys Med Rehabil* 79(6): 700-708.

Fritz, J.M., Erhard, R.E., et al. 1997a. A nonsurgical treatment approach for patients with lumbar spinal stenosis. *Phys Ther* 77(9): 962-973.

Fritz, J.M., Erhard, R.E., et al. 1997b. Preliminary results of the use of a two-stage treadmill test as a clinical diagnostic tool in the differential diagnosis of lumbar spinal stenosis. *J Spinal Disord* 10(5): 410-416.

Frymoyer, J.W. 1988. Back pain and sciatica. *N Engl J Med* 318(5): 291-300.

Fukusaki, M., Kobayashi, I., et al. 1998. Symptoms of spinal stenosis do not improve after epidural steroid injection. *Clin J Pain* 14(2): 148-151.

Gaines, W.G. Jr., Hegmann, K.T. 1999. Effectiveness of Waddell's nonorganic signs in predicting a delayed return to regular work in patients experiencing acute occupational low back pain. *Spine* 24(4): 396-400; discussion 401.

Garfin, S.R., Yuan, H.A., et al. 2001. New technologies in spine: Kyphoplasty and vertebroplasty for the treatment of painful osteoporotic compression fractures. *Spine* 26(14): 1511-1515.

Geraci, M.C., Alleva, J.T. 1997. Physical examination of the spine and its functional kinetic chain. In *The low back pain handbook*, 49-70. eds. A.J. Cole and S. A. Hering. Philadelphia: Hanley and Belfus.

Hall, S., Bartleson, J., et al. 1985. Lumbar spinal stenosis: Clinical features, diagnostic procedures, and results of surgical treatment in 68 patients. *Ann Intern Med* 103: 271-275.

Herring, S., Kibler, W. 1998. A framework for rehabilitation. In *Functional rehabilitation of sports and musculoskeletal injuries*, 1-8. eds. W.B. Kibler, S.A. Herring, J.M. Press, and P.A. Lee. Gaithersburg, MD: Aspen.

Herring, S.A., Weinstein, S.M. 1995. Assessment and nonsurgical management of athletic low back injury. In *The lower extremity and spine in sports medicine*. eds. J.A. Nicholas and E.B. Hershman. St. Louis: Mosby, 1171-1197.

Hodges, P.W., Richardson, C.A. 1997. Contraction of the abdominal muscles associated with movement of the lower limb. *Phys Ther* 77(2): 132-142; discussion 142-144.

Hosea, T., Gatt, C., et al. 1990. Biomechanical analysis of the golfer's back. *Science and golf*. A. Cochrane. London: Chapman and Hall, 43-48.

Hosea, T., C. Gatt, et al. 1994. Biomechanical analysis of the golfer's back. In *Feeling up to par: Medicine from tee to green*, 97-108. eds. C. Stover, J. McCarroll and W. Mallon. Philadelphia: F.A. Davis.

Inufusa, A., An, H.S., et al. 1996. Anatomic changes of the spinal canal and intervertebral foramen associated with flexion-extension movement. *Spine* 21(21): 2412-2420.

Jacobson, R.E. 1976. Lumbar stenosis: An electromyographic evaluation. *Clin Orthop* (115): 68-71.

Jenis, L.G., An, H.S. 2000. Spine update: Lumbar foraminal stenosis. *Spine* 25(3): 389-394.

Jenis, L.G., An, H.S., et al. 2001. Foraminal stenosis of the lumbar spine: A review of 65 surgical cases. *Am J Orthop* 30(3): 205-211.

Jensen, M.C., Brant-Zawadzki, M.N., et al. 1994. Magnetic resonance imaging of the lumbar spine in people without back pain [see comments]. *N Engl J Med* 331(2): 69-73.

Jensen, M.E., Evans, A.J., et al. 1997. Percutaneous polymethylmethacrylate vertebroplasty in the treatment of osteoporotic vertebral body compression fractures: Technical aspects. *AJNR Am J Neuroradiol* 18(10): 1897-1904.

Johnson, E.K., Chiarello, C.M. 1997. The slump test: the effects of head and lower extremity position on knee extension. *J Orthop Sports Phys Ther* 26(6): 310-317.

Johnsson, K.E., Rosen, I., et al. 1992. The natural course of lumbar spinal stenosis. *Clin Orthopaedics Related Res* (279): 82-86.

Johnsson, K.E., Uden, A., et al. 1991. The effect of decompression on the natural course of spinal stenosis: A comparison of surgically treated and untreated patients. *Spine* 16(6): 615-619.

Katz, J.N., Dalgas, M., et al. 1995. Degenerative lumbar spinal stenosis: Diagnostic value of the history and physical examination. *Arthritis Rheum* 38(9): 1236-1241.

Kaul, M., Herring, S. 1998. Rehabilitation of lumbar spine injuries. In *Functional rehabilitation of sports and musculoskeletal injuries*, 188-215. eds. W. Kibler, S. Herring, J. Press, and P. Lee. Gaithersburg, MD: Aspen.

Kirkaldy-Willis, W.H., Burton, C.V. 1992. *Managing low back pain*. New York: Churchill Livingstone.

Kirkaldy-Willis, W.H., Wedge, J.H., et al. 1978. Pathology and pathogenesis of lumbar spondylosis and stenosis. *Spine* 3(4): 319-328.

Kraft, G.H. 1990. Fibrillation potential amplitude and muscle atrophy following peripheral nerve injury. *Muscle Nerve* 13(9): 814-821.

Kraft, G.H. 1998. A physiological approach to the evaluation of lumbosacral spinal stenosis. *Phys Med Rehabil Clin N Am* 9(2): 381-389, viii.

Liang, M., Komaroff, A.L. 1982. Roentgenograms in primary care patients with acute low back pain: A cost-effectiveness analysis. *Archives of Internal Medicine* 142(6): 1108-1112.

Lindsay, D., Horton, J., et al. 2000. A review of injury characteristics, aging factors and prevention programmes for the older golfer. *Sports Med* 30(2): 89-103.

Lutz, G.E., Vad, V.B., et al. 1998. Fluoroscopic transforaminal lumbar epidural steroids: An outcome study. *Arch Phys Med Rehab* 79(11): 1362-1366.

Lyritis, G.P., Ioannidis, G.V., et al. 1999. Analgesic effect of salmon calcitonin suppositories in patients with acute pain due to recent osteoporotic vertebral crush fractures: A prospective double-blind, randomized, placebo-controlled clinical study. *Clin J Pain* 15(4): 284-289.

Magee, D.J. 2002. *Orthopedic physical assessment*. Philadelphia: Saunders.

Matheson, G., Macintyre, J., et al. 1988. Musculoskeletal injuries associated with physical activity in older adults. *Med Sci Sports Exerc* 21(4): 379-385.

McCarroll, J.R. 1996. The frequency of golf injuries. *Clin Sports Med* 15(1): 1-7.

McGill, S.M. 1998. Low back exercises: Evidence for improving exercise regimens. *Phys Ther* 78(7): 754-765.

McGill, S.M. 2001. Low back stability: From formal description to issues for performance and rehabilitation. *Exerc Sport Sci Rev* 29(1): 26-31.

Moreland, D., Landi, M., et al. 2001. Vertebroplasty: Techniques to avoid complications. *The Spine Journal* 1(1): 66-71.

Nachemson, A. 1960. Lumbar interdiscal pressure. *Acta Orthop Scand* 43.

Nachemson, A., Lewin, T., et al. 1970. In vitro diffusion of dye through the end-plates and the annulus fibrosus of human intervertebral discs. *Acta Orthop Scand* 41: 589-607.

Nadler, S.F., Malanga, G.A., DePrince, M., Stitik, T.P., Feinberg, J.H. 2000. The relationship between lower extremity injury, low back pain, and hip muscle strength in male and female collegiate athletes. *Clin J Sport Med* 10(2): 89-97.

Panjabi, M.M., White, A.A. 1990. Physical properties and functional biomechanics of the spine. *Clinical biomechanics of the spine*, 58-67. eds. M.M. Panjabi and A.A. White. Philadelphia: Lippincott-Raven.

Papageorgiou, A.C., Croft, P.R., et al. 1995. Estimating the prevalence of low back pain in the general population. Evidence from the South Manchester Back Pain Survey. *Spine* 20(17): 1889-1894.

Porter, R. 1996. Spinal stenosis and neurogenic claudication. *Spine* 21(17): 2046-2052.

Porter, R.W., Hibbert, C., et al. 1984. The natural history of root entrapment syndrome. *Spine* 9(4): 418-421.

Press, J.M., Young, J.L. 1997. Electrodiagnostic medicine. In *The low back pain handbook*, 213-226. eds. A.J. Cole and S.A. Herring. Philadelphia: Hanley and Belfus.

Ray, N., Chan, J., et al. 1997. Medical expenditures for the treatment of osteoporotic fractures in the United States in 1995: Report from the National Osteoporosis Foundation. *J Bone Miner Res* 12: 24-35.

Riew, K.D., Yin, Y., et al. 2000. The effect of nerve-root injections on the need for operative treatment of lumbar radicular pain: A prospective, randomized, controlled, double-blind study. *J Bone Joint Surg Am* 82-A(11): 1589-1593.

Rivest, C., Katz, J.N., et al. 1998. Effects of epidural steroid injection on pain due to lumbar spinal stenosis or herniated disks: A prospective study. *Arthritis Care Res* 11(4): 291-297.

Saal, J., Franson, R., et al. 1990. High level of inflammatory phospholipase A2 activity in lumbar disc herniations. *Spine* 15: 674-678.

Sapsford, R.R., Hodges, P.W., Richardson, C.A., Cooper, D.H., Markwell, S.J., Jull, G.A. 2001. Co-activation of the abdominal and pelvic floor muscles during voluntary exercises. *Neurourol Urodyn* 20(1): 31-42.

Schumacher, H., Klippel, J., et al., eds. 1993. *Primer on the rheumatic diseases*. Atlanta: Arthritis Foundation.

Schwarzer, A.C., Aprill, C.N., et al. 1994. The relative contributions of the disc and zygapophyseal joint in chronic low back pain. *Spine* 19(7): 801-806.

Schwarzer, A.C., Aprill, C.N., et al. 1995. The sacroiliac joint in chronic low back pain. *Spine* 20(1): 31-37.

Seppalainen, A.M., Alaranta, H., et al. 1981. Electromyography in the diagnosis of lumbar spinal stenosis. *Electromyogr Clin Neurophysiol* 21(1): 55-66.

Simotas, A.C. 2001. Nonoperative treatment for lumbar spinal stenosis. *Clin Orthop Related Res* (384): 153-161.

Simotas, A.C., Dorey, F.J., et al. 2000. Nonoperative treatment for lumbar spinal stenosis: Clinical and outcome results and a 3-year survivorship analysis. *Spine* 25(2): 197-203; discussions 203-204.

Sinaki, M. 1993. Osteoporosis. In *Rehabilitation medicine: Principles and practice*, 1018-1035. ed. J. Delisa. Philadelphia: Lippincott.

Slipman, C.W., Patel, R.K., et al. 2003. Epidemiology of spine tumors presenting to musculoskeletal physiatrists. *Arch Phys Med Rehabil* 84(4): 492-495.

Slipman, C.W., Sterenfeld, E.B., et al. 1998. The predictive value of provocative sacroiliac joint stress maneuvers in the diagnosis of sacroiliac joint syndrome. *Arch Phys Med Rehabil* 79(3): 288-292.

Spivak, J. 1998. Degenerative lumbar spinal stenosis. *J Bone Joint Surg* 80-A: 1053-1066.

Stucki, G., Daltroy, L., et al. 1996. Measurement properties of a self-administered outcome measure in lumbar spinal stenosis. *Spine* 21(7): 796-803.

Sturesson, B., Selvik, G., et al. 1989. Movements of the sacroiliac joints: A roentgen stereophotogrammetric analysis. *Spine* 14(2): 162-165.

Suarez-Almazor, M.E., Belseck, E., et al. 1997. Use of lumbar radiographs for the early diagnosis of low back pain. Proposed guidelines would increase utilization [see comments]. *JAMA* 277(22): 1782-1786.

Sullivan, W.J., Willick, S.E., et al. 2000. Incidence of intravascular uptake in lumbar spinal injection procedures. *Spine* 25(4): 481-486.

Von Korff, M., Deyo, R.A., et al. 1993. Back pain in primary care: Outcomes at 1 year. *Spine* 18(7): 855-862.

Waddell, G., McCulloch, J.A., et al. 1980. Nonorganic physical signs in low-back pain. *Spine* 5(2): 117-125.

Waddell, G., Newton, M., et al. 1993. A Fear-Avoidance Beliefs Questionnaire (FABQ) and the role of fear-avoidance beliefs in chronic low back pain and disability. *Pain* 52(2): 157-168.

Watts, N. 2000. Postmenopausal osteoporosis. *SpineLine* 1: 5-10.

Weinstein, S., Herring, S., et al. 1998. Rehabilitation of the patient with spinal pain. In *Rehabilitation medicine: Principles and practice*, 1423-1451. ed. J. DeLisa and B. Gans. Philadelphia: Lippincott-Raven.

White, A., Panjabi, M. 1990. *Clinical biomechanics of the spine*. Philadelphia: Lippincott-Raven.

Whitman, J.M., Flynn, T.W., Fritz, J.M. 2003. Nonsurgical management of patients with lumbar spine stenosis: A literature review and a case series of three patients managed with physical therapy. *Phys Med Rehabil Clin N Am* 14(1): 77101, vi-vii Review.

Wiesel, S. W., Tsourmas, N., et al. 1984. A study of computer-assisted tomography. I. The incidence of positive CAT scans in an asymptomatic group of patients. *Spine* 9(6): 549-551.

Willner, S. 1985. Effect of a rigid brace on back pain. *Acta Orthop Scand* 56(1): 40-42.

Yang, K., King, A. 1984. Mechanism of facet load transmission as a hypothesis for low-back pain. *Spine* 9(6): 557-565.

Young, J., Press, J., et al. 1997. The disc at risk in athletes: Perspectives on operative and nonoperative care. *Med Sci Sports Exerc* 29(7 Suppl): S222-S232.

Chapter 10

Brignall, C.G., Stainsby, G.D. 1991. The snapping hip. *J Bone Joint Surg Br* 73(2): 253-254.

Erb RE. 2001. Current concepts in imaging the adult hip. *Clin Sports Med* 20(4): 661-696.

Gray-Alistar, J.R., Villar, R.N. 1997. The ligamentum teres of the hip: An arthroscopic classification of its pathology. *Arthroscopy* 13(5): 575-578.

Healy, W.L., Iorio, R., Lemos, M.J. 2001. Athletic activity after joint replacement. *Am J Sports Med* 29(3): 377-388.

Jacobson, T., Allen, W.C. 1990. Surgical correction of the snapping iliopsoas tendon. *Am J Sports Med* 18(5): 470-474.

Kagan, A. 1999. Rotator cuff tears of the hip. *Clin Orthop* 368: 135-140.

Kandemir, U., Bharam, S., Philippon, M.J., Fu, F.H. 2003. Endoscopic treatment of calcific tendonitis of the gluteus medius and minimus: A case report. *Arthroscopy* 19(1): E4.

Kilgus, D.J., Dorey, F.J., Finerman, G.A., et al. 1991. Patient activity, sports participation, and impact loading on the durability of cemented total hip replacements. *Clin Orthop* 269: 25-31.

Kingzett-Taylor, A., Tirman, P.F., Feller, J., et al. 1999. Tendinosis and tears of gluteus medius and minimus muscles as a cause of hip pain, MR imaging findings. *Am J Roentgenol* 173(4): 1123-1126.

Lage, L.A., Patel, J.V., Villar, R.N. 1996. The acetabular labral tear: an arthroscopic classification. *Arthroscopy* 12(3): 269-272.

Mallon, W.J., Callaghan, J.J. 1992. Total hip arthroplasty in active golfers. *J Arthroplasty* 7(suppl): 339-346.

Meyers, W.C., Foley, B.P., Garrett, W.E., et al. 2000. Management of severe lower abdominal or inguinal pain in high-performance athletes. *Am J Sports Med* 28(1): 2-8.

Mont, M.A., LaPorte, D.M., Mullick, T., et al. 1999. Tennis after total hip arthroplasty. *Am J Sports Med* 27: 60-64.

Pelsser, V., Cardinal, E., Hobden, R., et al. 2001. Extraarticular snapping hip: Sonographic findings. *Am J Roentgenol* 176(1): 67-73.

Philippon, M.J. 2001. The role of arthroscopic thermal capsulorraphy in the hip. *Clin Sports Med 20*(4): 817-829.

Philippon, M.J. 2003. Hip arthroscopy in athletes. In *Operative arthroscopy*, 3rd ed. ed. McGinty JB, Philadelphia: Lipponcott Williams & Wilkins.

Steadman, J.R., Rodkey, W.G., Briggs, K.K., et al. 1999. The microfracture technique in the management of complete cartilage defects in the knee joint. *Orthope* 28(1): 26-32.

Wasielewski, R.C. 1998. The hip. In *The adult hip*. eds. Callaghan JJ, Rosenberg AG, Rubash HE, 57-73. Philadelphia: Lippincott-Raven.

Zoltan, D.J., Clancy, W.G. Jr., Keene, J.S. 1986. A new approach to snapping hip and refractory trochanteric bursitis in athletes. *Am J Sports Med* 14(3): 201-204.

Chapter 11

Adams, M.E., Atkinson, M.H., Lussier, A.J., Siminovitch, K.A., Wade, J.P., Zummer, M. 1995. The role of viscosupplementation with hylan G-F 20 (Synvisc) in the treatment of osteoarthritis of the knee: A Canadian multicenter trial comparing multicenter trial comparing hylan G-F 20 alone, hylan G-F20 with non-steroidal anti-inflammatory drugs (NSAIDs) and NSAIDs alone. *Osteoarthritis Cartilage* 3(4): 213-225.

Altman, R.D., Moskowitz, R., Hyalgan Study Group. 1998. Intra-articular sodium hyaluronate (Hyalgan) in the treatment of patients with osteoarthritis of the knee: A randomized clinical trial. *J Rheumatol* 25: 2203-2212.

Anderson, J.K., Goldstein, W.M. 1991. Arthroscopy in patients over the age of 50 years. *Am J Arthroscopy* 1:15-18.

Ayers, D.C., Dennis, D.A., Johanson, N.A., Pellegrini, V.D. Jr. 1997. Common complications of total knee arthroplasty. *J Bone Joint Surg* 79A: 278-311.

Balazs, E.A., Denlinger, J.L. 1993. Viscosupplementation: A new concept in the treatment of osteoarthritis. *J Rheum* 20(Suppl 39): 3-9.

Baumgaertner, M.R., Cannon, W.D., Vittori, J.M., Schmidt, E.S., Maurer, R.C. 1990. Arthroscopic debridement of the arthritic knee. *Clin Orthop* 253: 197-202.

Broughton, N.S., Newman, J.H., Baily, R.A.J. 1986. Unicompartmental replacement and high tibial osteotomy for osteoarthritis of the knee: A comparative study after 5-10 years' follow-up. *J Bone Joint Surg Br* 68: 447-452.

Corrado, E.M., Peluso, G.F., Gigliotti, S., et al. 1995. The effects of intra-articular administration of hyaluronic acid on osteoarthritis of the knee: A clinical study with immunological and biochemical evaluations. *Eur J Rheumatol Inflamm* 15: 47-56.

Das, A., Hammad, T.A. 2000. Efficacy of a combination of FCHG 49 glucosamine hydrochloride, TRH 122 low molecular weight sodium chondroitin sulfate and manganese ascorbate in the management of knee osteoarthritis. *Osteoarthritis Cartilage* 8(5): 343-350.

Dejour, J., Neyret, P., Boileau, P., Donnell, S.T. 1994. Anterior cruciate reconstruction combined with valgus tibial osteotomy. *Clin Orthop* 299: 220-228.

Delafuente, J.C. 2000. Glucosamine in the treatment of osteoarthritis. *Rheum Dis Clin N Am* 26(1): 1-11, vii. Review.

Dennis, D.A., Komistek, R.D., Northcut, E.J., Wood, A., Stiehl, J.B. 1999. An in vivo analysis of the effectiveness of the arthritic knee brace during heel strike of gait. Presented at American Academy of Orthopaedic Surgeons 1999 Annual Meeting, February 6, 1999.

Deyle, G.D., Henderson, N.E., Natekel, R.L., Ryder, M.G., Garber, M.B., Allison, S.C. 2000. Effectiveness of manual physical therapy and exercise in osteoarthritis of the knee: A randomized, controlled trial. *Ann Intern Med* 132: 173-181.

Dougados, M., Nguyen, M., Listrat, V., Amor, B. 1993. High molecular weight sodium hyaluronate (hyalectin) in osteoarthritis of the knee: A 1-year placebo controlled trial. *Osteoarthritis Cartilage* 1(2): 97-103.

Draper, E.R.C, Cable, J.M., Sanches-Ballester, J., Hunt, N., Robinson, J.R., Strachan, R.K. 2000. Improvement in function after valgus bracing of the knee: An analysis of gait symmetry. *J Bone Joint Surg Br* 82: 1001-1005.

Drovanti, A., Bignamini, A.A., Rovati, A.L. 1980. Therapeutic activity of oral glucosamine sulfate in osteoarthritis: A placebo-controlled double-blind investigation. *Clin Ther* 3: 260-272. Citation.

Engh, G.A., McAuley, J.P. 1999. Unicondylar arthroplasty: an option for high-demand patients with gonarthrosis. In *Instructional Course Lectures, American Academy of Orthopaedic Surgeons*. Vol. 48, pp.143-148. Rosemont, Illinois, American Academy of Orthopaedic Surgeons 1999.

Fife, R.S., Brandt, K.D., Braunstein, E.M., Katz, B.P., Shelbourne, K.D., Kalsinski, L.A., Ryan, S. 1991. Relationship between arthroscopic evidence of cartilage damage and radiographic evidence of joint space narrowing in early osteoarthritis of the knee. *Arthritis Rheum* 34(4): 377-382.

Fisher, N.M., Gresham, G.E., Abrams, M., Hicks, J., Horrigan, D., Pendergast, D.R. 1993. Quantitative effects of physical therapy on muscular and functional performance in subjects with osteoarthritis of the knees. *Arch Phys Med Rehabil* 74: 840-847.

Fleisch, A.M., Merlin, C., Imhoff, A., et al. 1997. A one-year randomized, double-blind, placebo controlled study with oral chondroitin sulfate in patients with knee osteoarthritis. *Osteoarthritis Cartilage* 5: 70.

Hanssen, A.D., Stuart, M.J., Scott, R.D., Scuderi, G.R. 2000. Surgical options for the middle-aged patient with osteoarthritis of the knee joint. *J Bone Joint Surg Am* 82: 1768-1781.

Healy, W.L., Iorio, R., Lemos, M.J. 2001. Athletic activity after joint replacement. *Am J Sports Med* 29(3): 377-388.

Jackson, R.W., Silver, R., Marans, H. 1986. Arthroscopic treatment of degenerative joint disease. *J Arthroscopy* 2: 114.

Johnson, L.L. 1986. Arthroscopic abrasion arthroplasty historical and pathological perspective: Present status. *Arthroscopy* 2: 54-69.

Katz, M.M., Hungerford, D.S., Krackow, K.A., Lennox, D.W. 1987. Results of total knee arthroplasty after failed proximal tibial osteotomy for osteoarthritis. *J Bone Joint Surg Am* 69: 225-233.

Kirkley, A., Webster-Bogaert, S., Litchfield, R., Macdonald, S., Amendola, A., McCalden, R., Fowler, P. 1999. The effect of bracing on varus gonarthrosis. *J Bone Joint Surg* 81(4): 539-547.

Lysholm, J., Hamberg, P., Gillquist, J. 1987. The correlation between osteoarthrosis as seen on radiographs and on arthroscopy. *J Arthroscopy* 3: 161-165.

Magnuson, P.B. 1941. Joint debridement: Surgical treatment of degenerative arthritis. *Surg Gynecol Obstetr* 73: 1-9.

Mankin, H.J. 1982. The response of articular cartilage to mechanical injury. *J Bone Joint Surg Am* 64: 460-466.

Mazieres, B., Loyau, G., Menkes, C.J., et al. 1992. Le chondroitine sulfate dans le traitment de la gonarthrose et de la coxarthrose. *Rev Rheum Mal Osteartic* 59: 466.

Minor, M.A., Hewett, J.E., Webel, R.R., Anderson, S.K., Kay, D.R. 1989. Efficacy of physical conditioning exercise in patients with rheumatoid arthritis and osteoarthritis. *Arthritis Rheum* 32: 1396-1405.

Morreale, P., Manopulo, R., Galati, M., Boccanera, L., Saponati, G., Bocchi, L. 1985. Comparison of the anti-inflammatory efficacy of chondroitin sulfate and diclofenac sodium in patients with knee osteoarthritis. *J Rheumatol* 23(8): 1835-1391.

Nagel, A., Insall, J.N., Scuderi, G.R. 1996. Proximal tibial osteotomy: A subjective outcome study. *J Bone Joint Surg Am* 78: 1353-1358.

Noyes, F.R., Barber, S., Simon, R. 1993. High tibial osteotomy and ligament reconstruction in varus angulated, anterior cruciate ligament-deficient knees. *Am J Sports Med* 21: 2-12.

Parker, R.D., Dimeff, R.J., Kolczun, M.C. 2001. Arthritis of the knee in the active person. Presented at AOSSM 27th Annual Meeting, Keystone, CO. June 2001.

Pelletier, J.P., Martel-Pelletier, J. 1993. The pathophysiology of osteoarthritis and the implication of the use of hyaluronan and hylan as therapeutic agents in viscosupplementation. *J Rheumatol* 20(39S): 19-24.

Pujalte, J.M., Llavore, E.P., Ylescupidez, F.R. 1980. Double-blind clinical evaluation of oral glucosamine sulfate in the basic treatment of osteoarthritis. *Curr Med Res Opin* 7(2): 110-114.

Rand, J.A. 1991. Role of arthroscopy in osteoarthritis of the knee. *J Arthroscopy* 7: 358-363.

Repicci, J.A. 2001. Minimally invasive arthroplasty. Presented at Orthopaedic Learning Center, Biomet, Inc. Unicondylar Workshop, February 16, 2001.

Rodeo, S.A., Forster, R.A., Weiland, A.J. 1993. Current concepts review. Neurological complications due to arthroscopy. *J Bone Joint Surg Am* 75: 917-926.

Salisbury, R.B., Nottage, W.M., Gardner, V. 1985. The effect of alignment on the results in arthroscopic debridement of the degenerative knee. *Clin Orthop* 198: 268-272.

Salter, R.B., Simmonds, D.R., Malcolm, B.W., Rumble, D.J., McMichael, D., Clements, N.D. 1980. The biological effect of continuous passive motion of healing of full-thickness defects in articular cartilage: An experimental investigation in the rabbit. *J Bone Joint Surg Am* 62: 1232-1251.

Schmalzried, T.P., Shepherd, E.F., Dorey, F.J. 2000. Wear is a function of use, not time. *Clin Orthop* 381: 36-46.

Shelbourne, K.D., Patel, D.V., Martini, D.J. 1996. Classification and management of arthrofibrosis of the knee after anterior cruciate ligament reconstruction. *Am J Sports Med* 24(6): 857-862.

Shelbourne, K.D., Stube, L.C.C. 1997. Anterior cruciate ligament-deficient knee with degenerative arthrosis: Treatment with an isolated autogenous patellar tendon ACL reconstruction. *Knee Surg Sports Traumatol* 5: 150-156.

Simon, L.S. 1999. Viscosupplementation therapy with intra-articular hyaluronic acid: Fact or fiction? *Rheum Dis Clin North Am* 25(2): 1-13.

Vaz, A. 1982. Double-blind clinical evaluation of the relative efficacy of ibuprofen and glucosamine sulfate in the management of osteoarthritis of the knee in out-patients. *Curr Med Res Opin* 8: 145.

Verbruggen, G., Goemaere, S., Veys, E.M. 1997. Chondroitin sulfate S/DMOAD (Structure/Disease Modifying Osteoarthritis (OA) Drug) in the treatment of OA of the finger joints. *Osteoarthritis Cartilage* 5: 70.

Weiss, C., Band, P. 1999. Basic principles underlying the development of viscosupplementation for the treatment of osteoarthritis. *J Clin Rheum* 5: S2-S11.

Chapter 12

Anderson, R.B., Davis, W.H. 2000. Management of the adult flatfoot deformity. In Myerson, M.S., ed., *Foot and ankle disorders*, 1017-1039. Philadelphia: WB Saunders.

Armagan, O., Shereff, M. 2000. Tendon injury and repair. In Myerson, M.S. ed., *Foot and ankle disorders*, 942-972. Philadelphia: WB Saunders.

Baxter, D.E. 1999. The foot in running. In Coughlin, M.J., Mann, R.A., eds., *Surgery of the foot and ankle*, 7th ed., 1210-1224. Philadelphia: Mosby.

Clanton, T.O. 1999. Athletic injuries to the soft tissues of the foot and ankle. In Coughlin, M.J., Mann, R.A., eds., *Surgery of the foot and ankle*, 7th ed. 1090-1209. Philadelphia: Mosby.

Coughlin, M.J. 1999a. Arthritides. In Coughlin, M.J., Mann, R.A., eds., *Surgery of the foot and ankle*, 7th ed., 560-650. Philadelphia: Mosby.

Coughlin, M.J. 1999b. Disorders of tendons. In Coughlin, M.J., Mann, R.A., eds., *Surgery of the foot and ankle*, 7th ed., 786-861. Philadelphia: Mosby.

Coughlin, M.J., Mann, R.A. 1999. Lesser toe deformities. In Coughlin, M.J., Mann, R.A., eds., *Surgery of the foot and ankle*, 7th ed., 320-391. Philadelphia: Mosby.

Daniels, T.R. 2000. Osteochondroses of the foot. In Myerson, M.S., ed., *Foot and ankle disorders*, 785-799. Philadelphia: WB Saunders.

Ferkel, R.D. 1999. Arthroscopy of the foot and ankle. In Coughlin, M.J., Mann, R.A., eds., *Surgery of the foot and ankle*, 7th ed., 1257-1297. Philadelphia: Mosby.

Hamilton, W.G., Hamilton, L.H. 1999. Foot and ankle injuries in dancers. In Coughlin, M.J., Mann, R.A., eds., *Surgery of the foot and ankle*, 7th ed., 1225-1256. Philadelphia: Mosby.

Horton, G.A. 2000. Hallux rigidus. In Myerson, M.S., ed., *Disorders of the foot and ankle*, 289-307. Philadelphia: WB Saunders.

Mann, R.A. 1999. Flatfoot in adults. In Coughlin, M.J., Mann, R.A., eds., *Surgery of the foot and ankle*, 7th ed., 733-767. Philadelphia: Mosby.

Mann, R.A., Coughlin, M.J. 1999. Adult hallux valgus. In Coughlin, M.J., Mann, R.A., eds., *Surgery of the foot and ankle*, 7th ed., 150-269. Philadelphia: Mosby.

Myerson, M.S., Mendelbaum, B. 2000. Disorders of the Achilles tendon and the retrocalcaneal region. In Myerson, M.S., ed., *Foot and ankle disorders*, 1367-1398. Philadelphia: WB Saunders.

Pfeffer, G.B. 2000. Plantar heel pain. In Myerson, M.S., ed., *Foot and ankle disorders*, 834-850. Philadelphia: WB Saunders.

Sanders, R. 1999. Fractures of the midfoot and forefoot. In Myerson, M.S., ed., *Surgery of the foot and ankle*, 7th ed., 1574-1605. Philadelphia: Mosby.

Schon, L.S. 2000. Decision-making for the athlete: The leg, ankle, and foot in sports. In Myerson, M.S., ed., *Foot and ankle disorders*, 1435-1476. Philadelphia: WB Saunders.

Scioli, M.W. 2000. Injuries about the ankle: Instability of the ankle and subtalar joint. In Myerson, M.S., ed., *Foot and ankle disorders*, 1399-1419. Philadelphia: WB Saunders.

Scranton, P.E. 2000. Lower extremity stress fractures. In Myerson, M.S., ed., *Foot and ankle disorders*, 1420-1434. Philadelphia: WB Saunders.

Toth, A.P., Easley, M.E. 2000. Ankle chondral injuries and repair. *Foot and Ankle Clinics* 5:799-840.

INDEX

Note: The italicized *f* and *t* following page numbers refer to figures and tables, respectively.

T

ABOUT THE EDITOR

Kevin Speer, MD, is an orthopedic surgeon from Raleigh, North Carolina. As a former team doctor for Duke University and through his own practice, Speer has extensive experience treating both athletes and older patients. Speer was head team physician for all Duke University athletic teams, assistant team physician for the New York Giants, the New York Mets, and St. John's University, and head team physician for the Durham women's professional fast-pitch softball team.

Speer has been listed in America's Registry of Outstanding Professionals and has received numerous awards and fellowships related to orthopedic research, publications, and education.

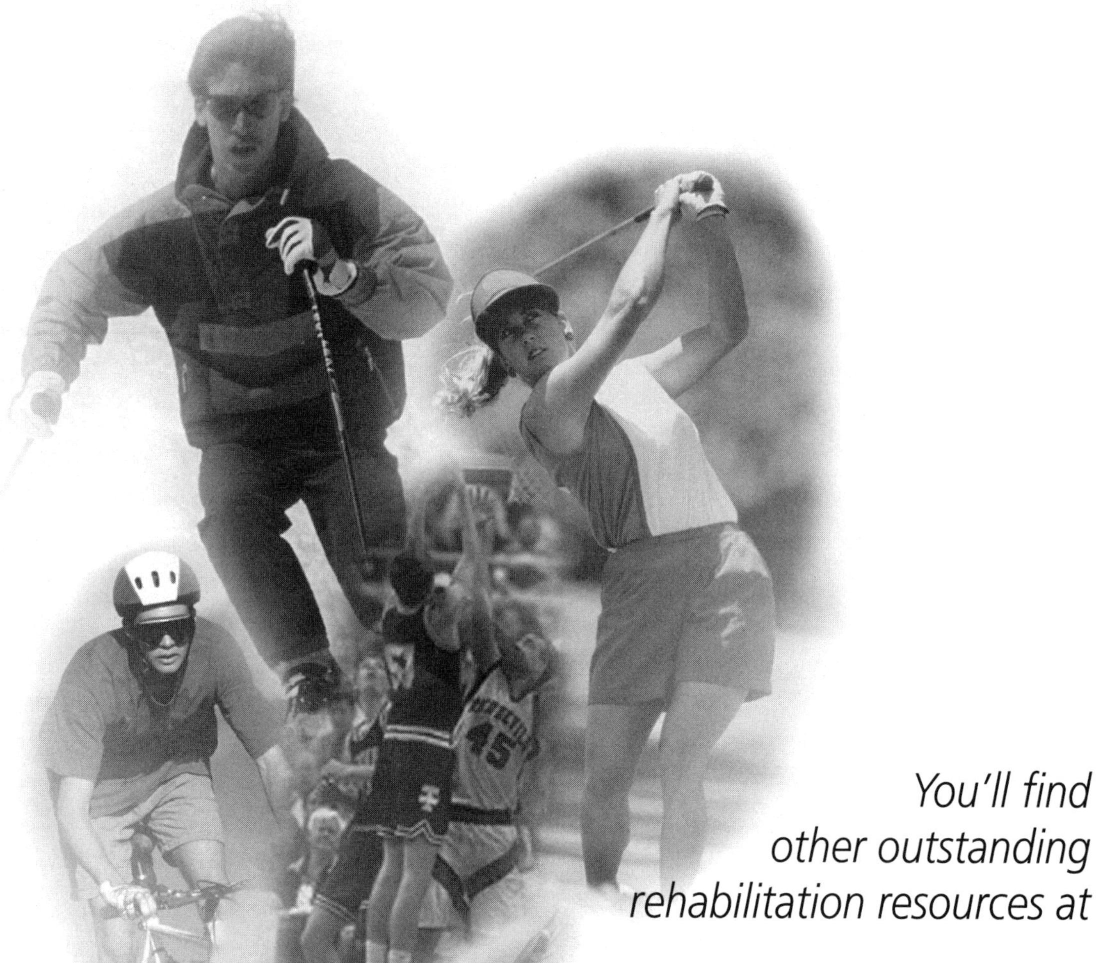